The Vulva

The Vulva

Anatomy, Physiology, and Pathology

Edited by

Miranda A. Farage
The Procter & Gamble Company
Cincinnati, Ohio, U.S.A.

Howard I. Maibach
University of California School of Medicine
San Francisco, California, U.S.A.

informa
healthcare

New York London

Informa Healthcare USA, Inc.
270 Madison Avenue
New York, NY 10016

Printed in the United States of America on acid-free paper
10 9 8 7 6 5 4 3 2

International Standard Book Number-10: 0-8493-3608-2 (Hardcover)
International Standard Book Number-13: 978-0-8493-3608-9 (Hardcover)

Library of Congress Cataloging-in-Publication Data

The vulva : anatomy, physiology, and pathology / edited by Miranda A. Farage, Howard I. Maibach.
p. ; cm.
Includes bibliographical references and index.
ISBN-13: 978-0-8493-3608-9 (hardcover : alk. paper)
ISBN-10: 0-8493-3608-2 (hardcover : alk. paper)
1. Vulva--Diseases. 2. Vulva--Pathophysiology. 3. Vulva--Anatomy. I. Farage, Miranda A. II. Maibach, Howard I.
[DNLM: 1. Vulva. 2. Vulvar Diseases. WP 200 V9913 2006]

RG261.V86 2006
618.1'6--dc22
2006044473

Visit the Informa Web site at
www.informa.com

and the Informa Healthcare Web site at
www.informahealthcare.com

To my adored Mother and Father: your countless sacrifices have formed my world and given me the gift of purpose and strength of will to succeed. Wherever you are, I am nourished and guided by your never-ending love.

M.A.F.

Foreword

This is a much needed book for the patient with vulvovaginal symptomatology too often faces the prospect of an incomplete evaluation and misdirected therapies. There are many reasons for this. Physicians with practice time constraints magnified by an office full of waiting patients too often begin their physical examination with the introduction of the vaginal speculum, bypassing the vulva. In addition, the record of diagnostic accuracy of vaginal infections by physicians shows a high error rate and inaccurate diagnoses lead to inappropriate therapeutic interventions, which only prolong and sometimes intensify patient's symptomatology. Finally, to a large extent, the care of patients with vulvovaginal problems requires dermatologic insights that are too often lacking for many practitioners.

The editors of this book, Miranda A. Farage and Howard I. Maibach, attempt to address these shortcomings and I applaud their efforts. They have selected experts who have both the knowledge and the ability to organize their prose that captures reader attention and accomplishes reader understanding. The underlying philosophy of this book is to provide an in-depth exposé of the anatomy and physiology: a basis for the understanding of the pathophysiology and one that sets a goal to achieve with appropriate therapy. This is followed by an exposition of the myriad presentations of patients with vulvovaginal disease, and current scientifically accepted treatment regimens. There is an excellent analysis of the menstrual cycle and the range of health care products that are now available to women. Since medicine is not practiced in a vacuum, the influences of race and societal norms on women are provided in detail. Finally, there is a fascinating section that provides an in-depth review of newer investigational techniques that will influence the future care of women.

This is a book for all readers. For me, it is a cover-to-cover joy to read. For others, it will be a valuable office reference to be opened every day to address problems of individual patient care. My congratulations to both the editors and the authors. Obviously, it is a labor of love that hits the mark.

William J. Ledger, M.D.
Professor and Chairman Emeritus
Department of Obstetrics and Gynecology
New York Presbyterian Hospital-Cornell Medical Center
New York, New York, U.S.A.

Preface

Few books are devoted exclusively to the vulva. The assumption that vulva skin is like the skin of external body surfaces is wrong. Vulvar tissue has many unique physiological properties and characteristics that differentiate it from the skin and tissue of other body sites. Researchers studying the vulva and clinicians treating patients with vulvar conditions know that there is a paucity of information about the vulva in the medical literature. Consequently, the unique physiology of the vulva, its normal and diseased states, pertinent cultural and hygiene practices that affect vulvar health, and the direction of current investigative research are not widely recognized. This insufficient body of information is responsible for the existing deficiencies in knowledge of the vulva, education and training of physicians about vulvar conditions, and appropriate diagnosis and treatment of vulvar pathology.

We attempt to redress these deficiencies with this new volume, *The Vulva*, a compilation of up-to-date clinical and research information collected in one comprehensive work. *The Vulva* was written primarily for medical and scientific audiences to underscore unique aspects of vulvar physiology, to highlight possible ethnic differences, to review vulvar diseases, to alert researchers and clinicians to cultural and hygiene practices that affect vulvar health, and to share the latest techniques in investigative research on vulvar tissue. *The Vulva* includes chapters on vulvar anatomy, physiology, microbiology, age-related changes, ethnicity, diseases, global cultural and hygiene practices, personal products used on the vulva, and toxicological and bioengineering research methods applied to vulvar research.

The information included in this book presents the current knowledge and understanding of vulvology. Although this work attempts to be a comprehensive and up-to-date resource, we acknowledge that research on the vulva lags behind other fields. Researchers and clinicians who have contributed to this volume hope to promote a better understanding of the unique physiology of the vulva and to encourage needed research.

This book is intended to increase awareness of the unique health concerns of the vulva and to be a valuable resource on the vulva region for the medical and scientific communities.

ACKNOWLEDGMENTS

Many appreciations and thanks are gratefully owed to the many people who contributed knowingly and indirectly to this book.

The following readers generously offered their time and expertise to peer-review relevant chapters: Drs. Kenneth W. Miller, Bruce E. Jones, Mr. John Blevins, Ms. Lisa Lennon, Drs. Tom Osborn, Brian Gray, Ray Warren, Mr. Ron Visscher and Mr. Kevin Johnson. In addition, Ms. Jan Tremaine, Drs. D. A. Hutchins, and T. L. Nusair have assisted with the review of this book. Their collective recommendations have vastly improved the texts assembled here. Many thanks go to the efforts and help of all the contributors of this book.

This book represents the fruits of a jointly conceived and executed venture and has benefited from partners. Many thanks and appreciations go to Drs. Sharon Mitchell and Bruce E. Jones who encouraged and supported the idea for this book from the start. My thanks go to Ms. Lisa Lennon for her help and support of this book. No praise is excessive for her efforts for which she has my heartfelt gratitude. My deepest and most sincere debt is owed to an exceptional person who shepherded the book from start to finish, Dr. Kenneth W. Miller without whose belief, support, help, encouragement, guidance and understanding, this book would not have seen the light of day.

Above all, my everlasting gratitude, thanks and love go to my family, husband and children who supported, helped and encouraged me all the way with their incredible patience. Your continuous care, unconditional love and sacrifice made all this possible, and easier to achieve.

Miranda A. Farage
Howard I. Maibach

Contents

Foreword William J. Ledger . . . . *v*
Preface . . . . *vii*
Contributors . . . . *xv*

PART I. ANATOMY AND PHYSIOLOGY

1. Anatomy of the Vulva *1*
Aikaterini Deliveliotou and George Creatsas
Introduction *1*
Embryology of Vulva *1*
Anatomy of the Vulva *2*
Conclusion *7*
References *7*

2. Tissue Structure and Physiology of the Vulva *9*
Miranda A. Farage and Howard I. Maibach
Introduction *9*
Variations in Epithelial Structure *12*
Blood Flow and Innervation *14*
Hormonal Responsiveness *16*
Immune Cell Populations *16*
Tissue Hydration and Barrier Function *17*
Permeability *18*
Skin Irritation *19*
Microbiology *20*
Conclusion *22*
References *22*

3. Changes in the Vulva and Vagina Throughout Life 27
Miranda A. Farage, Howard I. Maibach, Aikaterini Deliveliotou, and George Creatsas
Introduction *27*
Infancy and Early Childhood *30*
Puberty *32*
Reproductive Years *34*
Menopause and Older Age *36*
Conclusion *39*
References *39*

4. Microbial Ecology of the Vulva 43
Ronald W. Berg and Catherine C. Davis
Introduction *43*
Anatomical Structure of the Vulva *43*
Factors Controlling Microbial Growth and Diversity *44*
Microflora of the Vulva *48*
Conclusion *53*
References *54*

PART II. SYMPTOMS, DISEASES, AND THERAPIES

5. Are Vaginal Symptoms Ever Normal? 57
Matthew Anderson, Alison Karasz, and Sarah Friedland
Introduction *57*
Characteristics of Normal Vaginal Discharge *58*
Characteristics of Normal Vaginal Odor *59*
Normalcy of Irritative Symptoms *60*
Conclusion *60*
References *61*

6. Common Diseases of the Vulva 63
Diane Elas and Rudolph P. Galask
Introduction *63*
Assessment *63*
Physical Examination *64*
Diseases that Cause Vulvar Burning *66*
Diseases that Cause Vulvar Itching *71*
Diseases that Cause Vulvar Pain *77*
Diseases that Cause Vaginal Discharge *80*
Conclusion *81*
References *81*

7. Idiopathic Vulvodynia 85
Lauren D. Arnold and Gloria A. Bachmann
Introduction *85*
Symptoms *87*
Etiology *87*
Prevalence *88*
Demographics *89*
Comorbid Conditions *89*
Gynecologic History *90*
Psychosocial and Sexual Aspects *90*
Diagnosis *90*
Treatment *94*
Conclusion *96*
References *97*

8. Vulvar Vestibulitis Syndrome 101
Miranda A. Farage and Rudolph P. Galask
Introduction *101*
Definition and Disease Characteristics *101*
Prevalence and Patient Demographics *103*
Differential Diagnosis *104*
Etiology *105*
Management *107*
Conclusion *110*
References *111*

9. Vulvar Therapies: Evidence Vs. Testimony 115
Natalie Moulton-Levy and Howard I. Maibach
Introduction *115*
Vulvodynia *115*
Eczematous and Papulosquamous Vulvar Dermatoses *117*
Benign Vulvar Nodules or Tumors *123*
Infectious Diseases *123*
Vulvar Neoplasm *138*
Conclusion *142*
References *143*

PART III. MENSES, HYGIENE, AND PRODUCTS

10. The Menstrual Cycle, the Composition of Menses, and the Effect of Menses on the Skin 151
Miranda A. Farage, William H. Hood, and Paula J. Adams Hillard
Introduction *151*
The Menstrual Cycle *152*

Composition and Properties of Menses *155*
Effects of Menses and Venous Blood on the Skin *160*
Conclusion *163*
References *164*

11. The Menstrual Cycle and the Skin *167*
Birgit Drexler, Michael Landthaler, and Silvia Hohenleutner
Introduction *167*
Hormonal Changes in the Course of the Menstrual Cycle *167*
Influence of the Sex Hormones on the Skin *168*
Premenstrual Syndrome *171*
Menstrual Cycle and Associated Skin Disorders *172*
Conclusion *179*
References *179*

12. Genital Hygiene: Culture, Practices, and Health Impact *183*
Miranda A. Farage and Mario Bramante
Introduction *183*
Genital Hygiene of Infants *183*
Genital Hygiene Among Premenarchal Girls *184*
Genital Hygiene Among Women of Reproductive Age *188*
Genital Hygiene Among Older Women *204*
Conclusion *208*
References *208*

13. Products for Vulvar Hygiene *217*
Miranda A. Farage and Lisa Lennon
Introduction *217*
Cleanliness and Odor-Control Products *217*
Menstrual Protection Products *223*
Products for Incontinence Control *227*
Other Products Used on the Vulva *228*
Medications *229*
Conclusion *230*
References *230*

PART IV. ETHNICITY AND SOCIOLOGY

14. Vulva Ethnic Differences: An Overview *235*
Marina Goldovsky and Howard I. Maibach
Introduction *235*

Assessments of Variable Characteristics of Ethnically/Racially Different Skin *236*
Lipid Content *247*
Clinical Observations *249*
Conclusion *249*
References *252*

15. Female Genital Alterations: A Sociological Perspective *255*
Samar A. Farage
Introduction *255*
The Management of Sexuality as a Problem: Postmasturbation Disease *259*
Types of Female Genital Alterations *263*
Procedures of the 19th and 20th Centuries *264*
Contemporary Female Genital Alterations in North America *266*
Conclusion *267*
References *267*

PART V. INVESTIGATIONAL METHODS

16. Bioengineering Methods for the Vulva *271*
Sibylle Schliemann, Britta Opper, and Peter Elsner
Introduction *271*
Common Bioengineering Techniques *272*
Measuring Mechanical Properties *277*
Conclusion *277*
References *277*

17. Transepidermal Water Loss Dynamics of Human Vulvar and Thigh Skin *281*
Raphael Warren, Michaelle B. Jones, and Peter Elsner
Introduction *281*
Evaluation of Transepidermal Water Loss *282*
Transepidermal Water Loss Findings *283*
Conclusion *284*
References *285*

18. Vulvar Toxicology *287*
Christina Y. Wang and Howard I. Maibach
Introduction *287*
Irritation of the Vulva *288*
Bioengineering Methods of Assessment *290*

Behind the Knee Test *290*
Vulvar Dermatitis *291*
Contact Urticaria *294*
Conclusion *295*
References *295*

19. Consumer Research and In-Market Comments 297
Brigitte Nijs
Introduction *297*
What Do Women Want from a Feminine Hygiene Pad? *297*
Consumer Research Process for Feminine Hygiene Products *298*
Quality Assurance for Production of Feminine Hygiene Products *300*
Consumer Comments from Market Use *301*
Conclusion *302*
Reference *302*

Index *303*

Contributors

Matthew Anderson Department of Family and Social Medicine, Albert Einstein College of Medicine, Bronx, New York, U.S.A.

Lauren D. Arnold Douglass College, New Brunswick, New Jersey, U.S.A.

Gloria A. Bachmann Robert Wood Johnson Medical School, University of Medicine and Dentistry of New Jersey, New Brunswick, New Jersey, U.S.A.

Ronald W. Berg The Procter & Gamble Company, Cincinnati, Ohio, U.S.A.

Mario Bramante Central Product Safety Services, Procter & Gamble Service GmbH, Schwalbach am Taunus, Germany

George Creatsas Second Department of Obstetrics & Gynecology, University of Athens Medical School, Aretaieion Hospital, Athens, Greece

Catherine C. Davis The Procter & Gamble Company, Cincinnati, Ohio, U.S.A.

Aikaterini Deliveliotou Second Department of Obstetrics & Gynecology, University of Athens Medical School, Aretaieion Hospital, Athens, Greece

Birgit Drexler Clinic and Outpatient Clinic of Dermatology, Clinical Center of the University of Regensburg, Regensburg, Germany

Diane Elas Department of Obstetrics and Gynecology, Vulvar Vaginal Diseases Clinic, University of Iowa Hospitals and Clinics, Roy J. and Lucille A. Carver College of Medicine, Iowa City, Iowa, U.S.A.

Peter Elsner Department of Dermatology and Allergology, Friedrich-Schiller University, Jena, Germany

Miranda A. Farage Feminine Care Clinical Sciences, The Procter & Gamble Company, Cincinnati, Ohio, U.S.A.

Samar A. Farage Department of Sociology, Pennsylvania State University, State College, Pennsylvania, U.S.A.

Sarah Friedland Sarah Lawrence College, Bronxville, New York, U.S.A.

Rudolph P. Galask Department of Obstetrics and Gynecology, Vulvar Vaginal Diseases Clinic, University of Iowa Hospitals and Clinics, Roy J. and Lucille A. Carver College of Medicine, Iowa City, Iowa, U.S.A.

Marina Goldovsky Department of Dermatology, University of California School of Medicine, San Francisco, California, U.S.A.

Paula J. Adams Hillard Department of Pediatrics, Obstetrics, and Gynecology, University of Cincinnati College of Medicine, Cincinnati, Ohio, U.S.A.

Silvia Hohenleutner Clinic and Outpatient Clinic of Dermatology, Clinical Center of the University of Regensburg, Regensburg, Germany

William H. Hood Feminine Care Analytical Sciences, The Procter & Gamble Company, Cincinnati, Ohio, U.S.A.

Michaelle B. Jones The Procter & Gamble Company, Cincinnati, Ohio, U.S.A.

Alison Karasz Department of Family and Social Medicine, Albert Einstein College of Medicine, Bronx, New York, U.S.A.

Michael Landthaler Clinic and Outpatient Clinic of Dermatology, Clinical Center of the University of Regensburg, Regensburg, Germany

Lisa Lennon The Procter & Gamble Company, Cincinnati, Ohio, U.S.A.

Howard I. Maibach Department of Dermatology, University of California School of Medicine, San Francisco, California, U.S.A.

Natalie Moulton-Levy Jefferson Medical College, Philadelphia, Pennsylvania, U.S.A.

Brigitte Nijs The Procter & Gamble Company, Schwalbach am Taunus, Germany

Britta Opper Department of Dermatology and Allergology, Friedrich-Schiller University, Jena, Germany

Sibylle Schliemann Department of Dermatology and Allergology, Friedrich-Schiller University, Jena, Germany

Christina Y. Wang Department of Occupational and Environmental Medicine, University of California, and Kaiser Permanente, San Francisco, California, U.S.A.

Raphael Warren The Procter & Gamble Company, Feminine Care Innovation Center, Cincinnati, Ohio, U.S.A.

1

Anatomy of the Vulva

Aikaterini Deliveliotou and George Creatsas

Second Department of Obstetrics & Gynecology, University of Athens Medical School, Aretaieion Hospital, Athens, Greece

INTRODUCTION

The vulva, or pudendum, is a collective term for the external female genital organs that are visible in the perineal area. Knowledge of the basic anatomy of the vulva is necessary in order to understand its physiology and appropriately recognize the wide spectrum of vulvar pathology. To achieve these goals the vulvar embryology is first presented before describing the anatomy of the vulva in women of reproductive age. Lifetime changes in the vulva from birth to adulthood are described in Chapter 3.

EMBRYOLOGY OF VULVA

Early in the fifth week of embryonic life, the cloaca is divided by the urorectal septum, which gives rise to the perineum. Folds of tissue form on either side of the cloaca: the anterior folds are urogenital and the posterior folds are anal. The anterior folds meet at the midline to form the genital tubercle (1). The genital tubercle enlarges. In the male embryo, under the influence of androgens, the genital tubercle becomes the penis; in the female embryo, growth slows and it becomes the clitoris. On either side of the tubercle, the urogenital folds form the labia minora. In the indifferent stage, the labioscrotal swellings develop on either side of the urogenital folds. In the male embryo, under the influence of androgens, they differentiate into the scrotum; in the female, lacking androgenic stimulation, they remain largely unfused to become the labia majora. The definitive urogenital sinus gives rise to the vaginal vestibule, into which the urethra, vagina, and greater vestibular glands open.

ANATOMY OF THE VULVA

The vulva consists of the mons pubis, the labia majora, the labia minora, hymen, the clitoris, the vestibule of the vagina, the urethral orifice, Skene's glands, Bartholin's glands, and the vestibular bulbs (Fig. 1).

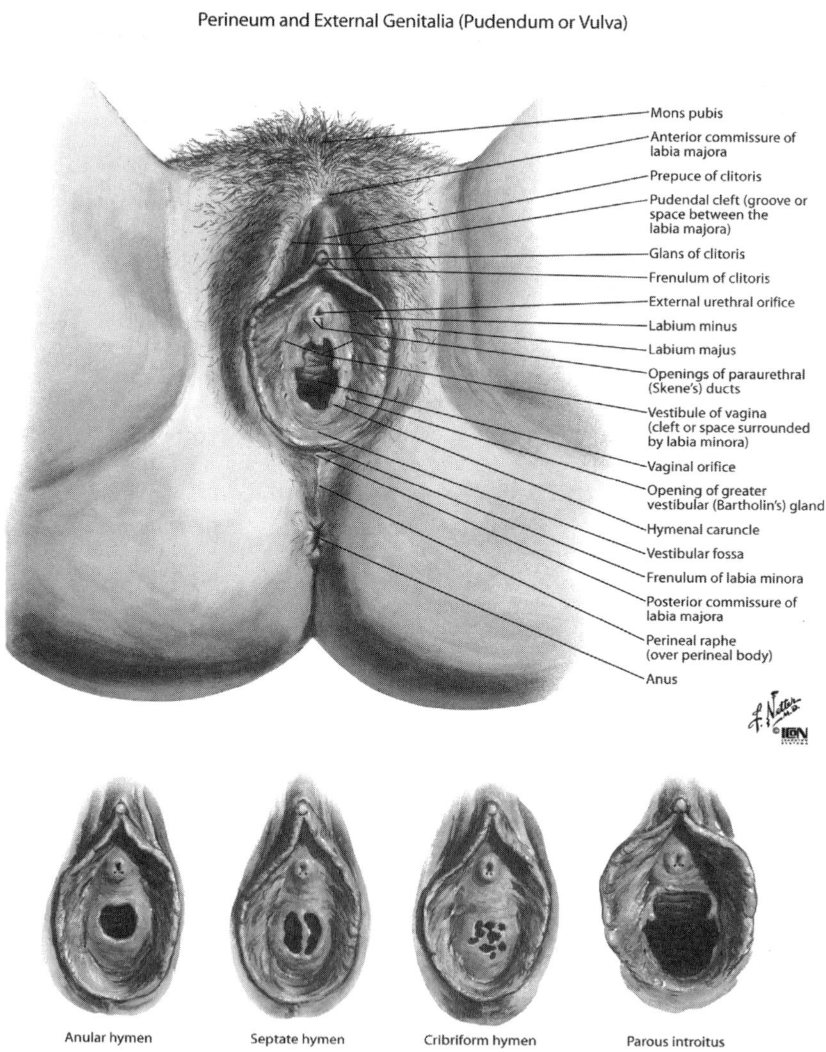

Figure 1 Anatomy of the adult vulva. *Source*: Courtesy of Elsevier. (*See color insert p. 1.*)

The anterior and posterior boundaries of the vulva extend from the mons pubis to the anus, respectively; its lateral boundaries lie at the genitocrural folds. The vulvar epithelium exhibits regional differences in tissue structure based on embryonic derivation. The skin-bearing mons pubis, perineum, and labia are derived from the embryonic ectoderm. Vulvar skin, like skin at other sites, has a keratinized, stratified, squamous epithelial structure with hair follicles, sebaceous glands, and sweat glands. The thickness degree of keratinization of vulvar skin decreases progressively from the labia majora, over the clitoris, to the labia minora. The vulvar vestibule, derived from the embryonic endoderm, is nonkeratinized. Chapter 2 describes in detail the regional tissue structure of the vulva.

Mons Pubis

The mons pubis (mons Veneris) is the rounded eminence in front of the pubic symphysis, which is formed by a collection of adipose tissue beneath the integument. During puberty, it becomes covered with hair up to its junction with the abdominal wall. The hair pattern, or escutcheon, of most women is triangular. Genetic and racial differences produce a variety of normal hair patterns, with approximately one in four women having a modified escutcheon with a diamond pattern.

Labia Majora

The labia majora are a pair of prominent longitudinal, cutaneous folds of fibroadipose tissue that are homologous to the scrotum in the male. The structures bear epidermal tissue resembling the dartos tunic of the scrotum, as well as adipose tissue, areolar tissue, blood vessels, nerves, and glands. The labia majora also include the terminal extension of the round ligament and, occasionally, a peritoneal diverticulum, the canal of Nuck.

The size of the labia majora is related to fat content. Each is approximately 7 to 8 cm in length and 2 to 3 cm in width. The labia majora extend downward and backward from the mons pubis, thus forming the lateral boundaries of a fissure or cleft (the pudendal cleft or rima) into which the vagina and urethra open.

Each labium majus has two surfaces: the outer surface is pigmented, rugose, and bears pubic hair, sebaceous glands, apocrine glands, and eccrine glands. The inner surface is smooth; it bears sebaceous, apocrine, and eccrine glands but no hair follicles. Vulvar apocrine glands are similar to those of the breast and axillary areas.

The labia majora are thicker in front. Anterior to the clitoris, they join to form the anterior boundary of the pudendal cleft, known as anterior labial commissure. The labia majora do not surround the pudendal cleft fully; laterally, they remain approximately parallel to it and posteriorly, they gradually merge with the neighboring integument below the juncture of the labia minora (fourchette). The posterior ends of the labia majora and the connecting skin between them form the posterior boundary of the pudendum, known as posterior labial commissure. The interval between the posterior commissure and the anus is 2.5 to 3 cm in length and constitutes the perineum.

Labia Minora

The labia minora (nymphae) are two small cutaneous folds that are situated between the labia majora and the vaginal orifice. The labia minora are homologous to the penile urethra and part of the skin of the penis in males. Laterally, they extend obliquely from the clitoris toward the rear for about 4 cm on either side of the vaginal orifice. They are shorter and thinner than the labia majora. At the clitoris, the anterior portion of each labium minus divides into two segments. Each upper segment passes anteriorly to the clitoris to meet its fellow of the opposite side, forming a fold, the preputium clitoridis, which overhangs the glans of the clitoris. Each lower segment passes beneath the clitoris, joining with its fellow to form the frenulum, which is attached to the inferior surface of the clitoris. The posterior portions of the labia minora surround the vestibule of the vagina. Their posterior juncture is the fourchette.

Histologically, the labia minora are composed of dense connective tissue, erectile tissue, and elastic fibers. Unlike the labia majora, they do not contain adipose tissue. The skin of the opposed surfaces of labia minora has numerous sebaceous glands but no hair follicles or sweat glands. Among women of reproductive age, there is significant variation in the size of the labia minora. They are relatively more prominent in children and postmenopausal women.

Clitoris

The clitoris is a short, cylindrical, erectile structure, 2 to 3 cm in length, at the superior portion of the vestibule. It is the female homologue of the penis. It is situated beneath the anterior labial commissure, partially hidden between the anterior segments of the labia minora. The clitoris consists of a base of two crura that attach to the periosteum of the symphysis pubis. Like the penis, the clitoris has a suspensory ligament and two small muscles, the ischiocavernosi, which are inserted into the crura of the clitoris. The body of the clitoris consists of two cylindrical corpora cavernosa composed of thin-walled, vascular channels that function as erectile tissue. The distal one-third of the clitoris is a small rounded tubercle (glans clitoridis) that consists of spongy erectile tissue with many nerve endings. Usually, only the glans is visible, with the body of the clitoris positioned beneath the skin surface. The normal glans clitoridis in adult women has a width less than 1 cm, with an average length of 1.5 to 2 cm. Age, weight, and oral contraceptive use do not change its anatomic dimensions. Childbearing may influence the size of the clitoris.

Hymen

The hymen is a thin fold of mucous membrane situated at the entrance to the vagina. Between the hymen and the frenulum of the labia minora is a shallow depression, the navicular fossa. The inner edges of the hymen may be in contact with each other, such that the vaginal orifice appears as a cleft between them. The hymen is usually perforated, with many variations in its structure and shape. The most common forms are that of a ring, which is broadest posteriorly, or that of a semilunar fold, with a hollow margin turned toward the pubes. The hymen is rarely cribriform or has inner edges that form a membranous fringe. It can be completely absent or can appear as a complete septum across the lower end of the vagina, a condition known as an imperforate hymen. Small tags or nodules of firm fibrous material, termed carunculae myrtiformes, are the remnants of the hymen in sexually active women. However, the hymen can persist after the first sexual intercourse, so its presence cannot be considered a sign of virginity. Histologically, the hymen is covered by stratified squamous epithelium on both sides and consists of fibrous tissue with a few small blood vessels.

Vestibule

The vestibule is derived from the endoderm, the lowest portion of the embryonic urogenital sinus. It is the cleft posterior to the glans clitoridis and between the labia minora. It can be visualized by holding the labia minora apart. The vestibule extends from the clitoris to the posterior fourchette. Hart's line marks the juncture of the nonkeratinized epithelium of the vulvar vestibule and the keratinized epithelium of the inner surface of the labia minora. The urethral and vaginal orifices as well as the ducts of the greater vestibular glands open into the vestibule. The remnants of the hymen and numerous small mucinous glands are located within the area of the vestibule.

Urethra

The female urethra, a membranous conduit for urine, runs from the urinary bladder to the vestibule and measures 3.5 to 5 cm in length. The mucosa of the distal one-third of the urethra is lined with stratified squamous epithelium, whereas the proximal two-thirds are lined with stratified transitional epithelium. The external urethral orifice is 4 to 6 mm in diameter and is immediately anterior to the vaginal orifice, approximately 2 to 3 cm beneath the glans clitoridis. Its mucosal edges grossly appear slightly everted, forming a short, sagittal cleft.

Vaginal Orifice

The vaginal orifice is a median slit below and posterior to the opening of the urethra; the hymen surrounds it, so that its size varies inversely with that of the hymen. It opens into the vagina, a neuromuscular vault connecting to the cervix of the uterus that unsheathes the penis during sexual intercourse and allows passage of the newborn infant during birth.

Skene's Glands

Skene's or paraurethral glands are homologous to the prostate in the male. They are branched, tubular glands, adjacent to the distal urethra. Usually, Skene's ducts run parallel to the long axis of the urethra for approximately 1 cm before opening into the distal urethra. Sometimes they open into the area just outside the urethral orifice. The duct of the Skene's gland presents an opening on its posterior surface. Skene's glands are the largest of the paraurethral glands; however, many smaller glands empty into the urethra.

Bartholin's Glands

The greater vestibular glands, or Bartholin's glands, are the homologues of the bulbourethral glands (Cowper's glands) in the male. They consist of two small, roundish, reddish-yellow bodies. Bartholin's glands are situated on the posterolateral aspect of the vaginal orifice, in contact with the posterior end of each lateral mass of the bulb of the vestibule. Histologically, the gland is composed of cuboidal epithelium. The duct from each gland is approximately 2 cm in length and is lined by transitional epithelium. Bartholin's ducts open immediately lateral to the hymen into the groove between the hymen and the labia minora. Their mucus secretion helps maintain adequate lubrication. Infection of these glands can result in an abscess.

Vestibular Bulbs

The vestibular bulbs are the homologues of the bulb and adjoining part of the corpus cavernosum urethrae of the male. They consist of two elongated masses of erectile tissue situated on either side of the vaginal orifice and are united to each other in front by a narrow median band termed the pars intermedia. Each lateral mass measures approximately 2.5 cm in length. The distal ends of the vestibular bulbs are adjacent to Bartholin's glands, whereas the proximal ends are tapered and joined to one another by the pars intermedia. Their deep surfaces are in contact with the inferior fascia of the urogenital diaphragm. Each bulb is immediately below the bulbocavernosus muscle.

Muscles of the Vulva

Three types of muscle exist in the vulva:

1. The ischiocavernosus muscle compresses the crura and lowers the clitoris. It originates from the ischial tuberosity and inserts at the ischiopubic bone.

2. The bulbocavernosus muscle compresses the vestibular bulb and dorsal vein of the clitoris. It originates from the perineal body and inserts into the posterior aspect of the clitoris; some fibers pass above the dorsal vein of the clitoris in a sling-like fashion.
3. The superficial transverse perineal muscle holds the perineal body fixed. It originates from the ischial tuberosity and inserts at the central perineal tendon.

Blood Supply of the Vulva

The vulva derives its blood supply from the femoral artery via the external and internal pudendal arteries. The venous drainage occurs via the internal pudendal veins.

Lymphatic Drainage of the Vulva

The vulva drains primarily to the superficial and deep inguinal nodes and along the dorsal vein of the clitoris, directly to the iliac nodes.

Innervation of the Vulva

The innervation of the vulva derives from branches of several nerves, including the ilioinguinal nerve, the genital branch of genitofemoral nerve, the perineal branch of the lateral femoral cutaneous nerve of the thigh, and the perineal branch of the pudendal nerve.

CONCLUSION

This chapter provided a review of the embryology and anatomy of the vulva in women of reproductive age. This knowledge is necessary in order to understand the vulva's physiology and recognize the wide spectrum of vulvar pathology.

REFERENCES

1. Anderson JR, Genardy R. Anatomy and embryology. In: Berek JS, ed. Novak's Gynecology. Chap. 5. Baltimore: Lippincott Williams & Wilkins, 2002.
2. Carpenter SK, Rock JA. Pediatric and Adolescent Gynecology. Chap. 3. 2nd ed. Baltimore: Lippincott Williams & Wilkins, 2000.
3. Creatsas G. Modern Gynecology and Obstetrics. Chaps. 2,10. 1st ed. Athens: Paschalidis, 1998.
4. Creatsas G. Neonatal, Pediatric and Adolescent Gynecology. Chap. 2. 2nd ed. Athens: 1987.
5. Creatsas G. Obstetrics and Gynecology of Childhood and Adolescence. Chaps. 5,6,9. 1st ed. Athens: Paschalidis, 2001.
6. Gray H. Anatomy of the Human Body. Chap. XI 3d.5. 1918.

7. Gardner JJ. Descriptive study of genitalia variation in healthy, non-abused premenarcheal girls. J Pediatr 1992; 120:251.
8. Huffmann JM. Examination of the newborn. In: Huffmann JM, Dewhurst J, Capraro V, eds. The Gynecology of Childhood and Adolescence. Philadelphia: W.B. Saunders Co., 1981:70.
9. Marshall WA, Tanner JM. Variations in pattern of pubertal changes in girls. Arch Dis Child 1969; 44:291.
10. Pokorny SF, Kozinetz CA. Configuration and other anatomic details of the prepubertal hymen. Adolesc Pediatr Gynecol 1998; 1:97.
11. Tribaud E. Gynecologic clinical examination of the child and adolescent. In: Sultan C, ed. Pediatric and Adolescent Gynecology. Evidence-Based Clinical Practice. Vol. 7. Switzerland: Karger, 2004:1.

2

Tissue Structure and Physiology of the Vulva

Miranda A. Farage
Feminine Care Clinical Sciences, The Procter & Gamble Company, Cincinnati, Ohio, U.S.A.

Howard I. Maibach
Department of Dermatology, University of California School of Medicine, San Francisco, California, U.S.A.

INTRODUCTION

The vulva is composed of specialized tissue with regional differences in embryonic derivation, structure, and morphology. The vulva comprises the mons pubis, the labia majora and minora, the clitoris, the vulvar vestibule surrounding the urethral orifice and vaginal introitus, and the hymen, a membrane at the juncture of the vulvar vestibule and the vagina. This chapter describes variations in epithelial structure, blood flow, hormonal and immune responsiveness, barrier function, permeability, irritant susceptibility, and microbial colonization of the vulva in women of reproductive age (Table 1).

Portions of this chapter appeared in Farage MA, Maibach HI. The vulvar epithelium differs from the skin: implications for cutaneous testing to address topical vulvar exposures. Contact Dermatitis 2004; 51:201. Reprinted with permission from Blackwell Publishing.

Table 1 Qualitative Differences Between Exposed Skin and Vulvovaginal Epithelia

Characteristic	Exposed skin	Vulvar skin	Vulvar vestibule	Vaginal epithelium
Embryonic derivation	Ectodermal		Endodermal	Mesodermal (estrogen dependent)
Tissue structure	Keratinized, stratified squamous epithelium		Nonkeratinized epithelium with less distinct stratification	
Blood flow	Depends on anatomical site	Higher blood flow than exposed forearm skin	No data	
Hydration	Depends on anatomical site	More hydrated than forearm skin (28,29)	Hydrated by cervicovaginal secretions	
Occlusion	Depends on anatomical site	Greater occlusion than forearm skin	Greater occlusion than exposed skin	
Friction	Depends on anatomical site	Higher coefficient of friction than forearm skin (31)	Not determined	
Hormonal influences	Menstrual cycle variability in water barrier function and susceptibility to irritants (53,54)	Thickness unchanged over the course of menstrual cycle (1) Menstrual cycle variability in barrier function and irritant susceptibility unknown	Not determined	Menstrual cycle variability in epithelial thickness, glycogen content, and nuclear pyknosis (13,15)

Permeability	Varies by site; influenced by skin thickness (33)	Permeability affected by increased hydration and occlusion (34,35)	Significantly more permeable than keratinized skin (45)	
Immune cell densities	Diverse population of immune cells	Langerhans cells most common No difference in Langerhans cell density between keratinized and nonkeratinized regions (16)		Langerhans cell densities lowest at fornix, highest at introitus (17)
Microbiology	Diverse population includes *Staphylococcus aureus*, coagulase-negative staphylococci, streptococci, diphtheroids, yeasts, etc.	Microflora affected by hydration, occlusion, and vaginal and perineal cross-colonization. Higher densities of *S. aureus*, streptococci, lactobacilli, *Candida*, than exposed skin (55)	Microflora influenced by cervicovaginal secretions, perineal and urethral cross-colonization	Highly diverse, mixed aerobic and anaerobic microflora. Acid-producing microbes are dominant in healthy women (83)

VARIATIONS IN EPITHELIAL STRUCTURE

The lower urogenital tract is the only portion of the female anatomy derived from all three embryologic layers (ectoderm, endoderm, and mesoderm) (Table 2). In the vulva, cutaneous epithelium derived from the embryonic ectoderm is juxtaposed closely with nonkeratinized epithelium derived from the embryonic endoderm (1,2).

The embryonic ectoderm gives rise to the keratinized cutaneous epithelium of the mons pubis, labia majora, clitoris, labia minora, and perineum. Like skin at other anatomical sites, the epidermis of the mons pubis, labia majora, and perineum has a keratinized, stratified squamous structure with sweat glands, sebaceous glands, and hair follicles (Fig. 1). Cutaneous thickness and degree of keratinization are relatively high on the mons pubis and labia majora, but decrease over the anterior portions of the clitoris and decline progressively from the outer surface to the inner surface of the labia minora (3).

The cutaneous epithelium consists of four layers:

1. A basal germinative layer (stratum basale), which rests on the basal lamina between the epidermis and the dermis.
2. A spinous or prickle cell layer, forming the bulk of the epidermal thickness (stratum spinosum).
3. A granular layer (stratum granulosum).
4. A surface layer of flattened, keratinized cells embedded in hydrophobic intercellular lipid (stratum corneum).

Three specialized cells—melanocytes, Langerhans cells, and Merkel cells—also reside in the epidermis. Melanocytes represent one-tenth to one-fifth of the cells in the cutaneous basal layer (4). They convert tyrosine to melanin pigment, which protects the basal cells from ultraviolet (UV) damage. Melanocytes respond regionally to hormones: at puberty, pigmentation of the mons pubis and labia majora increases; during pregnancy, steroid hormones stimulate

Table 2 Embryologic Derivation of the Female Lower Urogenital Tract

Origin	Structures
Ectoderm	Skin of the labia majora and part of the labia minora
Endoderm	Vulvar vestibule Bladder (except trigone) Anterior urethral wall
Mesoderm	Hymenal membrane Posterior urethral wall Bladder trigone

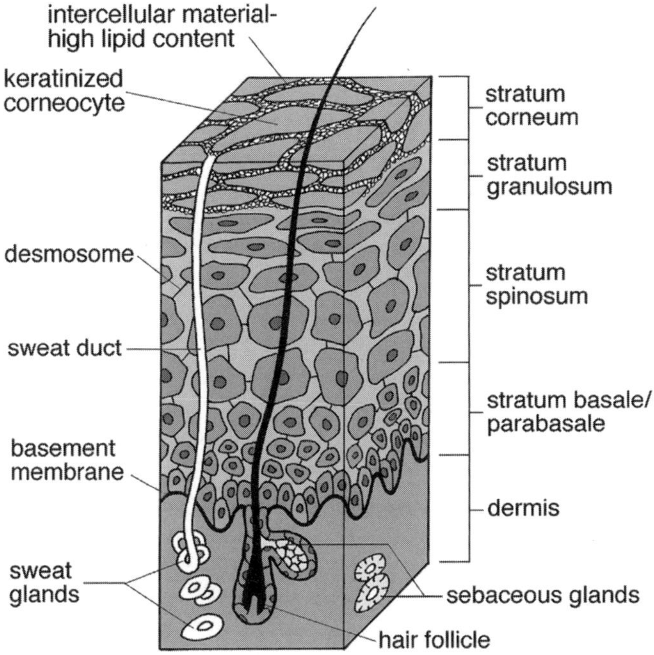

Figure 1 Epithelial structure of vulvar skin. *Source*: Adapted from Ref. 84. (*See color insert p. 2.*)

melanogenesis in the areola, nipples, and perineum and on the midline of the anterior abdominal wall.

Langerhans cells are dendritic cells found in the epidermis, in thymic and mucosal tissues, and in lymph nodes. Their chief function is to sample antigen at the epithelial surface, process it, and present it to circulating T lymphocytes, the activation of which initiates the cell-mediated immune response.

Merkel cells are found in the basal epidermal layer. Their cell bodies form synapse-like contacts with the terminal endings of myelinated nerve fibers. They release neurotransmitters in response to sensory excitation (5). Merkel cells serve as skin mechanoreceptors that shape sensitivity to soft touch.

The nonkeratinized epithelium of the vulvar vestibule is the only portion of the female genital tract of endodermal origin (2,6). The epithelial structure of the vulvar vestibule resembles that of the vagina and buccal mucosa (Fig. 2) (2,7). Its superficial stratum bears large, moderately flattened cells lacking keratin but containing glycogen granules and, frequently, pyknotic nuclei. Differentiation of the inner epithelial layers is indistinct: loosely packed, polyhedral cells alter in size and organelle density as they migrate upward from the generative basal layer, but do not form clearly demarcated strata as

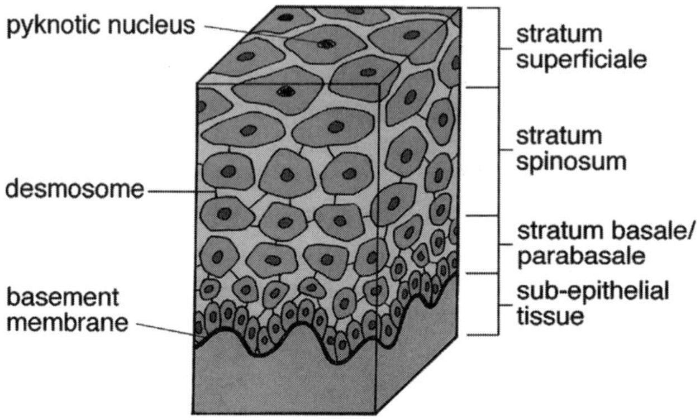

Figure 2 Epithelial structure of the vulvar vestibule. *Source*: Adapted from Ref. 84. (*See color insert p. 2.*)

observed in the skin. Langerhans cells are present in the epithelium of the vulvar vestibule.

BLOOD FLOW AND INNERVATION

The vulva is a highly vascularized and well-innervated structure (8). Arterial blood supplies the vulva bilaterally and derives from branches of the internal iliac and femoral arteries; venous drainage eventually reaches the femoral and internal iliac veins.

Blood flow in labia majora skin is more than twice that in forearm skin (Table 3) (9). Studies of vulvar skin have demonstrated increased blood flow in response to histamine at doses to which forearm skin is unresponsive (10).

Innervation of vulvar tissue reflects its role in the sexual response. The vulva has both somatic and autonomic innervation. Motor components mediate pelvic muscle contraction and vascular engorgement of clitoral and vaginal tissue. Sensory components convey touch, pain, itch, temperature, wetness, distention of the anal canal and vagina, and sensations related to sexual arousal. In the clitoris, nerve fibers from the small and large trunks of the dorsal nerve form extensive plexuses in the deeper regions of the dermis and subcutaneous layers (8). In the upper regions of the dermis, the nerve fibers display terminal fibrils with endings that penetrate the epidermis. These epidermal nerve endings vary from simple axon terminals to highly branched and encapsulated structures. Although such structures are found in other regions of the vulva, they decrease in number in a lateral direction from the clitoris.

Innervation of the labia majora differs from that of the rest of the vulva: although both superficial and deep neural nets are present, superficial nerves are reduced markedly. Most nerve endings in the labia majora are parafollicular and do not extend into the epidermis (8).

Table 3 Quantitative Comparison of Biophysical Variables, Permeability and Irritant Susceptibilities in Forearm and Vulvar Skin (Labia Majora)

Parameter assessed (units)	Forearm	Vulva	Statistical significance (n = number of subjects)	Reference
Transepidermal water loss (g/m^2 hr)	3.5 ± 0.3	14.5 ± 1.3	$p < 0.001$[a] ($n = 44$)	(31)
Friction coefficient (μ, unitless)	0.48 ± 0.01	0.66 ± 0.03	$p < 0.001$[a] ($n = 44$)	(31)
Blood flow (Absorbance units)	22.0 ± 3.0	59.5 ± 7.4	$p < 0.001$[a] ($n = 9$)	(9)
Hydrocortisone penetration (% of applied dose absorbed in 24 hr)	2.8 ± 2.4	8.1 ± 4.1	$p < 0.01$[b] ($n = 9$)	(35)
Testosterone penetration (% of applied dose absorbed in 24 hr)	20.2 ± 8.1	25.2 ± 6.8	NS[b,c] ($n = 9$)	(35)
Frequency of irritant reactions to 20% maleic acid solution (%)	62	76	Not determined ($n = 21$)	(49)
Mean intensity of irritant reactions to 20% maleic acid at 24 hr postapplication (0–3 visual scale)	0.86 ± 0.36	1.29 ± 0.83	$p = 0.036$[a] ($n = 21$)	(49)
Frequency of irritant reactions to 17% benzalkonium chloride solution (%)	9	57	Not determined ($n = 21$)	(49)
Mean intensity of irritant reactions to 17% benzalkonium chloride solution at 24 hr postapplication (0–3 visual scale)	0.19 ± 0.33	1.00 ± 0.88	$p = 0.0003$[a] ($n = 21$)	(49)
Irritant reactions to 1% sodium lauryl sulfate at day 2 postapplication (proportion of scores > 1 on 0–4 scale)	9/10	0/10	$p < 0.05$[d] ($n = 10$)	(51,52)

[a]Student *t* test.
[b]One-way analysis of variance followed by Neuman-Keuls multiple range test.
[c]Not significant.
[d]Wald-Wolfowitz two sample test.

HORMONAL RESPONSIVENESS

Vulvar skin has a higher concentration of epidermal androgen receptors than skin at nongenital sites (11). At puberty, androgens direct the maturation of vulvar sebaceous glands and hair follicles (12).

The vaginal epithelium has a high level of estrogen receptors and is responsive to ovarian hormone cycling. At midcycle, vaginal epithelial cell proliferation, glycogen content, and nuclear pyknosis increase in response to estrogen. A small but statistically significant increase in vaginal epithelial cell layers as been found at midcyle (13), but no significant difference in epithelial thickness has been observed between follicular and luteal phases (13,14). The concentration of estrogen receptors decreases progressively from the vagina to the vulva, with the lowest levels on keratinized vulvar skin (11). The thickness of the vulvar epithelium remains constant over the course of the menstrual cycle, but its surface cells are predominantly orthokeratotic (lacking nuclei) at the beginning and end of the cycle, and increasingly parakeratotic (bearing a degenerated nucleus) at midcycle (1,15).

Progesterone receptors are not found on vulvar skin; they are restricted to the transitional epithelium of the inner aspect of the labia minora and to the nonkeratinized epithelia of the vagina and vulvar vestibule (11).

IMMUNE CELL POPULATIONS

Immune cell infiltration of the vulva is most evident during the reproductive years (12). Langerhans cells are the most common immune cell type in the vulva; intraepithelial and perivascular lymphocytes are found infrequently (16). A gradient in Langerhans cell density exists along the lower female genital tract. In Rhesus macaques, for example, cell densities are lowest at the vaginal fornix and highest at the introitus (17). Human studies demonstrate a higher density of Langerhans cells in the vulva than in the vagina, with no difference between keratinized and nonkeratinized regions (16). Langerhans cell densities were estimated at 19 per 100 basal cells in the vulvar epithelium, 13 per 100 basal cells in the cervix, and 6 per 100 basal cells in the vagina.

By contrast, lymphocytes predominate in the vagina: the $CD8^+$ subtype, which dominates in human mucosal epithelia, is the most common vaginal immune cell (14). The $CD4^+$ subtype constitutes the second largest population of vaginal immune cells and tissue macrophages represent the third.

Growing evidence suggests that immune responsiveness is modulated differentially along the reproductive tract. Transplantation studies suggest that the cervix is immunologically privileged in order to protect the fetus from maternal alloresponses to antigens in ejaculate (18). Cervical mucus, which protects the entry to the uterus, contains secretory antibodies, particularly IgA. These secretory antibodies inactivate antigens by forming nonabsorbable complexes with them. They are bacteriocidal in the presence of lysozyme and complement, and can agglutinate bacteria and opsonize them for phagocytosis by macrophages.

Langerhans cells, the concentration of which varies in different regions of the genital tract, are part of the dendritic cell system. They serve as sentinels, sampling antigen at the epithelial surface, then transporting and presenting it in immunogenic form to responsive T lymphocytes in regional lymph nodes. The deficit in vaginal Langerhans cells relative to their vulvar concentrations may be one of several adaptations to the antigenic challenges posed by resident vaginal microflora and foreign proteins encountered during intercourse. Seminal fluid also contains a variety of inhibitors that suppress immune function in the vagina and cervix.

Different regions of the genital tract exhibit distinct responses to antigen. Antigen application to vulvar skin can result in sensitization; indeed, allergic contact dermatitis to topical agents is a prime contributor to persistent vulvar discomfort (19–21). By contrast, antigen application to nonkeratinized mucosa may induce tolerance. This phenomenon, best characterized in the oral mucosa, is not due to the phenotype of resident Langerhans cells, but results from altered responses at the level of the draining lymph nodes (22,23). Studies in animal models demonstrate that tolerance induction also occurs in the vagina, where the phenomenon is hormonally regulated (24). In mice, vaginally induced tolerance occurred only during the estrogen-dominant phase of the estrus cycle when sperm exposure would occur.

Conflicting data exist on the hormonal modulation of immune cell densities in the human vaginal epithelium. Langerhans cell densities are of particular interest, since these cells are involved in the mechanisms of sensitization and tolerance and have been suggested to be the major target of vaginally transmitted HIV infection in women (25,26). Several investigators reported the number and distribution of vaginal immune cells to be stable throughout the menstrual cycle (13,14). One study demonstrated an increase in the density of vaginal Langerhans cells in response to vaginally administered progesterone (27). However, no such effect was found in women using the synthetic, long-acting progestin contraceptives depot medroxyprogesterone acetate (DMPA) or levonorgestrel. DMPA caused a selective increase in $CD8^+$ T lymphocytes, levonorgestrel increased the $CD4^+$:$CD8^+$ ratio, and the combined oral contraceptive caused no cell population changes (14). Further research is needed to elucidate the mechanisms by which hormonal cycling may modulate the immune response of the lower genital tract.

TISSUE HYDRATION AND BARRIER FUNCTION

Vulvar tissue is more hydrated and has a lower barrier function than exposed skin, as assessed by transepidermal water loss (TEWL). Water diffuses across the stratum corneum of the labia majora at a higher rate than across the stratum corneum of forearm skin (Table 3) (28,29). To a degree, this reflects elevated skin hydration due to occlusion. However, vulvar skin also presents an intrinsically lower barrier to water loss: steady-state TEWL values remain higher on the vulva than on the forearm after equilibration with the environment or after the prolonged drying of both sites with a desiccant (29,30). The comparatively greater hydration of occluded vulvar skin raises its friction coefficient (Table 3), which may make vulvar skin more susceptible to mechanical damage (31).

PERMEABILITY

Predicting tissue permeability is complex. The phenomenon depends on the extent to which the penetrant partitions into the tissue, the rate at which the penetrant diffuses through the tissue, and the distance to be traversed (32). Consequently, vulvar penetration of exogenous agents is influenced by regional differences in epithelial structure and lipid composition, the physicochemical characteristics of the penetrants, and the nature of the applied vehicle.

Permeability of Labia Majora Skin

Table 4 illustrates skin permeability to hydrocortisone by anatomic site (33). Vulvar skin is substantially more permeable than forearm skin to this agent (34,35). Probable contributing factors include elevated vulvar skin hydration, the higher concentration of hair follicles and sweat glands on vulvar skin, and increased cutaneous blood flow. Tissue penetration rates also depend on the

Table 4 Relative Permeability to Hydrocortisone (% of Dose Absorbed) by Anatomical Site

Site	Permeability relative to forearm skin
Forearm (ventral)	1.0×
Forearm (dorsal)	1.1×
Foot arch (plantar)	0.14×
Ankle (lateral)	0.42×
Palm	0.83×
Back	1.7×
Scalp	3.5×
Axilla	3.6×
Forehead	6.0×
Vulva (labia majora)	2.8–7.0×
Jaw angle	13.0×
Scrotum	42×

Source: Adapted from Refs. 33, 34, 35.

properties of the penetrant. For example, there is no difference in the rate of testosterone penetration through vulvar and forearm skin (Table 3) (35). However, the skin at both sites is far more permeable to testosterone than to hydrocortisone. This is probably due to the greater hydrophobicity of testosterone and because of the presence of androgen receptors in the skin.

Permeability of the Vulvar Vestibule and Vaginal Epithelium

Nonkeratinized epithelia are more generally permeable to external penetrants. This has been described best in oral tissue which, like the vulva, displays regional differences in structure and keratinization (36,37). The nonkeratinized buccal mucosa, which resembles the vaginal epithelium morphologically, is tenfold more permeable to water than is keratinized skin (38). Buccal mucosa is more permeable than the skin to horseradish peroxidase, although absolute penetration rates of this large molecule are lower than those of water (36).

The heightened permeability of nonkeratinized tissue results from several factors. First, the absence of a stratum corneum removes a principal barrier to entry of external agents. Second, the more loosely packed cell layers create a structure with less resistance to paracellular movement, the principal route by which most penetrants traverse tissues (39,40). Third, such tissues have a less-structured lipid barrier with lower resistance to molecular diffusion (41,42). Finally, thinner epithelia (such as the buccal mucosa and vulvar vestibule) present a shorter path length to be traversed.

Nonkeratinized tissue is also more vulnerable to breaches in tissue integrity, which can augment tissue penetration. For example, buccal tissue was 40-fold more permeable than keratinized skin to the organic base nicotine, an irritant that increases the penetration of coadministered compounds (43,44).

The heightened permeability of the vulvar vestibule can be inferred from studies on vaginal and buccal epithelia, which serve as surrogate tissues. Vaginal and buccal epithelia have similar ultrastructural features and lipid composition. Moreover, comparable tissue penetration rates at coadministered sites have been observed for a range of model penetrants, including water, estradiol, vasopressin, and low molecular weight dextrans (45–48). Like these epithelia, the thin, non-keratinized vulvar vestibule may be more permeable than keratinized skin and more vulnerable to the effects of externally applied agents.

SKIN IRRITATION

Vulvar skin differs from exposed skin in its susceptibility to applied irritants. However, irritant effects are difficult to predict. The available evidence suggests that elevated skin hydration plays a role in vulvar susceptibility to polar irritants. For example, vulvar skin was more reactive than forearm skin to high aqueous concentrations of maleic acid (20% concentration) and benzalkonium chloride (17% concentration) (Table 3) (49). Because polar or charged materials do not penetrate the hydrophobic lipid barrier of the stratum corneum readily, the comparatively greater hydration of vulvar skin may have facilitated skin penetration of the polar irritants at this site.

The surfactant sodium lauryl sulfate (SLS) caused a different response. Vulvar skin was less reactive than forearm skin to low concentrations of this agent (Table 3) (50–52). This result may relate to the structure of the penetrant: the surfactant molecule bears both a charged head and a hydrophobic tail. Notably, hydrophobic molecules partition far more readily into the lipid barrier of the stratum corneum than do charged materials, and lipid partitioning is more favored when the applied medium is relatively polar. In the case of aqueous SLS, skin penetration of the charged head would be highly disfavored; therefore, lipid partitioning of the hydrophobic surfactant tail may have been a driving force for heightened effects on less hydrated forearm skin.

An effect of the menstrual cycle on vulvar skin reactions has not been documented. However, evidence from other anatomical sites suggests that skin barrier function and reactivity to irritants may exhibit cyclical variability. Water barrier function on the back and forearm (as measured by baseline TEWL values) was significantly lower on days just prior to menstruation compared to days just prior to ovulation (53). In women, forearm skin exhibited stronger reactions to SLS on day 1 than during days 9–11 of the menstrual cycle, while no difference was detected in a male control group evaluated over the same period (54).

MICROBIOLOGY

Until recently, most studies of vulvar and vaginal microbial colonization have employed traditional culture techniques. Using these techniques, higher cell densities of *Staphylococcus aureus*, coagulase-negative staphylococci, streptococci, diphtheroids, lactobacilli, and yeasts have been measured on the labia majora than on exposed skin (Table 5) (55).

Table 5 Microbial Cell Densities (cfu/cm^2) on Vulvar and Forearm Skin

Organism	Vulva	Forearm
Staphylococcus aureus	4.1×10^4	1.4×10
Coagulase negative staphylococci	5.7×10^5	1.8×10^2
Streptococci	3.7×10^2	0.48×10
Lipophilic diphtheroids	7.9×10^5	1.1×10^2
Non-lipophilic diphtheroids	4.6×10^5	1.1×10
Gram negative rods	1.8×10^3	0.12×10
Lactobacillus species	4.6×10^5	0.96×10
Yeasts	8.2×10	0.8×10

Source: From Ref. 55.

Traditional culture methods suggest that the vulva is the primary site of genital carriage of *S. aureus*; isolation frequencies as high as 60% to 70% have been found at this site (55). However, despite an epidemiological association between vulvar and vaginal carriage of *S. aureus* (56,57), lower vaginal isolation frequencies, in the range of 3–12%, have been found by these methods (58–61).

Modern detection techniques suggest that vaginal carriage of *S. aureus* may be more common than previously thought. For example, the technique of fluorescence in situ hybridization revealed the presence of *S. aureus* in 100% of 44 vaginal specimens obtained from 15 women, while standard microbial culture methods produced positive results in only 34% of the specimens (62).

Microbes derived from the intestinal tract are also part of the endogenous vulvovaginal flora. Nonpathogenic levels of such organisms can reside on the perineum, on the external labia majora, and in the vagina. Pathogenic strains of *Escherichia coli* cause urinary tract infections, but the mere presence of *E. coli* microbes on the vulva does not lead to urethral and bladder colonization; host factors and sexual activity play a more important role in determining individual susceptibility to infection (63–65). The most important risk factor for recurrent urinary tract infection in women of reproductive age is sexual intercourse (66,67), which promotes colonization of the introitus and urethra in susceptible women (68–70).

Candida species are found in the endogenous vulvovaginal microflora. These fungi exist as blastopheric spores or as germinative mycelia. The spore form can be associated with symptom-free vulvovaginal colonization, but adhesion, germination, and epithelial invasion are necessary for pathogenesis. Host predisposing factors play a role in the development of frank vulvovaginal candidiasis (VVC). Healthy women appear to possess an innate and noninflammatory form of local immunity that prevents symptomatic infection (71); suppression of this innate immunity is suspected of playing a role in recurrent VVC (72,73). Genetic polymorphisms in mannose binding lectins—surface recognition molecules involved in the immune defense against microorganisms—also play a role in individual susceptibility to *Candida* infection (74,75).

Elevated estrogen is another risk factor for symptomatic VVC. Use of high-estrogen oral contraceptives, for example, is linked epidemiologically to an elevated VVC risk (76). Acute episodes of VVC are more common during pregnancy and during the luteal phase of the menstrual cycle, when both estrogen and progesterone levels are elevated; experimental studies indicate that this link relates solely to the elevation of estrogen (77). The mechanism by which estrogen promotes symptomatic infection has not been elucidated fully. Estrogen raises the vaginal concentration of glycogen, which may serve as a nutritional source, and the hormone may act as a growth-promoting signal for some Candida strains (78).

People with diabetes mellitus and pregnant women are at elevated risk of developing symptomatic VVC. In these higher risk groups, the degree of glycemic control plays a role in the prevalence of *Candida* colonization at various body sites (79). In addition, *Candida* adherence to vaginal epithelial cells is enhanced in people with diabetes and during pregnancy (80).

Some studies link antibiotic therapy, which suppresses protective acid-producing microbes in the vagina, to an increased risk of subsequent VVC episodes (81); however, not all studies are consistent and the association of antibiotic use with clinical candidiasis remains controversial (82).

CONCLUSION

The vulva is a highly specialized tissue with regional distinctions in embryologic derivation and tissue structure. Unique physiological characteristics have been documented in blood flow, innervation, hormonal and immune responsiveness, skin friction, tissue hydration, permeability, and microbial populations. Most of these distinctions appear to represent adaptations to reproductive function. However, the characteristics of elevated skin friction and skin hydration, coupled with differences in tissue permeability, may also mediate genital susceptibility to various exogenous irritants and infectious agents.

REFERENCES

1. Nauth H. Anatomy and physiology of the vulva. In: Elsner P, Marius J, eds. Vulvovaginitis. New York, NY: Marcel Dekker, 1993:1.
2. Sargeant P et al. Ultrastructural study of the epithelium of the normal human vulva. J Submicrosc Cytol Pathol 1996; 28:161.
3. Jones IS. A histological assessment of normal vulval skin. Clin Exp Dermatol 1983; 8:513.
4. Hu F. Melanocyte cytology in normal skin. In: Ackerman AB, ed. Masson Monographs in Dermatology I. New York: Masson, 1981.
5. Haeberle H et al. Molecular profiling reveals synaptic release machinery in Merkel cells. Proc Natl Acad Sci USA 2004; 101:14503.
6. Woodruff JD, Friedrich EG, Jr. The vestibule. Clin Obstet Gynecol 1985; 28:134.
7. Thompson IO et al. A comparative light-microscopic, electron-microscopic and chemical study of human vaginal and buccal epithelium. Arch Oral Biol 2001; 46:1091.
8. Erickson KL, Montagna W. New observations on the anatomical features of the female genitalia. J Am Med Women's Assoc 1972; 27:573.
9. Elsner P, Wilhelm D, Maibach HI. Multiple parameter assessment of vulvar irritant contact dermatitis. Contact Dermatitis 1990; 23:20.
10. Britz M, Maibach HI. Normal vulvar skin: a model for specialized skin. In: Maibach H, Lowe N, eds. Models in Dermatology. Basel: Basel Karger, 1985:83.
11. Hodgins MB et al. An immunohistochemical study of androgen, oestrogen and progesterone receptors in the vulva and vagina. Br J Obstet Gynaecol 1998; 105:216.
12. Harper WF, McNicol EM. A histological study of normal vulval skin from infancy to old age. Br J Dermatol 1977; 96:249.

13. Patton DL et al. Epithelial cell layer thickness and immune cell populations in the normal human vagina at different stages of the menstrual cycle. Am J Obstet Gynecol 2000; 183:967.
14. Ildgruben AK, Sjoberg IM, Hammarstrom ML. Influence of hormonal contraceptives on the immune cells and thickness of human vaginal epithelium. Obstet Gynecol 2003; 102:571.
15. Nauth HF, Haas M. Cytologic and histologic observations on the sex hormone dependence of the vulva. J Reprod Med 1985; 30:667.
16. Edwards JN, Morris HB. Langerhans' cells and lymphocyte subsets in the female genital tract. Br J Obstet Gynaecol 1985; 92:974.
17. Miller CJ, McChesney M, Moore PF. Langerhans cells, macrophages and lymphocyte subsets in the cervix and vagina of rhesus macaques. Lab Invest 1992; 67:628.
18. Hoglund P, Karre K, Klein G. The uterine cervix—a new member of the family of immunologically exceptional sites? Cancer Immunol 2003; 3:6.
19. Fischer GO. The commonest causes of symptomatic vulvar disease: a dermatologist's perspective. Australas J Dermatol 1996; 37:12.
20. Marren P, Wojnarowska F, Powell S. Allergic contact dermatitis and vulvar dermatoses. Br J Dermatol 1992; 126:52.
21. Margesson LJ. Contact dermatitis of the vulva. Dermatol Ther 2004; 17:20.
22. van Wilsem EJ et al. Oral tolerance is determined at the level of draining lymph nodes. Immunobiology 1995; 194:403.
23. Van Wilsem EJ et al. Dendritic cells of the oral mucosa and the induction of oral tolerance. A local affair. Immunology 1994; 83:128.
24. Black CA et al. Vaginal mucosa serves as an inductive site for tolerance. J Immunol 2000; 165:5077.
25. Turville S et al. The role of dendritic cell C-type lectin receptors in HIV pathogenesis. J Leukoc Biol 2003; 74:710.
26. Turville SG et al. Bitter-sweet symphony: defining the role of dendritic cell gp120 receptors in HIV infection. J Clin Virol 2001; 22:229.
27. Wieser F et al. Progesterone increases the number of Langerhans cells in human vaginal epithelium. Fertil Steril 2001; 75:1234.
28. Britz MB, Maibach HI. Human labia majora skin: transepidermal water loss in vivo. Acta Derm Venereol Suppl 1979; 59:23.
29. Elsner P, Wilhelm D, Maibach HI. Physiological skin surface water loss dynamics of human vulvar and forearm skin. Acta Derm Venereol 1990; 70:141.
30. Elsner P, Maibach HI. The effect of prolonged drying on transepidermal water loss, capacitance and pH of human vulvar and forearm skin. Acta Derm Venereol 1990; 70:105.
31. Elsner P, Wilhelm D, Maibach HI. Frictional properties of human forearm and vulvar skin: influence of age and correlation with transepidermal water loss and capacitance. Dermatologica 1990; 181:88.
32. Potts RO, Guy RH. Predicting skin permeability. Pharm Res 1992; 9:663.
33. Feldmann RJ, Maibach HI. Regional variation in percutaneous absorption of [14C] cortisol in man. J Invest Dermatol 1967; 48:181.
34. Britz MB, Maibach HI, Anjo DM. Human percutaneous penetration of hydrocortisone: the vulva. Arch Dermatol Res 1980; 267:313.

35. Oriba HA, Bucks DA, Maibach HI. Percutaneous absorption of hydrocortisone and testosterone on the vulva and forearm: effect of the menopause and site. Br J Dermatol 1996; 134:229.
36. Squier CA, Hall BK. The permeability of skin and oral mucosa to water and horseradish peroxidase as related to the thickness of the permeability barrier. J Invest Dermatol 1985; 84:176.
37. Harris D, Robinson JR. Drug delivery via the mucous membranes of the oral cavity. J Pharm Sci 1992; 81:1.
38. Lesch CA et al. The permeability of human oral mucosa and skin to water. J Dent Res 1989; 68:1345.
39. Guy RH, Potts RO. Structure-permeability relationships in percutaneous penetration. J Pharm Sci 1992; 81:603.
40. Guy RH, Potts RO, Francoeur ML. Skin barrier function and the mechanism(s) of percutaneous penetration. Acta Pharm Nord 1992; 4:115.
41. Law S et al. Regional variation in content, composition and organization of porcine epithelial barrier lipids revealed by thin-layer chromatography and transmission electron microscopy. Arch Oral Biol 1995; 40:1085.
42. Squier CA, Cox P, Wertz PW. Lipid content and water permeability of skin and oral mucosa. J Invest Dermatol 1991; 96:123.
43. Du X et al. Penetration of N-nitrosonornicotine (NNN) across oral mucosa in the presence of ethanol and nicotine. J Oral Pathol Med 2000; 29:80.
44. Squier CA. Penetration of nicotine and nitrosonornicotine across porcine oral mucosa. J Appl Toxicol 1986; 6:123.
45. van der Bijl P, Thompson IO, Squier CA. Comparative permeability of human vaginal and buccal mucosa to water. Eur J Oral Sci 1997; 105:571.
46. van der Bijl P, van Eyk AD, Thompson IO. Penetration of human vaginal and buccal mucosa by 4.4-kd and 12-kd fluorescein-isothiocyanate-labeled dextrans. Oral Surg Oral Med Oral Pathol Oral Radiol Endod 1998; 85:686.
47. van der Bijl P, van Eyk AD, Thompson IO. Permeation of 17 beta-estradiol through human vaginal and buccal mucosa. Oral Surg Oral Med Oral Pathol Oral Radiol Endod 1998; 85:393.
48. van der Bijl P et al. Diffusion rates of vasopressin through human vaginal and buccal mucosa. Eur J Oral Sci 1998; 106:958.
49. Britz MB, Maibach HI. Human cutaneous vulvar reactivity to irritants. Contact Dermatitis1979; 5:375.
50. Elsner P, Wilhelm D, Maibach HI. Sodium lauryl sulfate-induced irritant contact dermatitis in vulvar and forearm skin of premenopausal and postmenopausal women. J Am Acad Dermatol 1990; 23:648.
51. Elsner P, Wilhelm D, Maibach HI. Effect of low-concentration sodium lauryl sulfate on human vulvar and forearm skin. Age-related differences. J Reprod Med 1991; 36:77.
52. Elsner P, Wilhelm D, Maibach HI. Irritant effect of a model surfactant on the human vulva and forearm. Age-related differences. J Reprod Med 1990; 35:1035.
53. Harvell J, Hussona-Saeed I, Maibach HI. Changes in transepidermal water loss and cutaneous blood flow during the menstrual cycle. Contact Dermatitis 1992; 27:294.
54. Agner T, Damm P, Skouby SO. Menstrual cycle and skin reactivity. J Am Acad Dermatol 1991; 24:566.

55. Aly R, Britz MB, Maibach HI. Quantitative microbiology of human vulva. Br J Dermatol 1979; 101:445.
56. Linnemann CC, Jr et al. The epidemiology of genital colonization with *Staphylococcus aureus.* Ann Intern Med 1982; 96:940.
57. Guinan ME et al. Vaginal colonization with *Staphylococcus aureus* in healthy women: a review of four studies. Ann Intern Med 1982; 96:944.
58. Chow AW et al. Vaginal colonization with Staphylococcus aureus, positive for toxic-shock marker protein, and *Escherichia coli* in healthy women. J Infect Dis 1984; 150:80.
59. Martin RR et al. Nasal and vaginal Staphylococcus aureus in young women: quantitative studies. Ann Intern Med 1982; 96:951.
60. Parsonnet J. Risk factors for TSS among European women: vaginal colonization with *S. aureus* and antibody to TSST-1. In: Arbuthnott J, Furman B, eds. International Congress and Symposium Series 229. European Conference on Toxic Shock Syndrome. London: The Royal Society of Medicine Press, Ltd, 1998:72.
61. Parsonnet J et al. Prevalence of toxic shock syndrome toxin-1 producing *Staphylococcus aureus* and the presence of antibodies to this superantigen in menstruating women. J Clin Microbiol 2005; 43:4628.
62. Veeh RH et al. Detection of *Staphylococcus aureus* biofilm on tampons and menses components. J Infect Dis 2003; 188:519.
63. Mulvey MA et al. Bad bugs and beleaguered bladders: interplay between uropathogenic *Escherichia coli* and innate host defenses. Proc Natl Acad Sci USA 2000; 97:8829.
64. Madersbacher S, Thalhammer F, Marberger M. Pathogenesis and management of recurrent urinary tract infection in women. Curr Opin Urol 2000; 10:29.
65. Funfstuck R et al. Pathogenetic aspects of uncomplicated urinary tract infection: recent advances. Clin Nephrol 1997; 47:13.
66. Scholes D et al. Risk factors for recurrent urinary tract infection in young women. J Infec Dis 2000; 182:1177.
67. Hooton TM et al. A prospective study of risk factors for symptomatic urinary tract infection in young women. N Engl J Med 1996; 335:468.
68. Russo TA et al. Chromosomal restriction fragment length polymorphism analysis of Escherichia coli strains causing recurrent urinary tract infections in young women. J Infect Dis 1995; 172:440.
69. Stamey TA. Periurethral or perineal bacteria in urinary tract infections? JAMA 1981; 245:127.
70. Stamey TA, Sexton CC. The role of vaginal colonization with enterobacteriaceae in recurrent urinary infections. J Urol 1975; 113:214.
71. Fidel PL, Jr. Immunity in vaginal candidiasis. Curr Opin Infect Dis 2005; 18:107.
72. Fidel PL, Jr. The protective immune response against vaginal candidiasis: lessons learned from clinical studies and animal models. Int Rev Immunol 2002; 21:515.
73. Giraldo P et al. Vaginal colonization by Candida in asymptomatic women with and without a history of recurrent vulvovaginal candidiasis. Obstet Gynecol 2000; 95:413.
74. Babula O et al. Relation between recurrent vulvovaginal candidiasis, vaginal concentrations of mannose-binding lectin, and a mannose-binding lectin gene polymorphism in Latvian women. Clin Infect Dis 2003; 37:733.

75. Babula O et al. Altered distribution of mannose-binding lectin alleles at exon I codon 54 in women with vulvar vestibulitis syndrome. Am J Obstet Gynecol 2004; 191:762.
76. Spinillo A et al. The impact of oral contraception on vulvovaginal candidiasis. Contraception 1995; 51:293.
77. Fidel PL, Jr, Cutright J, Steele C. Effects of reproductive hormones on experimental vaginal candidiasis. Infect Immunol 2000; 68:651.
78. Gujjar PR, Finucane M, Larsen B. The effect of estradiol on Candida albicans growth. Ann Clin Lab Sci 1997; 27:151.
79. Nowakowska D et al. Species distribution and influence of glycemic control on fungal infections in pregnant women with diabetes. J Infect 2004; 48:339.
80. Nwobu RA, Agbonlahor DE, Odugbemi TO. Adherence of *Candida albicans* to human vaginal epithelial cells. East Afr Med J 1997; 74:389.
81. Wilton L et al. Relative risk of vaginal candidiasis after use of antibiotics compared with antidepressants in women: postmarketing surveillance data in England. Drug Saf 2003; 26:589.
82. Xu J, Sobel JD. Antibiotic-associated vulvovaginal candidiasis. Curr Infect Dis Rep 2003; 5:481.
83. Zhou X et al. Characterization of vaginal microbial communities in adult healthy women using cultivation-independent methods. Microbiology 2004; 150:2565.
84. Farage M, Maibach HI. The vulvar epithelium differs from the skin: implications for cutaneous testing to address topical vulvar exposures. Contact Dermatitis 2004; 51:201.

3

Changes in the Vulva and Vagina Throughout Life

Miranda A. Farage
Feminine Care Clinical Sciences, The Procter & Gamble Company, Cincinnati, Ohio, U.S.A.

Howard I. Maibach
Department of Dermatology, University of California School of Medicine, San Francisco, California, U.S.A.

Aikaterini Deliveliotou and George Creatsas
Second Department of Obstetrics & Gynecology, University of Athens Medical School, Aretaieion Hospital, Athens, Greece

INTRODUCTION

The vulva and vagina change over the course of life. The most salient changes are hormonally mediated and are linked to the onset of puberty, the menstrual cycle, pregnancy, and menopause. This chapter reviews the morphology and physiology of the vulva and the vagina from infancy to old age (Table 1).

With kind permission of Springer Science and Business Media, portions of this review are reproduced from Farage M, Maibach H. Lifetime changes in the vulva and vagina. Arch Gynecol Obstet 2006; 273(4):195–202, online at http://dx.doi.org/10.1007/s00404-005-0079-x.

Table 1 The Vulva and Vagina from Infancy to Old Age

Life stage[a]	Pertinent physiology	Vulvar characteristics	Vaginal features
Newborn	Effects of residual, transplacental maternal estrogens	• Plump labia majora • Well-developed labia minora • Immature hair follicles and sebaceous glands	• Stratified squamous epithelium high in glycogen content • Lactic acid-producing microbes colonize the vagina shortly after birth • White or blood-tinged vaginal discharge may be present (3)
Early childhood	Lack of stimulation by adrenal or gonadal steroid hormones	• Mons pubis and labia majora lose fat • Benign labial adhesions, if present, normalize without treatment (8)	• The vaginal epithelium thins, is less stratified, and has a low glycogen content • Vaginal pH is neutral or alkaline • Cell densities of lactic acid-producing microbes decrease
Puberty	Adrenal and gonadal maturation ensue. Secondary sex characteristics are acquired and menstruation begins (1)	• Subcutaneous fat is deposited in the mons pubis and labia majora • The vulvar epithelium thickens • The labia minora and clitoris become more prominent • Pubic hair emerges	• The vaginal epithelium thickens and stratifies • Cyclical changes in intracellular glycogen content ensue • Cervico-vaginal secretions are produced • Cell densities of lactic acid-producing microbes rise (5)
Reproductive years	The menstrual cycle	• The morphology of the vulva is mature • Vulvar skin thickness remains constant throughout the menstrual cycle (33)	• Vaginal epithelial thickness, parakeratosis, and glycogen content rise at midcycle (32,33) • Lactic acid-producing microbes are numerically dominant in healthy women (35,36)

		• Parakeratosis of the vulvar stratum corneum rises at midcycle (32,33)	• Menstrual cyclicity becomes established (12,13) • Cervico-vaginal secretions become thicker, clearer and more elastic prior to ovulation
Pregnancy	Blood volume increases. The menstrual cycle ceases during gestation	• Hair may darken along the midline of the abdomen • Increased blood flow heightens vulvar coloration • Susceptibility to vulvar varicose veins increases (37) • Connective tissue relaxes • Flattening of the fourchette and perineal trauma may occur during delivery	• Connective tissue relaxes and vaginal muscle fibers thicken • The risk of Candida infection increases (38) • Following delivery, the morphology and dimensions of the vaginal tract are re-established
Postmenopause	Follicular function and the menstrual cycle cease. The prevalence of urinary and fecal incontinence rises. Physical health, immune function, tissue regeneration capacity, and cognition may be compromised with increasing age	• Pubic hair becomes sparse • Subcutaneous fat is lost • Vulvar tissue atrophies • The risk of perineal dermatitis rises in older women with incontinence	• The vaginal epithelium atrophies • Cervico-vaginal secretions become sparse • Vaginal pH rises; colonization by enteric microflora may rise • Atrophic vaginitis is common

[a]Because of inter-individual variations, the age definition of each life stage is approximate. The newborn period lies between birth and one month of age; early childhood refers to between one and eight years of age. Puberty usually occurs between eight and 15 years, although the age criteria for premature puberty are controversial. The reproductive years begin at menarche (mean age of about 12 years) and continue through the perimenopause. Menopause is defined to begin one year following the final menstrual period; menstruation ceases at a median age of 50 in Western industrialized countries.

Source: Adapted from Ref. 57.

INFANCY AND EARLY CHILDHOOD

The vulva and vagina of the newborn exhibit the effects of residual maternal estrogens (Fig. 1). At birth, the labia majora appear plump. The labia minora are well developed and may protrude beyond the labia majora. Similarly, the clitoris may appear disproportionately large. The vaginal introitus is visible but small (typically 4 to 5 mm in girls under the age of five). The hymen may appear thick and fibriated, a hymenal configuration common in girls under the age of three years. Bartholin's glands are visible and Skene's (paraurethral) glands are well formed. The urethral opening is not easily discerned. The vaginal epithelium is glycogen-rich and is colonized with lactic acid-producing microbes, such as *Lactobacillus* species, within the first 24 hours of birth (1). A physiologic, white mucoid vaginal discharge may be present. As residual levels of maternal estrogen diminish, this discharge may become tinged with blood from withdrawal endometrial bleeding (2,3).

These estrogenic effects dissipate between the fourth and eighth postnatal weeks. The labia majora lose fat and the prominence of the clitoris and labia minora diminishes (Fig. 2). The vaginal epithelium loses its stratification and glycogen content and becomes much thinner. The vaginal pH becomes neutral or

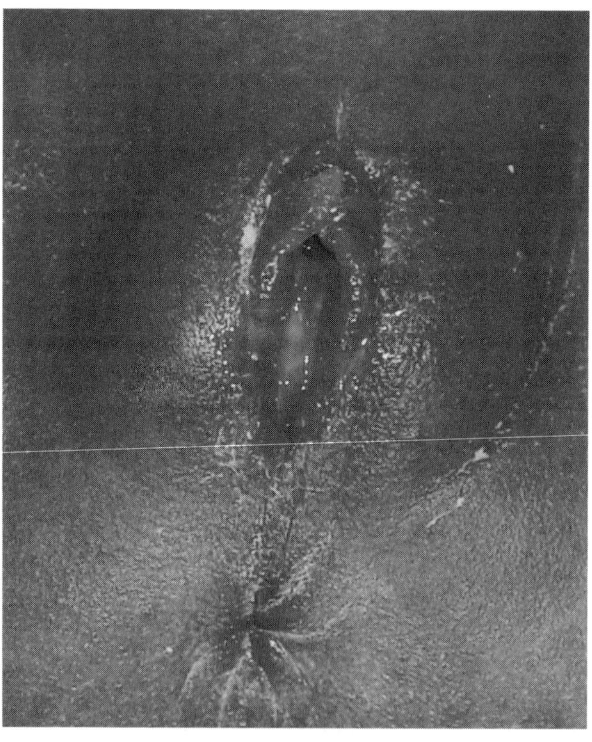

Figure 1 Anatomy of the newborn vulva. (*See color insert p. 2.*)

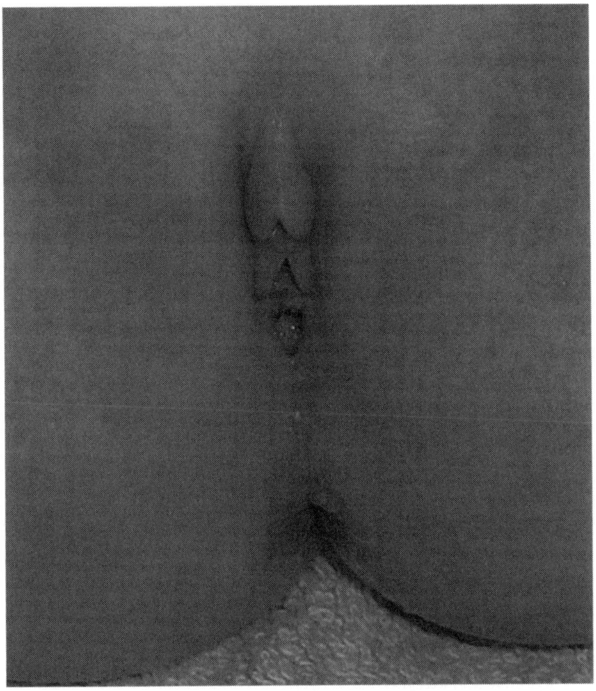

Figure 2 Anatomy of the prepubescent vulva. (*See color insert p. 3.*)

alkaline, presumably because of a relative deficiency of acid-producing vaginal microbes (4,5). Vulvar skin thickness decreases and the mons pubis and labia majora lose some of the subcutaneous fat present at birth (6,7). Although the full complement of vulvar hair follicles and sebaceous glands is thought to be present from birth, these structures do not mature until the adrenal glands are activated at puberty. The prepubescent labia minora have barely discernible vellus hair follicles that are lost at puberty when the follicles of the labia majora and mons pubis terminally differentiate (6). The appearance of the prepubescent hymen is variable. Two common forms in girls more than three years of age are:

1. The annular hymen that surrounds the introitus in a regular fashion, and
2. The crescentic hymen, a crescent-shaped conformation present along the posterior vaginal orifice only, the ends of which are attached to the lateral vaginal wall.

Labial adhesions occur more commonly in younger prepubertal girls (aged three months to six years, with a peak incidence at 13 to 23 months of age), creating a flat vulvar appearance (8). This acquired condition is the result of low estrogen levels in the prepubertal child and possibly of a chronic inflammatory process. First-line treatment with estrogen cream is recommended.

A failure to respond to medical therapy requires consideration of other options, which include in-office treatment with manual separation after topical anesthesia or, rarely, separation under sedation in an outpatient setting or surgical suite (9).

PUBERTY

Pubertal changes in the vulva and vagina are induced by adrenal and gonadal maturation. Puberty generally begins between ages 8 and 13 years. Physical changes associated with puberty are an accelerated growth rate, the appearance of pubic hair (pubarche), the appearance of axillary hair, breast development (telarche), and the onset of menstruation (menarche). The timing and stages of development of secondary sex characteristics were first defined in Marshall and Tanner's seminal study of 192 girls in a British orphanage (10).

Maturation of the adrenal glands and androgen secretion (adrenarche) begin at about age six, approximately two years before pituitary-gonadal maturation and the production of ovarian steroid hormones (gonadarche). Because adrenarche and gonadarche proceed independently, the appearance of pubic hair does not provide information about pituitary-ovarian maturation. Pubic hair development elicited by androgens proceeds in five stages as described by Tanner (Fig. 3) (10):

1. No pubic hair.
2. Sparse hair appears on the labia majora and the mons pubis along the midline.
3. Thickness and coarseness of the hair increase, with coverage of the lobes of the labia majora and increased lateral growth from the midline of the mons pubis.
4. Hair growth increases such that only the upper lateral corners of the mature triangular configuration are deficient.
5. Adult pattern, attained between the ages of 12 and 17 years, with a characteristic horizontal upper margin on the mons pubis just above the limit of the genitofemoral folds.

In most ethnic groups (except for women of Asian or Native American heritage), hair coverage extends from the labia to the upper aspects of the thighs.

Gonadal maturation usually occurs during the two years preceding menarche. During the maturation process, follicular development causes estrogen production

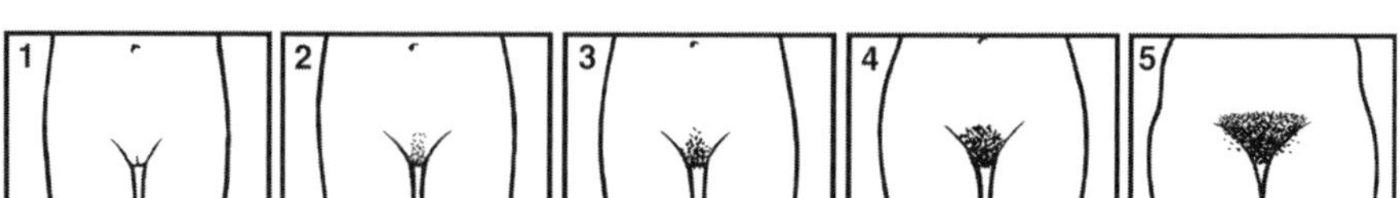

Figure 3 Tanner stages of pubic hair development. *Source*: Adapted from Ref. 57.

to rise. The vaginal epithelium thickens and intracellular glycogen production begins. The cervix and vagina increase in size, the vaginal fornices develop, cervicovaginal secretions are produced, and vaginal fluid becomes acidic.

Vulvar morphology matures at this time. Fat deposition occurs in the mons pubis and labia majora. The vulvar epithelium increases in thickness (7), labial skin becomes rugose, the clitoris becomes more prominent, the vestibular glands become active, the introitus increases in diameter, and the urethral orifice is more discernible. Vaginal discharge may be evident between the anterior folds.

Breast development, influenced by estrogens, is also described by five Tanner stages, from no development (Stage 1) to the mature adult breast (Stage 5) (10). Menarche occurs near the end of the Tanner sequence of breast changes, typically sometime between the ages of 11 and 15 years (1). The mean age of menarche worldwide is between 12 and 13 years (11). The sequence from the first appearance of pubic hair through breast development and menarche takes about four years. Normative menstrual cycle length is established by the sixth gynecologic year (i.e., the sixth year following menarche), usually around the chronologic age of 19, although this may occur anytime between the ages of 17 and 21, depending on menarcheal age (12,13).

Idiopathic Precocious Puberty

Historically, puberty had been defined as precocious in girls when secondary sex characteristics (particularly breast development) appeared prior to the age of eight. However, an apparent advance in the age of onset of pubertal changes has been observed in the United States and in girls from developing countries who have migrated to Western Europe for foreign adoption (reviewed in Ref. 14). Two large studies in the U.S. found that pubertal signs may appear before the age of eight, especially in African American as compared to Caucasian girls (Tables 2 and 3) (15–17). Between the 1970s and 1990s, the average age of menarche in the U.S. fell from 12.75 years to 12.54 years (17).

Table 2 Mean Onset of Secondary Sex Characteristics (Tanner Stage 2) and Menarche in Caucasian and African-American Girls from North American Suburban Medical Practices (1997)

Ethnicity	Mean age of onset (years): Menarche	Breast development	Pubic hair	% with Pubertal signs by age 8
African American	12.16 (SD 1.21)	8.87 (SD 1.93)	8.78 (SD 2.00)	48.3
Caucasian	12.88 (SD 1.20)	9.96 (SD 1.82)	10.52 (SD 1.67)	14.7

Abbreviation: SD, standard deviation.
Source: Adapted from Refs. 10, 15, 57.

Table 3 Mean Age of Menarche and Median Age of Onset of Secondary Sex Characteristics (Tanner Stage 2) (10) by Race from the U.S. Third National Health and Nutrition Examination Survey (NHANES III) (1988–1994)

	Age (years)		
Ethnicity	Menarche[a]	Breast development[b]	Pubic hair[b]
African American	12.14 (SE: 11.87–12.39)	9.48 (FL: 9.14–9.76)	9.43 (FL: 9.05–9.74)
Caucasian	12.60 (SE: 12.48–12.71)	10.38 (FL: 10.11–10.65)	10.57 (FL: 10.29–10.85)

[a]Mean age of menarche. From Ref. 17.
[b]Median age at which 50% of the sample entered Stage 2 of pubertal development. FL based on probit analysis for multiple race comparisons at the 95% confidence level (16).
Abbreviation: FL, fiducial limit.
Source: Adapted from Ref. 57.

Controversy surrounds the clinical significance of these findings. Most cases of early pubertal development are idiopathic and probably do not represent precocious puberty unless bone maturation and developmental characteristics are so accelerated that diminished adult height is likely (18,19). However, because true endocrine pathology may be overlooked if early pubertal signs are dismissed, vigilant longitudinal follow-up of girls with early pubertal onset is advised (20). Several risk factors (genetics, low birth weight, higher body mass index, exposure to endocrine disruptors) are correlated statistically with earlier pubertal onset, but the biological mechanisms of accelerated onset are unknown (17,21–31).

REPRODUCTIVE YEARS

Changes in the vulva and vagina during the reproductive years are linked to the menstrual cycle and pregnancy.

Vulvar and Vaginal Effects of the Menstrual Cycle

Vulvar epithelial thickness is at its highest in the reproductive years (Fig. 4). Vulvar skin thickness remains constant over the menstrual cycle, but its surface cells are predominantly orthokeratotic (lacking nuclei) at the beginning and end of the cycle, and increasingly parakeratotic (bearing a degenerated nucleus) at midcycle (32). These cytological changes are thought to be mediated by estrogen: parakeratosis of vulvar epithelial cells is rare in postmenopausal women but rises dramatically in response to systemic estrogen supplementation (32). The vaginal epithelium is sensitive to ovarian steroid hormone cycling. Estrogen stimulation causes the thickness, glycogen content, and parakeratosis of the vaginal epithelium to peak approximately at midcycle (Fig. 5) (33).

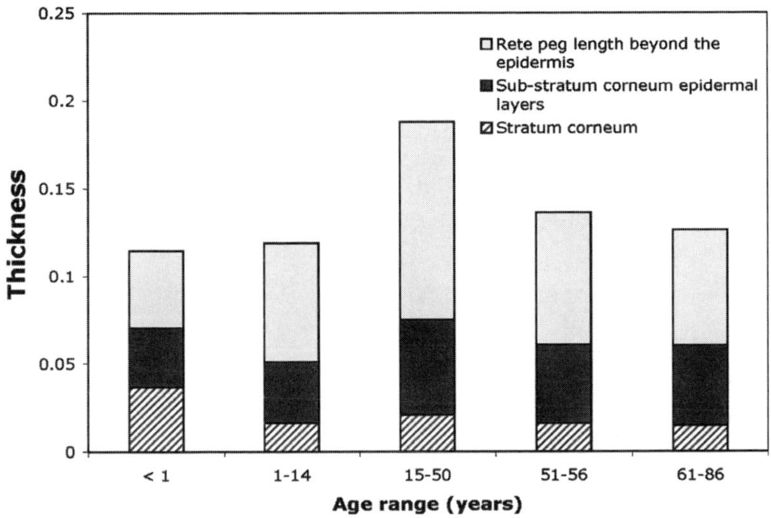

Figure 4 Epithelial thickness of the labia majora with age. *Source*: Based on data in Ref. 7. (*See color insert p. 3.*)

During menstruation, vaginal pH rises as high as six on day 2 and drops to approximately five by day 4 (34). The impact of the menstrual cycle on the microbial ecology of the vagina is not well understood. Studies using traditional culture techniques suggest that *Lactobacillus* species predominate in the vaginal flora of healthy women and that their cell densities remain relatively constant over the menstrual cycle (35). However, such techniques typically identify only the most readily cultivated microbial populations, which may represent but a subset of the extant community. Emerging data obtained by analysis of total microbial community DNA indicate that lactic acid-producing species such as *Atopobium*, *Megasphaera*, and *Leptotrichia*, rather than *Lactobacillus*, are numerically dominant in some women (36). Consequently, genera besides *Lactobacillus* may contribute to the acidity of vaginal tract, but the impact of the menstrual cycle on these genera has not been studied.

Vulvar and Vaginal Effects of Pregnancy and Delivery

During pregnancy, an increase in total blood volume heightens the coloration of the vulva and the vagina. The connective tissue of the vulva, vagina, and perineum relaxes and the muscle fibers of the vaginal wall increase in size in preparation for delivery. Progesterone elevates venous distensibility, which may cause varicose veins in the vulva (37). Pregnancy is associated with a 10- to 20-fold increased incidence of vulvovaginal candidiasis (38).

During delivery, the perineal and the vaginal musculature relax; the vaginal rugae flatten to allow expansion of the vaginal tract, accommodating passage for

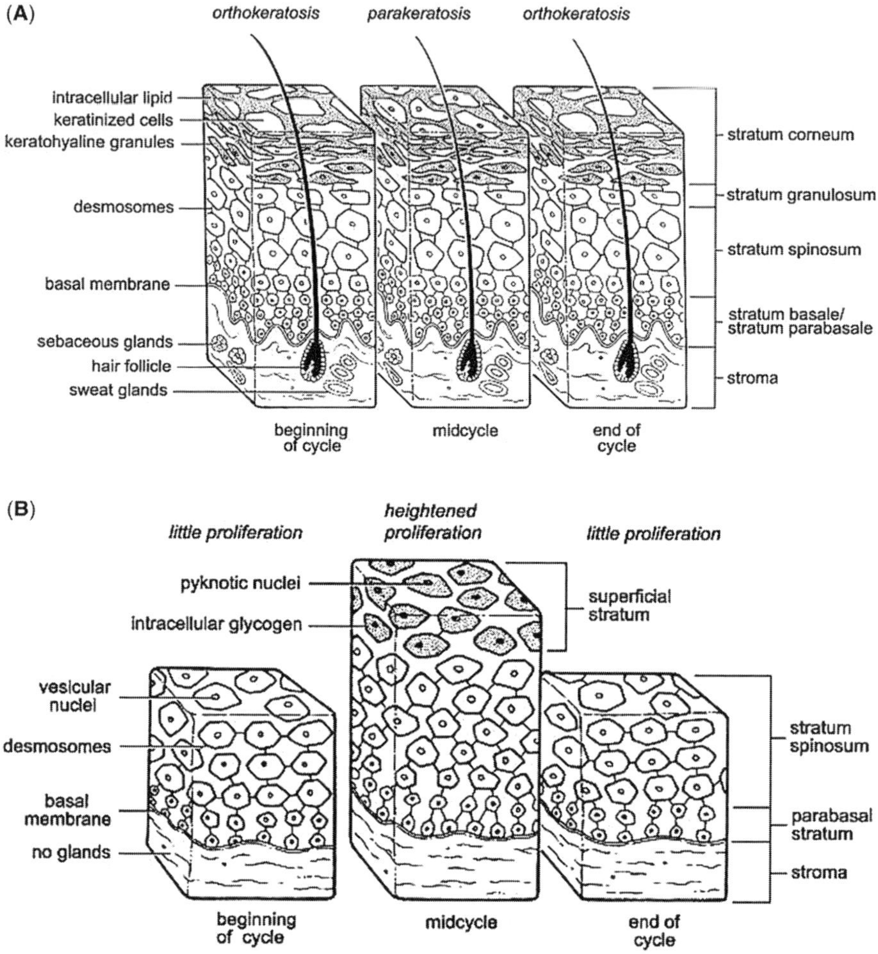

Figure 5 Menstrual cycle variations in **(A)** vulvar skin and **(B)** vaginal mucosa. *Source*: Adapted from Ref. 33.

the infant. Injury to the perineum can occur spontaneously or because of episiotomy. After delivery, the vaginal introitus is wider and the fourchette appears more flattened. Over the next 6 to 12 weeks, the morphology and dimensions of the vaginal tract are reestablished (39).

MENOPAUSE AND OLDER AGE

Menopause is the permanent cessation of menstruation due to the loss of follicular activity. A constellation of symptoms emerges during the perimenopause, the transition period to menopause. The most notable is menstrual cycle irregularity, reflecting an increase in the number of anovulatory cycles and cycles with a prolonged follicular phase. Some women experience cramps, bloating, or breast tenderness; symptoms of estrogen depletion, such as vasomotor symptoms (hot flashes), migraine, and vaginal dryness, can ensue. The perimenopause commences typically after the age of 45 and lasts about four years. Menstruation ceases at a median age of 50 in Western industrialized societies (40). Menopause is considered established one year after the final menstrual period (41).

Following menopause, pubic hair grays and becomes sparse, the labia majora lose subcutaneous fat, and the labia minora, vestibule, and vaginal epithelium atrophy (7,42). At the cytological level, estrogen-induced parakeratosis of vulvar stratum corneum is highest in the third decade of life, but rarely seen by the eighth decade (43).

Postmenopausal atrophic vulvovaginitis is a common condition. Vaginal secretions decrease, reducing lubrication and increasing coital discomfort. Thinned tissue is irritated more easily and may be more susceptible to infection. The vaginal pH rises and the prevalence of colonization by enteric organisms associated with urinary tract infections increases (44). In addition to these physiologically induced changes, certain vulvar dermatoses, such as lichen sclerosus, are most prevalent in peri- and postmenopausal women (45).

Vulvar skin differs from exposed skin in the characteristics of skin hydration, friction, permeability, and visually discernible irritation (reviewed in Ref. 46). It is assumed commonly that aged skin is intrinsically less hydrated, less elastic, more permeable, and more susceptible to irritation. As discussed later in this chapter, however, assessments of the vulvar skin of pre- and postmenopausal women by means of bioengineering techniques did not reveal large age-related changes in these characteristics (Table 4).

For example, the skin of the labia majora is more hydrated than forearm skin as measured by transepidermal water loss and its coefficient of friction is higher (47,48). Although small age-related changes in these parameters were measured on the forearm of pre- and postmenopausal women, the impact of the menopause on the water barrier function and friction coefficient of vulvar skin was negligible (Table 4) (48).

Vulvar skin is more permeable to hydrocortisone than forearm skin, but comparable testosterone penetration rates have been measured at both sites. In postmenopausal women, skin permeability to hydrocortisone drops on the forearm but not on the vulva, and no age-related differences in testosterone penetration were found at either site (Table 4) (49). (For perspective, penetration of testosterone but not hydrocortisone may be mediated by androgen receptors.)

Exposed forearm skin was more susceptible than vulvar skin to the model irritant, aqueous sodium lauryl sulfate (1% w/v). This agent caused intense erythema on the forearms of premenopausal women, but no visually discernable response on the vulva in either pre- or postmenopausal women (Table 4) (50).

Table 4 Physiologic Skin Parameters in Pre- and Postmenopausal Women

Parameter	Site	Age group[a]	Measured value	Significance[b]	Reference
Water barrier function (TEWL, g/m^2.hr)					
	Forearm	Premenopausal	3.7 ± 0.4	$P < 0.05$	(48)
		Postmenopausal	2.6 ± 0.3		
	Vulva	Premenopausal	14.8 ± 1.5	NS	(48)
		Postmenopausal	13.5 ± 1.8		
Skin hydration (capacitance, AU)					
	Forearm	Premenopausal	93.3 ± 2.3	NS	(48)
		Postmenopausal	91.9 ± 2.8		
	Vulva	Premenopausal	116.8 ± 4.1	NS	(48)
		Postmenopausal	118.0 ± 8.2		
Friction coefficient, μ					
	Forearm	Premenopausal	0.49 ± 0.02	$P < 0.05$	(48)
		Postmenopausal	0.45 ± 0.01		
	Vulva	Premenopausal	0.60 ± 0.04	NS	(48)
		Postmenopausal	0.60 ± 0.06		
Hydrocortisone penetration (% dose absorbed)					
	Forearm	Premenopausal	2.8 ± 2.4	NS	(49)
		Postmenopausal	1.5 ± 1.1		
	Vulva	Premenopausal	8.1 ± 4.1	$P < 0.01$	(49)
		Postmenopausal	4.4 ± 2.8		
Testosterone penetration (% dose absorbed)					
	Forearm	Premenopausal	20.2 ± 8.1	NS	(49)
		Postmenopausal	14.7 ± 4.2		
	Vulva	Premenopausal	26.7 ± 8.0	NS	(49)
		Postmenopausal	24.6 ± 5.5		
Number of positive visual erythema scores (on day 2, after 24-hr exposure to 1% SLS)					
	Forearm	Premenopausal	9	$P = 0.03$	(50)
		Postmenopausal	5		
	Vulva	Premenopausal	0	NS	(50)
		Postmenopausal	0		

[a]Group sizes (water barrier function, skin hydration and friction parameters): premenopausal—34 subjects, postmenopausal—10 subjects. Group sizes (hydrocortisone and testosterone penetration): 9 subjects in each group. Visual erythema score to sodium lauryl sulfate (SLS) application: 10 subjects per age group.

[b]Level of statistical significance of age-group difference.

Abbreviation: n.s., not significant.

Source: Adapted from Ref. 57.

Although large age-related differences in skin vulvar permeability and intrinsic susceptibility to irritants have not been demonstrated, dermatitis of the vulva, perineum, and buttocks can be a substantial problem in older people with incontinence. A mechanistic understanding of the etiology of incontinence dermatitis was first developed from studies on diapered infants and then extended to older adults. Chapter 12 provides a detailed explanation of the mechanistic factors that contribute to incontinence dermatitis. The etiology is multifactorial. In brief, exposure to urinary moisture under occlusion makes the skin more susceptible to friction damage; urinary ammonia elevates the local pH, which alters skin barrier function and activates fecal enzymes; these enzymes further compromise skin integrity and increase skin susceptibility to microbial infection (51–55). Incontinence dermatitis is particularly debilitating in older adults because urine and feces exert their effects against a background of atrophied tissue, immobility, a potentially weakened immune response, and often compromised physical health and cognition. Several factors exacerbate the deleterious effects of skin wetness, occlusion, and fecal enzyme action in elders. Although the baseline skin wetness level does not differ significantly in aged skin, the excess hydration induced by occlusion is significantly greater and dissipated more slowly in older skin than in young skin (56). Although the coefficient of friction of vulvar skin is unchanged in older women, reduced mobility subjects atrophied genital tissue to higher shear forces than those encountered by infants. Moreover, atrophied genital tissue may be more susceptible to pH changes and enzymatic action, while immune function and tissue regeneration capacity also may be compromised. Lastly, elders may not receive the same degree of attentiveness as infants and those with impaired cognition may be unable to alert caregivers to incontinent episodes. These factors underscore the need for vigilant care and proper hygiene to help maintain healthy urogenital skin in older women with incontinence.

CONCLUSION

In summary, the vulva and vagina undergo characteristic age-related changes in morphology and physiology over the course of a lifetime. At birth, these tissues exhibit the effects of residual maternal estrogens. During puberty, the vulva and vagina mature under the influence of adrenal and gonadal steroid hormones. During the reproductive years, the vagina responds to ovarian steroid hormone cycling and both tissues adapt to the needs of pregnancy and delivery. Following menopause, the vulva and vagina atrophy. A rise in the prevalence of incontinence among older women increases the risk of vulvar and perineal dermatitis. Vigilant care is needed to avoid dermatitis in the older person with incontinence, as the condition is particularly debilitating at this stage of life.

REFERENCES

1. Marshall WA, Tanner JM. Puberty. In: Davis JA, Dobbing J, eds. Scientific Foundations of Paediatrics. 2nd ed. London: Heinemann, 1981.
2. Altchek A. Vulvovaginitis, vulvar skin disease, and pelvic inflammatory disease. Pediatr Clin North Am 1981; 28:397.

3. Elvik SL. Vaginal discharge in the prepubertal girl. J Pediatr Health Care 1990; 4:181.
4. Gerstner GJ et al. Vaginal organisms in prepubertal children with and without vulvovaginitis. A vaginoscopic study. Arch Gynecol 1982; 231:247.
5. Hammerschlag MR et al. Microbiology of the vagina in children: normal and potentially pathogenic organisms. Pediatrics 1978; 62:57.
6. Harper WF, McNicol EM. A histological study of normal vulval skin from infancy to old age. Br J Dermatol 1977; 96:249.
7. Jones IS. A histological assessment of normal vulval skin. Clin Exp Dermatol 1983; 8:513.
8. Williams TS, Callen JP, Owen LG. Vulvar disorders in the prepubertal female. Pediatr Ann 1986; 15:588.
9. Bacon JL. Prepubertal labial adhesions: evaluation of a referral population. Am J Obstet Gynecol 2002; 187:327.
10. Marshall WA, Tanner JM. Variations in pattern of pubertal changes in girls. Arch Dis Child 1969; 44:291.
11. WHO, World Health Organization multicenter study on menstrual and ovulatory patterns in adolescent girls. I. A multicenter cross-sectional study of menarche. World Health Organization Task Force on Adolescent Reproductive Health. J Adolesc Health Care 1986; 7:229.
12. Flug D, Largo RH, Prader A. Menstrual patterns in adolescent Swiss girls: a longitudinal study. Ann Hum Biol 1984; 11:495.
13. Widholm O, Kantero RL. A statistical analysis of the menstrual patterns of 8,000 Finnish girls and their mothers. Acta Obstet Gynecol Scand Suppl 1971; 14(suppl 14):1–36.
14. Parent AS et al. The timing of normal puberty and the age limits of sexual precocity: variations around the world, secular trends, and changes after migration. Endocr Rev 2003; 24:668.
15. Herman-Giddens ME et al. Secondary sexual characteristics and menses in young girls seen in office practice: a study from the Pediatric Research in Office Settings network. Pediatrics 1997; 99:505.
16. Sun SS et al. National estimates of the timing of sexual maturation and racial differences among US children. Pediatrics 2002; 110:911.
17. Anderson SE, Dallal GE, Must A. Relative weight and race influence average age at menarche: results from two nationally representative surveys of US girls studied 25 years apart. Pediatrics 2003; 111:844.
18. Lee PA, Kulin HE, Guo SS. Age of puberty among girls and the diagnosis of precocious puberty. Pediatrics 2001; 107:1493.
19. Root AW. Precocious puberty. Pediatr Rev 2000; 21:10.
20. Midyett LK, Moore WV, Jacobson JD. Are pubertal changes in girls before age 8 benign? Pediatrics 2003; 111:47.
21. Treloar SA, Martin NG. Age at menarche as a fitness trait: nonadditive genetic variance detected in a large twin sample. Am J Hum Genet 1990; 47:137.
22. Ibanez L et al. Precocious pubarche in girls and the development of androgen excess. J Pediatr Endocrinol Metab 2000; 13:1261.
23. Charkaluk ML, Trivin C, Brauner R. Premature pubarche as an indicator of how body weight influences the onset of adrenarche. Eur J Pediatr 2004; 163:89.
24. Kaplowitz PB et al. Earlier onset of puberty in girls: relation to increased body mass index and race. Pediatrics 2001; 108:347.

25. Wang Y. Is obesity associated with early sexual maturation? A comparison of the association in American boys versus girls. Pediatrics 2002; 110:903.
26. Dimartino-Nardi J. Premature adrenarche: findings in prepubertal African-American and Caribbean-Hispanic girls. Acta Paediatr Suppl 1999; 88:67.
27. Demerath EW. Recent decline in age at menarche: the Fels Longitudinal Study. Am J Hum Biol 2004; 16:453.
28. Colon I et al. Identification of phthalate esters in the serum of young Puerto Rican girls with premature breast development. Environ Health Perspect 2000; 108:895.
29. Larriuz-Serrano MC et al. Natural history and incidence of premature thelarche in Puerto Rican girls aged 6 months to 8 years diagnosed between 1990 and 1995. P R Health Sci J 2001; 20:13.
30. McKee RH. Phthalate exposure and early thelarche. Environ Health Perspect 2004; 112:541.
31. Krstevska-Konstantinova M et al. Sexual precocity after immigration from developing countries to Belgium: evidence of previous exposure to organochlorine pesticides. Hum Reprod 2001; 16:1020.
32. Nauth HF, Haas M. Cytologic and histologic observations on the sex hormone dependence of the vulva. J Reprod Med 1985; 30:667.
33. Nauth H.Anatomy and physiology of the vulva. In: Elsner P, Marius J, eds. Vulvovaginitis. Vol 1. New York: Marcel Dekker, 1993.
34. Wagner G, Ottesen B. Vaginal physiology during menstruation. Ann Intern Med 1982; 96:921.
35. Eschenbach DA et al. Influence of the normal menstrual cycle on vaginal tissue, discharge, and microflora. Clin Infect Dis 2000; 30:901.
36. Zhou X et al. Characterization of vaginal microbial communities in adult healthy women using cultivation-independent methods. Microbiology 2004; 150:2565.
37. Gallagher PG. Varicose veins of the vulva. Br J Sex Med 1986; 13:12.
38. Wallenburg HC, Wladimiroff JW. Recurrence of vulvovaginal candidosis during pregnancy. Comparison of miconazole vs nystatin treatment. Obstet Gynecol 1976; 48:491.
39. Stewart EG, Spencer P. The V Book: a doctor's guide to complete vulvovaginal health. Bantam Trade Paperbacks. New York: Bantam Dell Publishing Group, 2002.
40. Ginsberg J. What determines the age at the menopause? BMJ 1991; 302:1288.
41. Burger HG. The menopausal transition. Baillieres Clin Obstet Gynaecol 1996; 10:347.
42. Erickson KL, Montagna W. New observations on the anatomical features of the female genitalia. J Am Med Womens Assoc 1972; 27:573.
43. Nauth HF, Boger A. New aspects of vulvar cytology. Acta Cytol 1982; 26:1.
44. Fischer BK, Margesson LJ. Normal anatomy of the vulva. Genital Skin Disorders. Diagnosis and Treatment. St Louis: Mosby Publishing, 1998:99.
45. Kamarashev JA, Vassileva SG. Dermatologic diseases of the vulva. Clin Dermatol 1997; 15:53.
46. Oriba HA, Elsner P, Maibach HI. Vulvar physiology. Semin Dermatol 1989; 8:2.
47. Elsner P, Maibach HI. The effect of prolonged drying on transepidermal water loss, capacitance and pH of human vulvar and forearm skin. Acta Derm Venereol 1990; 70:105.
48. Elsner P, Wilhelm D, Maibach HI. Frictional properties of human forearm and vulvar skin: influence of age and correlation with transepidermal water loss and capacitance. Dermatologica 1990; 181:88.

49. Oriba HA, Bucks DA, Maibach HI. Percutaneous absorption of hydrocortisone and testosterone on the vulva and forearm: effect of the menopause and site. Br J Dermatol 1996; 134:229.
50. Elsner P, Wilhelm D, Maibach HI. Effect of low-concentration sodium lauryl sulfate on human vulvar and forearm skin. Age-related differences. J Reprod Med 1991; 36:77.
51. Buckingham KW, Berg RW. Etiologic factors in diaper dermatitis: the role of feces. Pediatr Dermatol 1986; 3:107.
52. Berg RW, Buckingham KW, Stewart RL. Etiologic factors in diaper dermatitis: the role of urine. Pediatr Dermatol 1986; 3:102.
53. Berg RW. Etiology and pathophysiology of diaper dermatitis. Adv Dermatol 1988; 3:75.
54. Andersen PH et al. Faecal enzymes: in vivo human skin irritation. Contact Dermatitis 1994; 30:152.
55. Faria DT, Shwayder T, Krull EA. Perineal skin injury: extrinsic environmental risk factors. Ostomy Wound Manage 1996; 42:28.
56. Roskos KV, Guy RH. Assessment of skin barrier function using transepidermal water loss: effect of age. Pharm Res 1989; 6:949.
57. Farage MA, Maibach HI. Lifetime changes in the vulva and vagina. Arch Gynecol Obstet 2006; 273(4):195–202, online at http://dx.doi.org/10.1007/s00404-005-0079-x.

4

Microbial Ecology of the Vulva

Ronald W. Berg and Catherine C. Davis
The Procter & Gamble Company, Cincinnati, Ohio, U.S.A.

INTRODUCTION

Although there is a considerable body of literature regarding the composition of the vaginal microflora, remarkably little is known of the microbiology of the vulva. A comprehensive understanding of vulvar microbial ecology is hindered by the anatomical reality that the vulva is likely not a single ecological niche, but rather a structure that includes many unique and diverse microbial habitats. From an ecological perspective, the vulva can be best thought of as a transitional zone between the arid desert of external skin surfaces and the tropical rainforest of the vagina. Thus, the microbial ecology of the vulva is not a single entity but a complex construction, the nature of which is likely to be revealed in interwoven yet distinctive parts, depending on: (i) the anatomical areas sampled, (ii) the methodology used to analyze the samples, and (iii) the ability to describe the evenness, composition, and richness of the microbial communities.

ANATOMICAL STRUCTURE OF THE VULVA

The vulva consists of the mons pubis, the labia majora and minora, the clitoris, and the vestibule of the vagina. The external urethral orifice is situated in the vestibule, as are the ducts of the mucus-secreting paraurethral and Bartholin's glands.

The mons pubis and the outer aspects of the labia majora are covered with hairy skin that is similar to that of the scalp and axillae. The labia majora contain numerous sebaceous glands, along with apocrine glands and eccrine sweat

Table 1 Anatomical Features of Vulvar Skin Relevant to Microbial Ecology

Structure	Epithelium type	Hair	Eccrine sweat glands	Apocrine sweat glands	Sebaceous glands
Mons pubis	Keratinized	+	+	−	+
Clitoris	Nonkeratinized	−	−	−	−
Labia majora	Keratinized	+	+	+	+
Labia minora	Nonkeratinized	−	+/−	−	+
Vestibule—outside Hart's line	Keratinized	−	−	−	+
Vestibule—inside Hart's line	Nonkeratinized	−	−	−	−

glands. The labia minora, in contrast, are free from hair, and are covered with stratified squamous epithelium, which can have a thin layer of keratinized cells at its surface. Sebaceous glands are present, but as the skin is glabrous, these glands open directly at the surface. Eccrine sweat glands are found occasionally on the labia minora but apocrine glands are absent. The clitoris is covered with a thin, nonkeratinized, stratified squamous epithelium and contains nerve bundles and erectile tissue. From the innermost surface of the labia majora to the vagina, the epidermis gradually changes from the keratinized epithelium typical of other external body surfaces to the mucosal epithelium typical of the vagina and other mucous membranes. The vulvar vestibule extends laterally from the hymenal ring to a line of more keratinized skin on the labia minora (Hart's line). The overall structural diversity of the vulva is summarized in Table 1. An organ with this degree of structural diversity is unlikely to harbor a single microbial ecosystem, as the diverse habitats that result create unique ecological pressures that are likely to shape unique populations of microorganisms.

FACTORS CONTROLLING MICROBIAL GROWTH AND DIVERSITY

Although the environment of the vulva has some unique properties as compared to other skin sites, there are a number of ecological factors in common with other sites that can affect microbial populations. Relatively few studies have addressed vulvar skin directly, but there is a wealth of information from these other similar sites that can be instructive in understanding the factors that control vulvar microbial ecology.

Moisture

It has long been known that the availability of water is the primary rate-limiting factor for growth of bacteria on skin. The largest populations of microorganisms are found in those regions where high humidity results in high skin hydration, for example, perineum, axillae, and between the toes. The primary source of water on the skin is eccrine sweat. Transepidermal water loss (TEWL) also can contribute to skin hydration, particularly if the skin is occluded to limit evaporation. Studies have shown that TEWL is higher on labia majora skin than on forearm skin (1) or inner thigh skin adjacent to the vulva (2). Other sources of moisture unique to the vulvar area include vaginal secretions and urine. Increased skin hydration has been shown to result in both increases in microbial density and changes in the relative ratios of microorganisms (3,4). Adult forearms occluded tightly with plastic film showed increases in microbial populations from a baseline of approximately $10^2/cm^2$ to almost $10^8/cm^2$ over the course of several days. The relative population of micrococci decreased, Gram-negative rods emerged, and lipophilic diphtheroids became the dominant microflora. Although occlusion of the vulvar area resulting from tight-fitting clothing or nonbreathable fabrics is unlikely to approach the level provided by plastic film, it is readily apparent that increased moisture availability can have a dramatic effect on the quantitative and qualitative nature of microbial populations on skin.

pH

Most skin bacteria can grow under all pH conditions normally found on skin, but many bacteria possess individual pH optima for growth; therefore, small changes in pH have the potential to provide an ecological advantage to those finding more favorable conditions with regard to hydrogen ion concentration. Studies have shown that increased skin hydration resulting from occlusion is accompanied by an increase in pH, from its normal slightly acidic condition to near neutrality (5). pH can also exert an effect on microbial populations by altering the antimicrobial properties of fatty acids on the skin. The protonated form of the acid is more active than the unprotonated form, so as the pH approaches the pKa of the acid, antimicrobial activity increases. As microorganisms vary in their susceptibility to fatty acids, relatively small changes in pH can influence the numbers and kinds of organisms that thrive in a population.

Microbial Nutrients and Inhibitors

Nutrients on the skin surface are derived mainly from eccrine sweat, apocrine and sebaceous gland secretions, and the stratum corneum. These materials supply a rich mixture of proteins, peptides, amino acids, carbohydrates, nucleic acids, lipoidal material, and inorganic salts that provide ample nutrition to support large microbial populations. However, the epithelium also secretes a range of antimicrobial compounds that are able to kill microorganisms or inhibit their growth. The differential activity against various microbes provides additional ecological pressure to shape the resulting population. In areas where sebaceous glands are present, skin surface lipids are quantitatively the most important class of substances occurring on adult human skin. Sebum, as synthesized in the sebaceous gland, contains little or no free fatty acid (6). However, sebum triglycerides are hydrolyzed subsequently to liberate these acids. Generally, this hydrolysis is accepted to be the work of bacterial lipases, especially those of lipophilic diphtheroids (7). The antimicrobial properties of fatty acids have been known for many years. For example, the saturated free fatty acid fraction of skin lipids was shown to inhibit the growth of *Streptococcus pyogenes, Staphylococcus aureus*, and skin micrococci, whereas Gram-negative species such as *Pseudomonas aeruginosa* and *Escherichia coli* are resistant (8). In addition to the physiological products and microbial metabolites that influence microbial growth, the vulvar area also contributes vaginal secretions and urine to the nutrient pool. Therefore, the overall microbial nutrition picture of the vulva that emerges is dynamic, and the resulting variability further contributes to the dynamic nature of the microbial ecosystem.

Microbial Interactions

The interactions among the members of microbial populations on skin are undoubtedly important, but poorly understood. Some may involve more or less direct interactions via competition for available nutrients. It is generally accepted that free fatty acids on the skin surface are products of microbial metabolism and that they are inhibitory to some organisms, particularly potential pathogens. Corynebacteria are among the most active lipase producers on skin (9), but micrococci have also been shown to be important contributors of lipolytic activity (10). It has been suggested that fatty acids are an important mechanism by which Gram-positive bacteria on skin exert an inhibitory effect over Gram-negative bacteria (11). Conversely, it has been shown that suppressing Gram-positive skin populations with antibiotics can be followed by overgrowth of Gram-negative bacteria (12). Antagonism also can occur via excretion of bacteriocins, which are a chemically diverse group of substances produced by many microorganisms that inhibit the growth of other species. Bacteriocins produced by Gram-positive organisms tend to have activity against closely related strains or species, whereas those produced by Gram-negative bacteria have broader activity. Bacterial interference is likely to be an important natural phenomenon that is helpful in understanding the forces that shape microbial populations, but this concept also has been applied in a clinical setting for infection control. For example, artificial colonization of nasal mucosa and umbilical sites with a nonvirulent strain of *S. aureus* has been shown to result in a decreased incidence of infection at those sites (13). Not all microbial interactions are inhibitory in nature. In vitro studies of growth enhancement or satellitism have been reported between bacterial isolates from normal healthy skin (14). The mechanism of satellitism is not clearly understood, but could involve production of growth factors by one organism that are stimulatory to another, or perhaps by destruction of inhibitory materials. All of these interactions contribute to the composition of the skin microbiome, and it is apparent that the type and nature of the inhabitants, as well as the nature of the substrate, are important attributes that shape its composition.

Adherence

The ability of a microorganism to colonize a surface is generally proportional to the ability of the organism to adhere to that surface. This specific binding results from the interaction between the surface and specific cell receptors, and provides an ecological advantage by assuring that organisms can successfully colonize a surface that allows them to thrive. It has been suggested that fimbriae in Gram-positive bacteria and pili in Gram negatives may be involved in binding organisms to surfaces (15) and that teichoic acid is a major adhesin of *S. aureus* for epithelial cells (16). Human epithelial cells have been shown to bind specifically with *P. aeruginosa*, *S. epidermidis*, *S. aureus*, *S. pyogenes*, and diphtheroids, but not with viridans streptococci and *Candida albicans* (4). Microbial adhesion to the vulva per se has not been studied satisfactorily, in part because this environment contains several cell types and is, thus, ecologically complex. However, some microbial adherence properties of the labia majora and minora have been studied and the results demonstrate that labia majora cells generally are more amenable to microbial adherence than are labia minora cells (17).

Host Immune Mechanisms

Both innate and acquired host antimicrobial defense systems are operative on skin. Humoral and cell-mediated immune responses derive from Langerhans cells, keratinocytes, and endothelial cells that produce cytokines and lymphocytes. The skin-associated lymphoid tissue forms a protective barrier that can capture virtually any antigen that enters the skin. IgA and IgG antibodies are secreted by the eccrine sweat glands and are spread over the skin surface where they can exhibit antimicrobial effects and interfere with microbial adherence. The immunological factors important in the lower genital tract have been reviewed by Bulmer and Fox (18). Cervical mucus contains antibodies, in particular, secretory IgA, which are bactericidal in the presence of lysozyme and complement and can agglutinate bacteria and opsonize them for phagocytosis. Circulating antibodies to specific microorganisms can be demonstrated to result from many genital infections, but there is scant evidence of any resulting protective effect. For example, recurring episodes of chlamydial infection, genital herpes, trichomoniasis, and gonorrhea can take place in spite of high titers of circulating antibodies. Thus, a variety of immune mechanisms is operative on or in vulvar skin, but their role in shaping microbial populations is largely unknown.

Exogenous Microflora

As a result of its anatomical proximity to the anal, vaginal, and urethral orifices, the vulva is easily subject to contamination by resident microorganisms from these sites. These exogenous sources have different microbiota from one another and the impact of these populations on the microflora of the vulva is influenced not only by their diverse nature, but also by a number of other factors including personal hygiene practices, the occlusive properties of clothing, and individual anatomy. Continuous seeding of diverse microorganisms contributes heavily to the dynamic diversity of vulva microbial populations.

MICROFLORA OF THE VULVA

Few studies have been conducted to understand microbial populations on the vulva, and most of the results reported have been from traditional culture-based studies. Newer molecular methods may bring more clarity to issues such as resident versus transient microflora, and the prevalence of organisms that are difficult or impossible to isolate and identify by plating methods.

Resident Vs. Transient Microflora

It is generally accepted that resident microorganisms are those that multiply at a specific site, rather than simply survive. Transient organisms, on the other hand, arrive from an outside source, and are unable to compete successfully for a permanent home. While simple to state in principle, this difference is not easy to demonstrate in practice. There is an extensive body of literature concerning the microflora of the skin, but relatively little is known about the quantitative relationships among various microorganisms on various skin surfaces. Moreover, given the dichotomy between resident and transient microflora, quantitative data become difficult to interpret vis-à-vis the "normal" flora of a given site. Culturing a skin surface gives no indication whether the isolate represents resident or transient flora. It can be inferred from prevalence studies that an organism that is recovered repeatedly in large numbers is indeed a resident. However, minor residents are unlikely to be distinguishable from transients. Distinguishing residents from transients on the vulva is likely to be even more difficult because of the large number of transients contributed continuously by exogenous sources from the anus, urethra, and vagina. Thus, determining exactly what comprises the normal resident flora of the vulva will be difficult or impossible using traditional culture-based microbiological methods.

Culture-Based Studies

One of the first studies of vulvar microflora attempted to understand the relationship between urinary tract infections and the microflora of the vestibule (19). These researchers found that women with recurrent infections were more likely to be colonized with Gram-negative bacteria and speculated that the vestibule could serve as a reservoir for these potential pathogens. Moreover, the vestibules of normal healthy women were generally free from Gram-negative bacilli and were also found to have acidic pH more similar to the vagina than to that of other skin surfaces; the researchers suggested that this low pH might serve to inhibit the growth of Gram-negative enteric bacteria. Lactobacilli and corynebacteria were reported to constitute the predominant flora of the vestibule in this study. A more recent report (20) has shown a gradient in populations of enteric organisms from the perineum, through the vestibule, to the vagina. The pioneering study aimed at gaining an overall understanding of vulvar microflora was reported in 1979 (21), and remains the most comprehensive investigation to date. Eighteen normal healthy women with a mean age of 39 participated in this study, which compared vulvar skin with forearm skin, using the cup-scrub sampling method (22). Microbial counts were higher on the vulva ($2.8 \times 10^6/cm^2$) than on the forearm ($6.4 \times 10^2/cm^2$). Lipophilic diphtheroids, coagulase-negative staphylococci, micrococci, nonlipophilic diphtheroids, and lactobacilli were the dominant microflora of the vulva, and streptococci, Gram-negative rods, and yeasts were also present. Most categories of bacteria found on the vulva were present at higher density and prevalence as compared with the forearm microflora. Exceptions were noted for micrococci and *Bacillus*, which tended to occur more frequently on forearm skin. This may reflect the better adaptation of these organisms to the drier environment found on the forearm. This study also reported a surprisingly higher incidence of *S. aureus* on the vulva (67%) than on the forearm (11%). Quantitative results from this study are shown in Table 2.

A more recent study (23) investigated the bacterial population of the epithelial surface of the labia majora during the menstrual cycle. Samples were obtained at days 2, 4, and 21 of the menstrual cycle, and the results essentially confirmed those of the earlier study with regard to incidence and densities of the microorganisms isolated and identified. While the authors expected vulvar counts of vaginally derived organisms (lactobacilli and *Gardnerella vaginalis*)

Table 2 Microbial Counts on Vulva and Forearm Skin (Mean of 18 Subjects)

Organisms	Vulva (cfu/cm^2)	Forearm (cfu/cm^2)
Staphylococcus aureus	4.1×10^4	1.4×10
Coagulase-negative staphylococci	5.7×10^5	1.8×10^2
Micrococci	5.1×10^5	2.9×10^2
Streptococci	3.7×10^2	0.48×10
Lipophilic diphtheroids	7.9×10^5	1.1×10^2
Nonlipophilic diphtheroids	4.6×10^5	1.1×10
Lactobacillus spp.	4.6×10^5	0.96×10
Bacillus spp.	Not detected	1.2×10
Gram-negative rods	1.8×10^3	0.12×10
Yeasts	8.2×10	0.8×10
Total count	2.8×10^6	6.4×10^2

Source: Adapted from Ref. 21.

Table 3 Bacterial Populations on Vulvar Skin (cfu/cm^2) During the Menstrual Cycle (Mean of 20 Subjects)

Organisms	Day 2	Day 4	Day 21
Staphylococcus aureus	5.6×10^3	4.0×10^3	6.1×10^3
Coagulase-negative staphylococci	2.2×10^5	1.2×10^5	6.9×10^5
Micrococci	5.7×10^4	2.0×10^4	6.5×10^3
Lipophilic diphtheroids	3.1×10^5	3.3×10^5	4.5×10^5
Nonlipophilic diphtheroids	8.9×10^5	1.5×10^5	9.0×10^3
Beta hemolytic streptococci	1.0×10^2	Not detected	6.5×10
Alpha hemolytic streptococci	7.1×10^2	6.9×10^2	3.6×10^3
Nonhemolytic streptococci	3.1×10^5	1.6×10^2	1.2×10^2
Gram-negative rods	1.9×10^2	Not detected	3.5×10^2
Gram-positive rods	1.0×10^4	5.5×10	8.5×10^3
Nonpathogenic neisseria	Not detected	Not detected	1.9×10^3
Lactobacilli	1.8×10^5	2.9×10^3	3.4×10^5
Gardnerella vaginalis	5.7×10^2	2.2×10^5	8.0×10^4
Yeasts	Not detected	1.0×10	Not detected
Total count	2.0×10^6	8.9×10^5	1.6×10^6

Source: Adapted from Ref. 23.

to increase during menstruation, no significant changes in the microflora occurred at any of the three time points (Table 3).

A larger study involving 224 participants compared the frequencies and semiquantitative densities of selected microflora from the posterior vaginal fornix and the inner labial groove of the vulva (24). This study focused on aerobic and facultative species that are potentially pathogenic or otherwise have a known association with vaginal, vulvar, or urinary tract infections. Results (Table 4) revealed that the same organisms were generally found at both sites, but frequencies were significantly higher in the labial groove for a number of species, including *S. aureus* and other staphylococci, coliforms, and Gram-negative nonlactose fermenters, and Group D streptococci. *G. vaginalis*, in contrast, was more common in the vagina. The researchers also addressed the question whether daily wear of panty liners would increase the prevalence and/or density of clinically important species. No changes were detected that would suggest any adverse clinical outcomes. Similarly, more recent studies (25,26) have also concluded that tight-fitting underwear and panty liners are unlikely to increase microbial risk.

Nonculture-Based Studies

The microflora of a microbial community play many roles, such as resisting colonization by pathogens and nutritional interactions that shape and control the population (27). Adding to this complexity are the ecological pressures that the

Table 4 Comparison of the Frequencies and Densities of Selected Microorganisms Isolated from the Vagina and Vulva in 224 Women

	Vagina		Vulva	
Microorganisms	% Culture positive	Density[a]	% Culture positive	Density[a]
Candida albicans	12.1	1.3	8.5	1.3
Other yeasts	3.1	1.2	2.7	1.4
Gardnerella vaginalis	12.9	2.2	4.0[b]	1.5
Staphylococcus aureus	2.2	1.1	6.3[b]	1.8
Other *Staphylococcus* spp.	35.3	1.2	87.1[b]	1.9
Coliforms	17.0	1.7	37.9[b]	1.3
Gram-negative nonlactose fermenters	2.7	1.2	7.1[b]	1.0
Proteus spp.	1.3	1.0	3.1	1.2
Pseudomonas spp.	Not detected	—	Not detected	—
Streptococcus Group A	0.9	1.0	1.3	1.5
Streptococcus Group B	8.9	1.8	10.3	1.7
Streptococcus Group D	19.6	1.5	30.8[b]	1.9
Streptococcus beta hemolytic, non-A,B,D	Not detected	—	0.4	1.0
Viridans strep	15.2	1.8	19.6	1.7

[a]Semiquantitative 0–4 scale.
[b]Significantly different from vaginal site, $p < 0.05$.
Source: Adapted from Ref. 24.

host brings to bear on the community, which vary from one individual to another and over time. Understanding the diversity and role of individual microbes in the various human niches has, thus, been hampered severely by existing culture-based microbiological methodologies. The recent advent of molecular methodologies has been a boon to understanding the complex nature of the oro-gastrointestinal microflora (28,29). Future refinement and expansion of these molecular approaches potentially will unveil intricate details of the various ecological niches of the human.

Although tremendous strides have been made in community analyses of microbial populations, our knowledge of the ecology of the human microflora is largely still in its infancy. Many studies of environmental microbial communities have demonstrated clearly the limitations of culture-dependent techniques for analyses. Surprisingly, it has been estimated that more than 90% of the microbial communities are not amenable to culture-based analyses and thus, the composition (which species), species richness (number of species), and evenness (relative abundance of species) of microbial communities have been subjected to biased analyses using culture-dependent techniques for community analyses. Moreover, culture-based studies are limited fundamentally by their ability to grow and enumerate microorganisms on artificial culture media, where complex ecological and nutritional interactions found in natural habitats may be impossible to duplicate, even if such interactions were not so poorly understood.

The introduction of culture-independent technologies—in particular, those based on ribosomal RNA (rRNA) and their genes (rDNA)—are rapidly replacing conventional detection and enumeration methods and can provide insights into the phylogenetic diversity of communities. At present, the 16S rRNA molecule is the measure of diversity used most commonly because it is most amenable to DNA sequence analyses. By simply retrieving rDNA sequences from microbial samples, for example, using 16S rRNA-specific oligonucleotide primers and the polymerase chain reaction, the biodiversity and population dynamics of the ecosystem can be investigated rapidly. Large-scale cloning and sequencing of 16S rRNA from feces has revealed that microbial diversity has been grossly underestimated (29). Designing of specific probes to the 16S rRNA sequences allows estimation of the microbiota diversity by dot-blot hybridization techniques (30). More accurate enumeration of the microbiota can be achieved by fluorescent in situ hybridization (31).

Fingerprinting techniques for complex communities including denaturing/temperature gradient gel electrophoresis have been applied to human intestinal samples. A recent study that analyzed 13,355 prokaryotic rRNA gene sequences from multiple intestinal sites revealed that each individual's microbiota is remarkably stable and unique (29). Further improvements in molecular methods will involve the analysis of larger numbers of samples with greater speed and ease using high-throughput techniques such as DNA arrays. Table 5 provides a brief comparison of some culture-independent techniques used for analysis of microbial communities.

Table 5 Diversity Indices for a Hypothetical Community

Method	Richness	Evenness
LH-PCR	26	0.814
ARISA	68	0.951
DGGE	32	0.900
T-RFLP (*Rsa*I)	42	0.904
T-RFLP (*Msp*I)	40	0.885
T-RFLP (*Hha*I)	38	0.881
Ideal species level	41	1.00

Note: Calculations for the ideal values were based on a model community with all populations at equal abundances.

Abbreviations: LH-PCR, length heterogeneity polymerase chain reaction; ARISA, automated ribosomal intergenic spacer analysis; DGGE, denaturing gradient gel electrophoresis; T-RFLP, terminal restriction fragment length polymorphism with restriction enzymes *Rsa*I, *Msp*I, and *Hha*I.

Source: Adapted from Ref. 32.

Culture-Independent Analyses of Vaginal-Vulvar Communities

Some of these molecular techniques for community analyses have been applied to analyze samples obtained from the urogenital tracts of healthy female participants. Results indicated that the diversity and kinds of organisms that comprise the vaginal microbial community varied among women studied (33,34). Species of *Lactobacillus* dominated the communities in most of the vaginal samples analyzed. However, as an unexpected and surprising result, *Atopobium* sp. was identified as a dominant member in one woman and appreciable numbers of *Megasphaera* spp. and *Leptotrichia* spp. were identified in two women; none of these species has been shown previously to be common members of this ecosystem (34). Some progress has been made regarding the analysis of human vulvar microbial communities by molecular techniques (35). The results indicate that the microbial communities are more complex than previously thought and the complexity of the microbial communities of the labia majora and minora varies among women. In some cases, the communities are comparatively simple and contain few numerically dominant populations, whereas others are more complex. A further analysis of vulvar samples via nonculture-based techniques will undoubtedly provide more insight into these complex bacterial communities. Moreover, molecular techniques may open the door to the discovery of entirely new groups of microorganisms, independently of whether they can be cultured in the laboratory.

An unusual group of organisms was described in the late 1970s and was noted for its ability to grow at extreme temperatures (36). DNA sequence analyses showed that these organisms, which as a group exist typically at high temperatures and/or produce methane, clustered together well away from known bacteria (eubacteria) and eukaryotes. This observation led to the proposal that life be divided into three domains: eukaryotes, eubacteria, and archaea. Not only have these organisms been isolated from extreme environments (such as icebergs or hot sulfur springs), they have also been identified in human clinical samples. The methanogenic *Archaea* subsequently have been isolated from the human oral cavity (37) as well as from the human gut (38) and the vagina (39). Their potential presence on the vulva and their overall role in human microbial ecology are yet to be determined.

CONCLUSION

The vulva provides a complex microbiological environment. Its ecological characteristics range from zones of relative dryness to regions with high degrees of moisture and varying nutrient availability. Because of these variable characteristics, the vulva can be described as an anatomical structure with many diverse microbial habitats. Older culture-based studies have only hinted at the resulting microbial diversity. More recently, analyses of vulvovaginal samples using molecular techniques have indicated that microbial communities in this region are more complex than previously believed. As a result of using these improved tools, future research studying vulvar microbial ecology will likely yield a much more complete picture of the vulva's complex microbial communities.

REFERENCES

1. Elsner P, Wilhelm D, Maibach HI. Physiological skin surface water loss dynamics of vulvar and forearm skin. Acta Derm Venereol 1990; 70:141.
2. Warren R et al. Transepidermal water loss dynamics of human vulvar and thigh skin. Skin Pharmacol Physiol 2005; 18:139.
3. Marples RR. The effect of hydration on the bacterial flora of the skin. In: Maibach HI, Hildick-Smith G, eds. Skin Bacteria and their Role in Infection. New York: McGraw-Hill Book Co., 1963:33.
4. Aly R et al. Effect of prolonged occlusion on the microbial flora, pH, CO_2 and transepidermal water loss. J Invest Dermatol 1978; 71:378.
5. Aly R, Maibach H. Factors controlling skin bacterial flora. In: Maibach HI, Aly R, eds. Skin Microbiology: Relevance to Clinical Infection. New York: Springer-Verlag, 1981:29.
6. Kellum RE. Human sebaceous gland lipids. Analysis by thin-layer chromatography. Arch Dermatol 1967; 95:218.
7. Freinkel RK, Shen Y. The origin of free fatty acids in sebum. II. Assay of the lipases of the cutaneous bacteria and effects of pH. J Invest Dermatol 1969; 53:422.
8. Ricketts CR, Squire JR, Topley E. Human skin lipids with particular reference to the self-sterilizing power of the skin. Clin Sci 1951; 10:89.
9. Freinkel RK. The origin of free fatty acids in sebum. I. Role of coagulase negative staphylococci. J Invest Dermatol 1968; 50:186.
10. Marples RR et al. The role of the aerobic microflora in the genesis of fatty acids in human surface lipids. J Invest Dermatol 1970; 55:173.
11. Marples MJ. The normal microbial flora of the skin. In: Skinner FA, Carr JG, eds. The Normal Microbial Flora of Man. New York: Academic Press, 1974.
12. Taplin D. The use of antibiotics in dermatology. Adv Biol Skin 1972; 12:315.
13. Aly R, Maibach HI, Shinefield HR. Bacterial interference among strains of *S. aureus* in man. J Infect Dis 1974; 129:720.
14. Selwyn S, Ellis H. Skin bacteria and skin disinfection reconsidered. Br Med J 1972; 1:36.
15. Costerton JW, Geesey GG, Cheng K-J. How bacteria stick. Sci Am 1978; 238:86.
16. Aly R et al. Role of teichoic acid in the binding of *S. aureus* to nasal epithelial cells. J Infect Dis 1980; 141:463.
17. Bibel DJ et al. Importance of the keratinized epithelial cells in bacterial adherence. J Invest Dermatol 1987; 79:250.
18. Bulmer JN, Fox H. Immunopathology of the female genital tract. In: Fox H, ed. Haines and Taylor Obstetrical and Gynecological Pathology. London: Churchill Livingstone, 1995.
19. Fair WR et al. Bacteriologic and hormonal observations of the urethra and vaginal vestibule in normal, premenopausal women. J Urology 1970; 101:426.

20. Hochwalt AE et al. Site-specific prevalence and cell densities of selected microbes in the lower reproductive tract of menstruating tampon users. Infect Dis Obstet Gynecol 2002; 10:141.
21. Aly R, Britz MB, Maibach HI. Quantitative microbiology of human vulva. Br J Dermatol 1979; 101:445.
22. Williamson P, Kligman AM. A new method for the quantitative investigation of cutaneous bacteria. J Invest Dermatol 1965; 45:498.
23. Elsner P, Maibach HI. Microbiology of specialized skin: the vulva. Semin Dermatol 1990; 9:300.
24. Farage MA et al. Labial and vaginal microbiology: effects of extended panty liner use. Infect Dis Obstet Gynecol 1997; 5:252.
25. Runeman B et al. The vulvar skin microenvironment: impact of tight-fitting underwear on microclimate, pH and microflora. Acta Derm Venereol 2005; 85:118.
26. Runeman B et al. The vulvar skin microenvironment: influence of different panty liners on temperature, pH and microflora. Acta Derm Venereol 2004; 84:277.
27. Mackowiak PA. The normal microflora. New Engl J Med 1982; 307:83.
28. Kroes I, Lepp PW, Relman DA. Bacterial diversity within the subgingival crevice. Proc Nat Acad Sci 1999; 96:14547.
29. Eckburg PB et al. Diversity of the human intestinal microbial flora. Science 2005; 38:1635.
30. Smoot LM et al. DNA microarrays as salivary diagnostic tools for characterizing the oral cavity's microbial community. Adv Dent Res 2005; 18:6.
31. Veeh RH et al. Detection of *Staphylococcus aureus* biofilm on tampons and menses components. J Infect Dis 2003; 188:519.
32. Crosby LD, Criddle CS. Understanding bias in microbial community analysis techniques due to *rrn* operon copy number heterogeneity. Biotechniques 2003; 34:790.
33. Zhou X et al. Characterization of vaginal microbial communities in adult healthy women using cultivation-independent methods. Microbiology 2004; 150:2565.
34. Coolen MJL et al. Characterization of microbial communities found in the human vagina by analysis of terminal restriction fragment length polymorphisms (T-RFLPs) of 16S rRNA genes. Appl Env Micro 2005; 71:8729.
35. Coolen MJL et al. Characterization of the microbial flora of the human vulva by analysis of terminal restriction fragment length polymorphisms (T-RFLPs) of 16S rDNA genes, Abstract. Orlando: American Society for Microbiology, May 2001.
36. Kulik EM et al. Identification of archael rDNA from subgingival dental plaque by PCR amplification and sequence analysis. FEMS Microbiol Letters 1996; 196:129.
37. Lepp PW et al. Methanogenic *Archaea* and human periodontal disease. Proc Natl Acad Sci USA 2004; 101:6176.
38. Miller TL, Wolin MJ. Enumeration of *Methanobrevibacter smithii* in human feces. Arch Microbiol 1982; 13:14.
39. Belay N et al. Methanogenic bacteria in human vaginal samples. J Clin Microbiol 1990; 28:1666.

5

Are Vaginal Symptoms Ever Normal?

Matthew Anderson and Alison Karasz
Department of Family and Social Medicine, Albert Einstein College of Medicine, Bronx, New York, U.S.A.

Sarah Friedland
Sarah Lawrence College, Bronxville, New York, U.S.A.

INTRODUCTION

Vaginal symptoms are among the most common reasons for gynecologic consultation in primary care (1). In current practice, the evaluation of vaginal complaints among premenopausal women is based primarily on the diagnosis of one of the three conditions: bacterial vaginosis (BV), trichomoniasis, and vaginal candidiasis (2–4). Despite the general acceptance of this approach, studies in a variety of settings have demonstrated that neither BV nor any pathogenic microbe can be found in approximately one-third of symptomatic women (5,6). Furthermore, asymptomatic women can be infected with *Candida* (7) and *Trichomonas* (8), whereas *Gardnerella vaginalis* is considered part of the normal vaginal flora (9). Thus, the presence or absence of a microbe corresponds poorly with the presence or absence of symptoms.

Clinicians often encounter patients with symptoms for which there is no obvious cause. One possible explanation may be that the patient is interpreting normal physiologic processes as evidence of disease. This explanation, in turn, raises the question of how patients and physicians decide what is normal and what is disease.

There is little agreement among patients with vaginitis about the characteristics of normal vaginal discharge (10). Although most women think that some vaginal discharge is normal, an important minority believe that a healthy vagina should be dry. Even among women who accept vaginal wetness as normal, there can be little agreement about the characteristics of this discharge, such as its timing or color. Physicians also disagree and tend to base their opinions about normal versus abnormal discharge more on clinical experience than on textbooks.

Textbooks also disagree about what constitutes normal vaginal discharge and offer a variety of conflicting terms to describe the color of normal discharge (white, gray, yellow, clear) and its consistency (clumpy, floccular, semisolid, cream, high viscosity, nonhomogeneous, thin) (11–14). Although most textbook authors state that vaginal fluids were either odorless, minimally odorless, or did not have an unpleasant odor (12,13,15–17), one source mentioned the possibility that the normal vaginal odor might be unpleasant (18). Textbooks, however, generally agreed that irritative symptoms—itching, irritation, redness, and swelling—normally should not be present (12,15,17).

CHARACTERISTICS OF NORMAL VAGINAL DISCHARGE

In 1959, investigators examined a group of 113 New York City women, an unknown number of whom showed evidence of cervical or vaginal infection (19). The researchers quantified the discharge by swabbing the entire vagina during the course of an examination and measuring the weight change in the swab. The mean vaginal discharge was 0.76 g for all patients, 1.0 g for women with vaginal infection, and 0.50 g for women who had douched the day before the examination. The mean weight of vaginal discharge increased among women who were periovulational.

Another study evaluated a group of 27 women who had no vaginal symptoms and considered their discharge normal (20). The investigator provided the women with tampons to wear for eight hours and then mail to the investigator in a plastic container. Discharge was quantified by the weight change in the tampon. In this study, mean discharge was 1.55 g/8 hr, with a standard deviation of 0.6. Lowest values for discharge weight were obtained on day 7 of the cycle (1.38 g/8 hr) and day 26 (1.37 g/8 hr), and the highest value was on day 14 (1.96 g/8 hr); there was also a midcycle increase in discharge.

Another study of multiple aspects of the menstrual cycle evaluated 10 women who had undergone a thorough medical examination to exclude both medical and gynecologic disease (21). The researchers studied the subjects throughout the menstrual cycle and evaluated cervical mucus production during a speculum examination in terms of quantity (measured in milliliters), viscosity, and spinnbarkheit. Cervical mucus increased from 2.68 mL during the follicular cycle to 3.97 mL during midcycle and declined to 2.13 mL during the luteal phase. Viscosity showed an inverse pattern, decreasing at midcycle and increasing to a maximum in the luteal phase. Spinnbarkheit was maximal at midcycle, specifically on the day before the luteinizing hormone surge, dropping dramatically in the luteal phase.

The observation that variation in cervical secretions was associated with changes in vaginal discharge led the Australian physician John Billings to study vaginal secretions as a way of predicting ovulation (22,23). Billings studied several hundred women using self-report, often correlated with biochemical markers of ovulation, and described a typical pattern of vaginal discharge based on the changes in cervical mucus. The pattern began with a postmenses "dry period" followed by a period of discharge attributable to increasing production of cervical mucus. The discharge resulting from this mucus was initially opaque and sticky. At the time of ovulation, the discharge was stretchy, wet, and slippery (reflecting spinnbarkheit), becoming opaque and tacky later on in the cycle. The typical pattern might be altered by infection or semen. The "ovulation method" or "Billings ovulation method" is promoted either for the purpose of family planning or for that of infertility treatment (24).

A more recent study did not find a periovulational increase in vaginal fluid (25). The researchers studied 74 women (24 with evidence of "asymptomatic BV") by evaluating symptoms and physical examination findings at days 1 to 5, 7 to 12, and 19 to 24 of the menstrual cycle. They estimated the amount of vaginal discharge by instilling the vagina with 3 mL of phosphate-buffered saline using a pipette, removing all fluid, and estimating the increase in the aspirate. Discharge was graded as scant (<1 mL), normal (1 to 3 mL), or copious (>3 mL). Discharge volume increased over the three phases of the study; cervical mucus was greatest during days 1 to 5. "Most" subjects had white or clear discharge; women with yellow discharge were excluded from the study, but about 10% of the women had yellow discharge later. The discharge from 65 women had a "normal" consistency, the discharge from eight women was judged homogenous, and one woman had a curdy discharge. Forty-eight subjects had a discharge that was pooled; 24 had a diffuse discharge, and two had a patchy discharge.

CHARACTERISTICS OF NORMAL VAGINAL ODOR

There is an extensive body of literature discussing the biochemical composition and odor of vaginal fluid. This literature demonstrates clearly that there are malodorous components to vaginal fluids (26). In one study (27), investigators examined four women who collected samples of their vaginal secretions on a tampon every other day (excluding weekends) for four cycles. The researchers presented bottles containing tampons from 15 ovulatory cycles to 73 blinded volunteers (37 were men) who rated the odor of the bottles on scales of intensity and pleasantness. The majority of raters found the odors unpleasant. There was a wide variation in pleasantness and intensity of odor, both among individual women throughout the cycle and between different women at the same stages of the cycle. Several of the blinded observers remarked that the substances they smelled were "either deodorizing products, cheeses, or preservatives for food such as turkey or fish."

NORMALCY OF IRRITATIVE SYMPTOMS

Irritative symptoms have been reported to occur in normal women. Twenty-six volunteer health-care workers took vaginal swabs periodically throughout an eight-week period and maintained symptom diaries (28). The investigators divided the women into four groups on the basis of microscopy and cultures: a normal group (eight subjects), a *Candida* group (eight subjects), a BV group (10 subjects), and an ureaplasma group (10 subjects); an individual woman might change groups during the study depending upon the results of her smears. Of the eight normal patients, six had some symptoms of irritation, discharge, or odor during the course of the study. Intriguingly, there was no significant difference noted between the groups with regard to the number of women who had symptoms more than two days per week.

Another study found that 6 of 74 subjects (8%) experienced pruritus during the premenstrual period (days 19 to 24 of the cycle); four of these had positive *Candida* cultures (25).

CONCLUSION

There is a wide variation in what women and physicians consider normal vaginal discharge. Many of the symptoms associated with vaginal abnormality are present in healthy women, and healthy women experience vaginal discharge. The quantity of discharge appears to vary from woman to woman, as well as throughout an individual woman's menstrual cycle. Normal vaginal fluid may have an unpleasant odor. There is some evidence that healthy women can experience irritative symptoms.

It is troubling that these conclusions challenge some of what is written in textbooks. Physicians who are misinformed about the nature of vaginal wetness, odor, and irritation may impose the diagnosis of vaginitis on healthy women who would then be subject to needless worry and unnecessary medication. If true, this would be consistent with medicine's historical tendency to interpret the normal functions of the female reproductive system as diseased (29).

Although vaginal discharge, odor, and irritation may be normal, they may also be legitimate indicators of disease. Given the prevalence of vaginal symptoms, it is important for primary care researchers to develop clinically useful ways of making the distinction between normal and pathologic discharge and establish some criteria for "normality." Existing studies typically classify women as normal if either they had been examined thoroughly and no disease was found ("clinically normal") or if they declared themselves normal ("self-report"). There are other possible definitions of normality, including those based on a statistically derived norm or on a threshold value beyond which diagnosis and treatment become beneficial (30).

In addition, future studies will require more clinically useful measures. Measuring grams of discharge or milliliters of cervical mucus is not practical during a pelvic examination. If there is a wide variation in normal, it may be impossible to provide precise measures of normality for measures such as quantity of discharge. Alternative definitions of normal, such as change from usual pattern (31) or functional difficulties, may be more useful. Indeed, for patients, social factors may play a key role in determining what is or is not normal. Some patients with vaginal symptoms seek medical consultation when the discharge interferes with function, either during sexual relations or in the ability to perform activities of daily living. "Symptoms" are a nearly ubiquitous human experience, yet the decision to seek medical consultation is often triggered by some social difficulty (32).

Although vaginal symptoms portend serious disease only rarely, they are distressing to patients. Unfortunately, a good evidence base upon which to decide when discharge indicates pathology is lacking. Both clinicians and their patients would benefit from a better understanding of the range of normal as well as what constitutes a meaningful departure from that range.

REFERENCES

1. Kent HL. Epidemiology of vaginitis. Am J Obstet Gynecol 1991; 65:1168.
2. Anonymous. Technical Bulletin No. 226 Vaginitis, Washington, DC, American College of Obstetricians and Gynecologists, 1996.
3. Mou S. Vulvovaginitis. In: Rakel RE, Bope ET, eds. Conn's Current Therapy 2003. Philadelphia: W.B. Saunders, 2003.
4. Mulley AG. Approach to the patient with a vaginal discharge. In: Goroll AH, Mulley AG, eds. Primary Care Medicine: Office Evaluation and Management of the Adult Patient. Philadelphia: Lippincott Williams & Wilkins, 2000:702.
5. Schaaf VM, Perez-Stable EJ, Borchardt K. The limited value of symptoms and signs in the diagnosis of vaginal infections. Arch Intern Med 1990; 150:1929.
6. Berg AO et al. Establishing the cause of genitourinary symptoms in women in a family practice. Comparison of clinical examination and comprehensive microbiology. JAMA 1984; 251:620.
7. Bergman JJ, Berg AO. How useful are symptoms in the diagnosis of Candida vaginitis? J Fam Pract 1983; 16:509.
8. Blake DR et al. Evaluation of vaginal infections in adolescent women: can it be done without a speculum? Pediatrics 1998; 102(4 Pt 1):939.
9. Sobel JD. Vaginitis. N Engl J Med 1997; 337:1896.
10. Karasz A, Anderson M. The vaginitis monologues: women's experiences of vaginal complaints in a primary care setting. Soc Sci Med 2003; 56:1013.
11. Soper DE. Genitourinary infections and sexually transmitted diseases. In: Berek J, ed. Novak's Gynecology. Philadelphia: Lippincott Williams & Wilkins, 2002:453.
12. Thompson LC, Ryden J, McGregor JA. Vaginitis and sexually transmitted diseases. In: Ryden J, Blumenthal PD, eds. Practical Gynecology: a Guide for the Primary Care Physician. Philadelphia: American College of Physicians—American Society of Internal Medicine, 2002:198.
13. Carey JC. Pelvic inflammatory disease and vaginitis. In: Noble J, ed. Textbook of Primary Care Medicine. St. Louis: Mosby, Inc., 2001.

14. Smith RP. Vulvitis and Vaginal Infections. Gynecology in Primary Care. Baltimore: Williams & Wilkins, 1997.
15. Di Saia PJ. Vulvar and vaginal diseases. In: Scott JR, Di Saia PJ, Hammond CB, Spellacy WN, eds. Danforth's Obstetrics and Gynecology. Philadelphia: Lippincott Williams & Wilkins, 1999:779.
16. Swartz MH. Textbook of Physical Diagnosis, History and Examination. 4th ed. Philadelphia: W.B. Saunders, 2002.
17. Burke AE, Smith JM. Nonmalignant vulvovaginal and cervical disorders and chronic pelvic pain. In: Barker LR, Burton JR, Zieve PD, eds. Principles of Ambulatory Medicine. Philadelphia: Lippincott Williams & Wilkins, 2003:1591.
18. Ingalls RR, Rice PA. Sexually transmitted diseases. In: Manning S, ed. Textbook of Primary Care Medicine. St. Louis: Mosby-Year Book, Inc., 1996:855.
19. Stone A, Gamble CJ. The quantity of vaginal fluid. Am J Obstet Gynecol 1959; 78:279.
20. Godley MJ. Quantitation of vaginal discharge in healthy volunteers. Br J Obstet Gynaecol, 1985; 92:739.
21. Moghissi KS, Syner FN, Evans TN. A composite picture of the menstrual cycle. Am J Obstet Gynecol 1972; 114:405.
22. Billings EL et al. Symptoms and hormonal changes accompanying ovulation. Lancet 1972; 1:282.
23. Billings JJ. Cervical mucus: the biological marker of fertility and infertility. Int J Fertil 1981; 26:182.
24. Klaus H. Natural family planning: a review. Obstet Gynecol Surv 1982; 37:128.
25. Eschenbach DA et al. Influence of the normal menstrual cycle on vaginal tissue, discharge, and microflora. Clin Infect Dis 2000; 30:901.
26. Dravnieks A et al. Odor threshold and gas-chromatographic assays of vaginal odors: changes with nitrofurazone treatment. J Pharm Sci 1970; 59:495.
27. Doty RL et al. Changes in the intensity and pleasantness of human vaginal odors during the menstrual cycle. Science 1975; 190:1316.
28. Priestley CJ et al. What is normal vaginal flora? Genitourin Med 1997; 73:23.
29. Martin E. The Woman in the Body: A Cultural Analysis of Reproduction. Boston: Beacon Press, 2001.
30. Sackett DL et al. Evidence-based Medicine: How to Practice and Teach EBM. 1st ed. San Francisco: Churchill Livingstone, 1997.
31. Willard M. Vulvovaginitis and cervicitis. In: Taylor RB, ed. Family Medicine: Principles and Practice. New York: Springer Verlag, New York, Inc., 2002:867.
32. Zola IK. Socio-cultural factors in the seeking of medical care. Transcultural Psychiatry Res 1963; 14:62.

6

Common Diseases of the Vulva

Diane Elas and Rudolph P. Galask

Department of Obstetrics and Gynecology, Vulvar Vaginal Diseases Clinic, University of Iowa Hospitals and Clinics, Roy J. and Lucille A. Carver College of Medicine, Iowa City, Iowa, U.S.A.

INTRODUCTION

All females, regardless of age, are vulnerable to vulvar irritation and disease. Sometimes the irritation is short lived and may not cause the individual to seek treatment. Symptoms can be mild to severe, intermittent to constant, and predictable or unpredictable. Typically, a woman decides to see a health-care provider when she has begun to experience a disruption in her daily activities, which, most likely, has begun to affect her sexual life as well as her self-esteem (1–4).

This chapter identifies and describes common vulvovaginal symptoms and their associated conditions that health-care providers encounter frequently in clinical practice. This chapter also provides the clinician with a practical approach for assessment, diagnosis, and treatment of these conditions. Treating vulvovaginal disorders appropriately requires the health-care provider to incorporate his or her knowledge and skills in gynecology, dermatology, infectious diseases, and psychology.

ASSESSMENT

As with any diagnosis, taking a careful and focused history and performing a detailed physical examination are essential. Women can present with symptoms, such as vulvar burning, itching, pain with day-to-day activities, coital discomfort, and/or discharge/bleeding, or any combination of these symptoms as their chief complaint. Patients may also describe a sore, ulcer, or lump. The assessment should seek information about the onset of symptom and duration as well as information regarding aggravating factors (e.g., contact irritants and activities) and the response to any prior treatment. It is useful to obtain subjective and objective information when assessing symptoms. Clinicians can use a simple subjective symptom scale such as, "Are your symptoms better, unchanged, or worse?" An objective scale, such as a Likert 0 to 10 scale (with 0 being absence of symptoms and 10 being the most severe symptom) is also useful. In addition, it is important to identify any correlation of symptom change with the menstrual cycle (e.g., whether the symptoms improve or worsen before, during, or after menses). Identifying any correlation with the circadian cycle can help in disease identification; some symptoms can be less severe upon awakening and worsen as the day progresses. With some conditions, symptoms worsen at nighttime, disrupting sleep and leading to problems associated with sleep deprivation. Coital discomfort can be assessed by determining if the symptom occurs with insertion, thrusting, and/or irritation after coital activity. Evaluating the partner's symptoms with regard to coital activity can provide additional useful information as well.

Vulvar hygiene practices also can contribute to symptoms. Thus, clinicians must identify any chemical, mechanical, and moisture irritant(s) to which the vulva is exposed. Chemical irritant exposures include laundry detergents, fabric softeners, body soaps and washes, perfumes, depilatory creams, various hygiene wipes and douches, lubricants/spermicides with sexual activity, topical prescription and nonprescription medications, and activities such as swimming in a chlorinated pool or using a hot tub. Mechanical exposures include tight-fitting clothing, such as exercise clothing, swim suits, and thong-type undergarments. Also, daily sanitary pad wear can cause mechanical irritation. The clinician should assess other forms of mechanical irritation, which include scrubbing the vulva with a wash cloth, shaving to remove pubic hair, piercing the labia or the clitoris, exercises such as bicycling, and sexual practices including the use of vibrators.

Moisture (e.g., urine, perspiration, or aquatic activities) can exacerbate symptoms. Endogenous moisture exposure can result from normal or abnormal vulvovaginal discharge, normal urination, and perspiration, or urinary and fecal incontinence; thus, the assessment of any associated bladder and bowel symptoms is also important (5). Exogenous excess moisture can result from prolonged bathing or swimming. A complete assessment requires that the clinician obtain the patient's medical history and any family history of dermatologic and immunologic conditions as well.

PHYSICAL EXAMINATION

To perform an adequate physical examination, the clinician must identify the normal anatomic structures of the vulva (Fig. 1). The clinician should identify

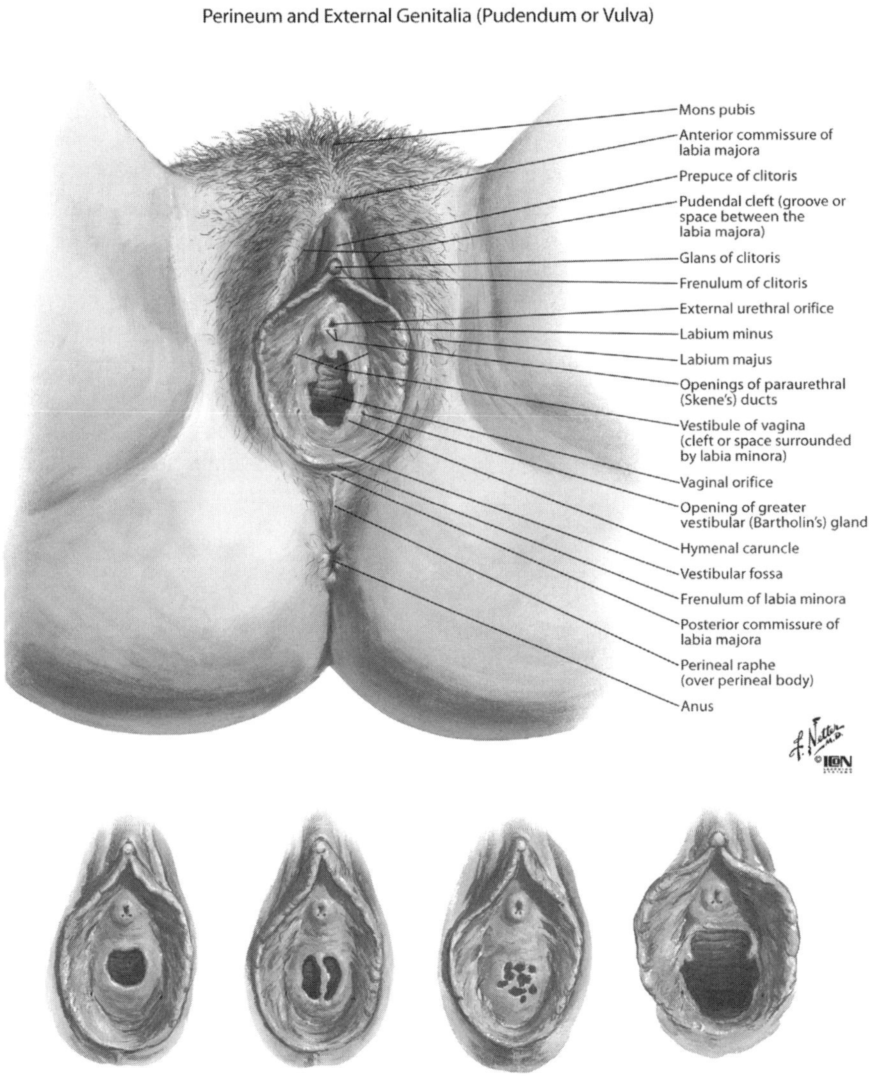

Figure 1 Anatomy of the vulva. *Source*: Courtesy of Elsevier. (*See color insert p. 1.*)

and examine the mons pubis, the labia majora and minora, and the clitoris, as well as the vulvar vestibule for Hart's line, the major vestibular ducts (Bartholin's glands), and the lesser vestibular ducts, including the periurethral ducts, Skene's ducts, and the hymenal ring.

After identifying the normal anatomy, the clinician should inspect the vulva visually to identify any primary lesions, such as macules, papules, plaques, nodules, pustules, vesicles, bullae, or hives, as well as any secondary lesions, such as scaling, crusting, erosions, ulcerations, fissures, atrophy tissue, and scars. Frequent changes of the vulva include erythema, edema, atrophy, hyperkeratosis, and/or hypo- and hyper-pigmented areas/lesions.

Next, the vaginal discharge should be evaluated microscopically. This is accomplished with a wet-smear preparation of the vaginal discharge. From this sample, a maturation index is performed to identify maturity of squamous cells to determine whether an atrophic or erosive condition is occurring. The sample should be evaluated microscopically for the presence or the absence of white blood cells (WBCs), red blood cells, Lactobacilli, budding yeast, hyphae, or Trichomonads. A yeast culture of vaginal discharge is useful either for identification of a subclinical yeast infection or for yeast strain identification.

In addition, a biopsy of any vulvar lesions may be necessary to identify a precancerous condition. Based on the patient's history and physical examination, additional cultures, hematologic, and/or serologic testing may be indicated as well.

DISEASES THAT CAUSE VULVAR BURNING

Vulvar diseases that present with burning as the predominant symptom are contact dermatitis of the vulva, atrophic vaginitis, vulvar intraepithelial neoplasia (VIN), and *Candida glabrata* yeast infection (6).

Contact Dermatitis of the Vulva

Contact dermatitis of the vulva is an inflammatory condition that can occur at any time during a woman's life in response to primary exposure to an irritant or from an allergic response to an irritant. Contact dermatitis also can occur secondary to another condition, such as a vaginal yeast infection or urinary and/or fecal incontinence. Common causes of irritative contact dermatitis of the vulva include laundry detergent, fabric softeners, body soaps, perfumes, hygienic wipes, and douches. In addition, many over-the-counter topical treatments as well as medications that have alcohol in the base, such as creams, can be chemical irritants. Typically, a patient describes vulvar/vaginal burning that is at its lowest intensity upon awakening in the morning but increases as the day goes on. Symptoms can be aggravated during and after urination and by touching or wiping the area. There may be an associated discharge, which is from "weeping" of the vulvar tissue rather than discharge from the vagina.

On examination, the vulvar vaginal area has uniform, symmetrical, and well-demarcated erythema, with or without edema (Figs. 2–4). Treatment for contact dermatitis of the vulva requires that the patient follow strict vulvar hygiene guidelines. This includes removing all contact irritants and exposure to chemicals such as laundry products and personal hygiene products. It is also important to decrease friction to the vulvar skin by avoiding

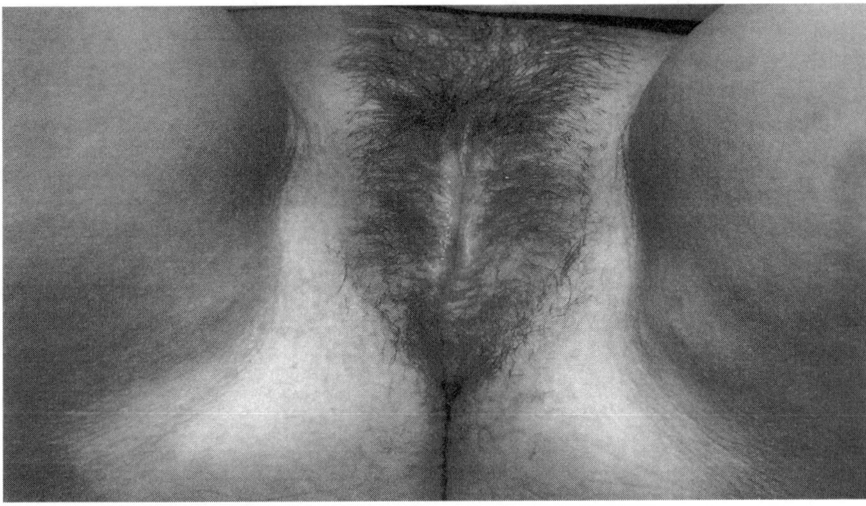

Figure 2 Contact dermatitis: uniform, well-demarcated erythema of the labia majora and labia minora. (*See color insert pp. 4 and 5.*)

tight-fitting/restrictive clothing. Also, decreasing moisture to the irritated area is helpful. Patients should avoid wearing synthetic fabric clothing and wear cotton undergarments to help promote air circulation and, thus, decrease the effects of perspiration and moisture on the vulvar skin. Normal vaginal discharge,

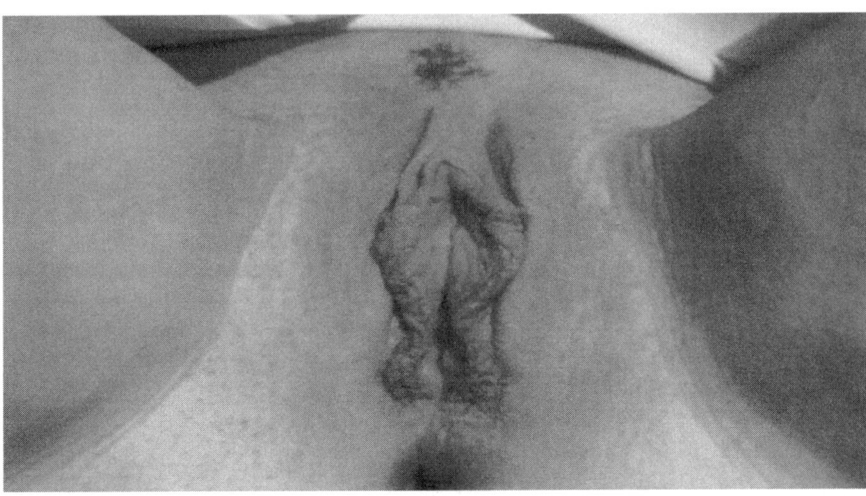

Figure 3 Contact dermatitis: uniform erythema and edema of the labia minora and introitus (same patient as in Fig. 2). (*See color insert pp. 4 and 5.*)

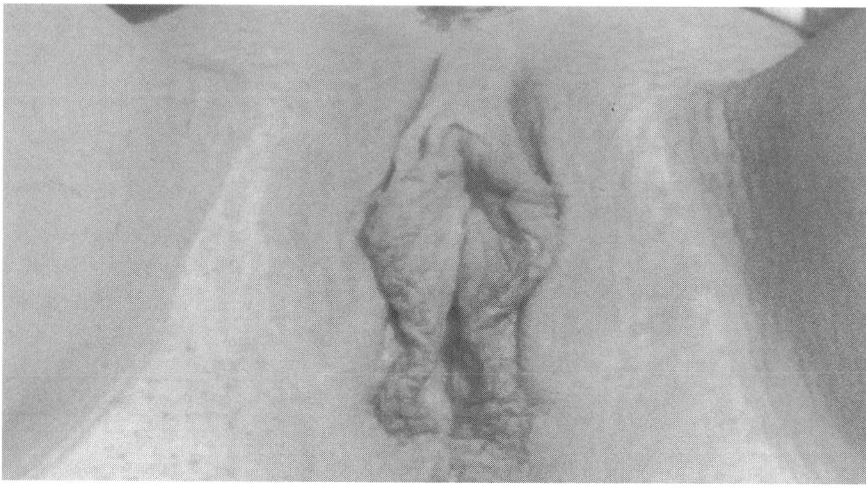

Figure 4 Same patient as Fig. 3 showing contact dermatitis: vulva is shaved, erythema is present in uniform distribution from daily pad wear. (*See color insert pp. 4 and 5.*)

menstrual flow, and normal urine also irritate the affected vulvar tissues; therefore, a bland occlusive dressing helps provide a moisture barrier to protect irritated vulvar skin. Products such as zinc oxide ointment, vegetable oil, or olive oil have proven to be useful for this purpose. A + D ointment can also be useful, but care needs to be taken with the use of this product as it contains lanolin, which can be a potent skin sensitizer for some patients.

The application of a low-to-moderate potency topical steroid ointment can hasten the resolution of the symptoms of contact dermatitis of the vulva. However, the patient must be cautioned that using steroids on the genital tissue can cause steroid atrophy. In addition, of lukewarm water soaks with either baking soda or colloidal oatmeal is useful to decrease inflammation and provide symptom relief.

Atrophic Vaginitis

Atrophic vaginitis is a condition that occurs when the vulvar vaginal tissue lacks estrogen. It occurs most commonly in postmenopausal females, but can also occur in situations that induce a hypoestrogenic state, such as when women are breastfeeding or taking medications such as depomedroxyprogesterone or tamoxifen. Atrophic vaginitis does not affect all women. Typically, women with atrophic vulvovaginitis experience burning that can range from intermittent to constant. Symptoms can be exacerbated with urination or with wiping after urination. In addition, some patients experience urinary urgency, frequency, and nocturia, and some patients also experience vaginal dryness and pain with

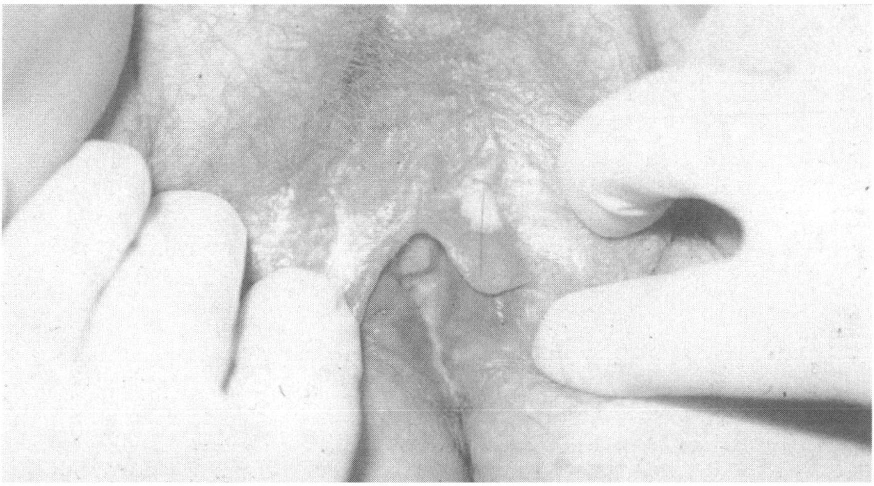

Figure 5 Atrophic vaginitis: thin, pale erythematous tissue. (*See color insert pp. 4 and 5.*)

sexual activity. In advanced cases, the skin is so thin and fragile that it is injured easily and can bleed with minimal trauma.

Examination of the vulvar tissue demonstrates a pale to erythematous mucosa. A urethral caruncle can be present (Fig. 5). The maturation index from microscopic evaluation of vaginal discharge demonstrates a decrease in the number of mature squamous epithelial cells and an increase in the number of basal and parabasal epithelial cells. Frequently, there is an increase in WBCs seen microscopically in the wet preparation sample.

Treatment for atrophic vaginitis is estrogen replacement. Intravaginal topical estrogen, either prescribed as vaginal cream or vaginal tablet, is effective. Systemic estrogen replacement, prescribed as either an oral tablet or a topical patch, can also be used. If systemic estrogen replacement is used and the patient still has her uterus, a progestin is also needed. Adhering to strict vulvar skin care hygiene guidelines, as well as using an occlusive, bland dressing to eliminate potential insult to the delicate skin as it heals, are important. Also, lukewarm water soaks can be quite soothing to these women.

Vulvar Intraepithelial Neoplasia

VIN or vulvar squamous dysplasia is a common cause of vulvar burning that is often missed by the health-care provider. VIN is categorized as VIN I (mild dysplasia), VIN II (moderate dysplasia), and VIN III (severe dysplasia, carcinoma in situ) (7). Women with VIN can present clinically with the predominate symptom of vulvar burning (6), which can be intermittent or constant. Women may or may not have a prior documented history of human papilloma virus infection. Frequently, the vulvar examination is normal or there may be unifocal

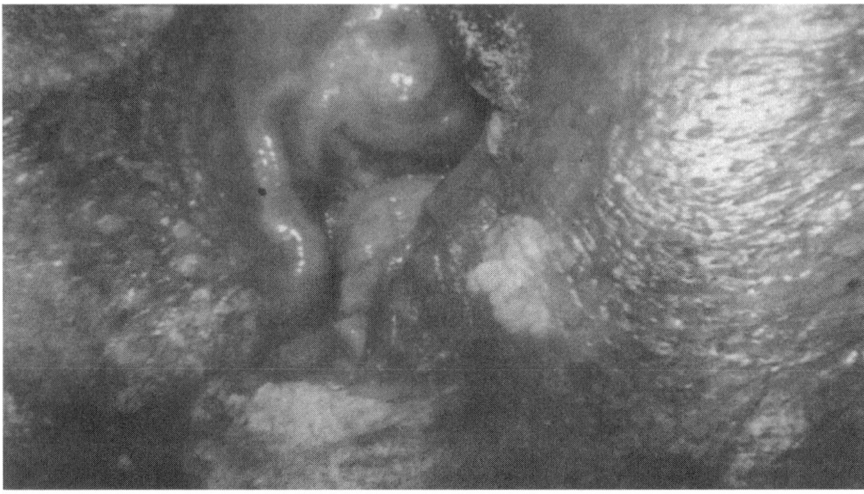

Figure 6 VIN I and II: acetowhite changes in the posterior fourchette and the left labia. *(See color insert pp. 4 and 5.)*

or multifocal lesions present. When lesions are present, as is seen typically in VIN III, their appearance can vary. They can be hypo- or hyper-pigmented, flesh colored, and can be hyperkeratotic. A 3% solution of acetic acid-soaked cotton balls, when applied to the vulvar area for three to five minutes, will cause abnormal skin to turn white. An excisional biopsy of a representative acetowhite area or suspicious lesion is required for pathological confirmation of the diagnosis of VIN (Figs. 6 and 7).

VIN I and II can be treated topically with 1% 5-fluorouracil cream (Fluoroplex®, Allergan, Inc., Irvine, CA, U.S.A.) or 5% imiquimod cream (Aldara™, 3M, St. Paul, MN, U.S.A.). During treatment with topical therapy, it is useful to have the patient adhere to strict vulvar skin care hygiene guidelines, as the topical medications used are known chemical irritants. VIN III lesions require surgical excision or laser ablation.

Candida (Torulopsis) glabrata

C. (Torulopsis) glabrata is a vaginal yeast infection that causes vulvar burning. Typically, women describe constant vulvar burning without an associated increase in vaginal discharge. Usually, these women have seen multiple providers and tried many over-the-counter as well as prescription medications without relief.

On vulvar examination, the genitalia can appear normal or there can be generalized erythema. Microscopic evaluation of the vaginal discharge may be normal or numerous budding yeasts may be present. A yeast culture is necessary to identify that *C. (T.) glabrata* is present. Treatment can be challenging, as it is resistant to all azoles used typically for Candidal infections (8–11). Boric acid

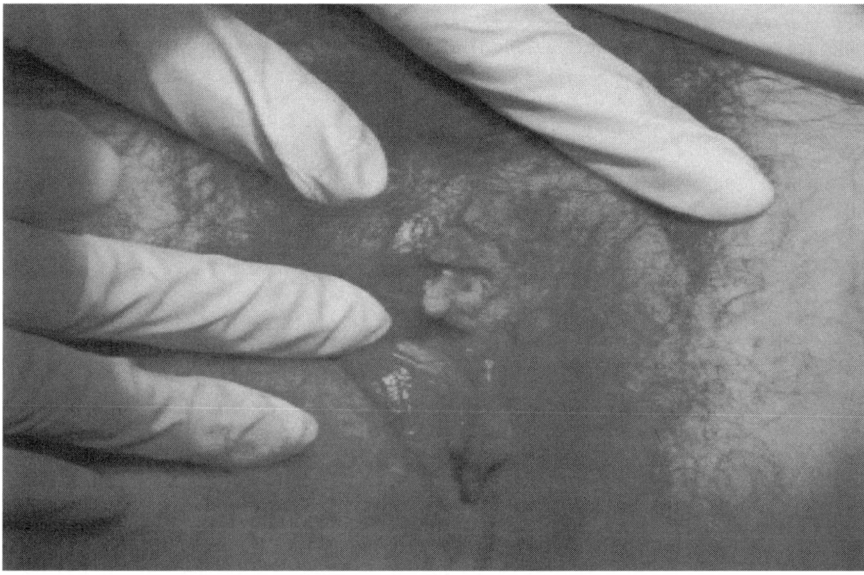

Figure 7 VIN III: periclitoral dysplastic disease. (*See color insert pp. 4 and 5.*)

capsules or suppositories have shown some efficacy for the treatment of *C.* (*T.*) *glabrata* vaginal infections (boric acid 600 mg, in either a gelatin capsule or suppository, inserted intravaginally twice daily for 14 days). The application of 1% or 2% gentian violet intravaginally prior to initiation of the boric acid capsules has been helpful for some women. A single course of boric acid capsules may not be curative and, therefore, retreatment may be required. Other treatment regimens for *C.* (*T.*) *glabrata* cited in the literature include boric acid with flucytosine or combined with flucytosine and amphotericin B topically (12–14).

Additional Diseases

There are other less common causes of vulvar burning. Some women with Sjögren's syndrome commonly experience vulvar/vaginal dryness and burning. Sjögren's syndrome is an autoimmune disease characterized by ocular and oral dryness. Also, women with a history of vulvar laser treatment or surgical vestibulectomy can experience vulvar burning.

DISEASES THAT CAUSE VULVAR ITCHING

Lichen Simplex Chronicus

Lichen simplex chronicus (LSC) of the vulva is a dermatologic condition that causes pruritus. Women may have mild to intense itching, which can occur during the day or night. If the LSC is severe, a woman may commonly scratch

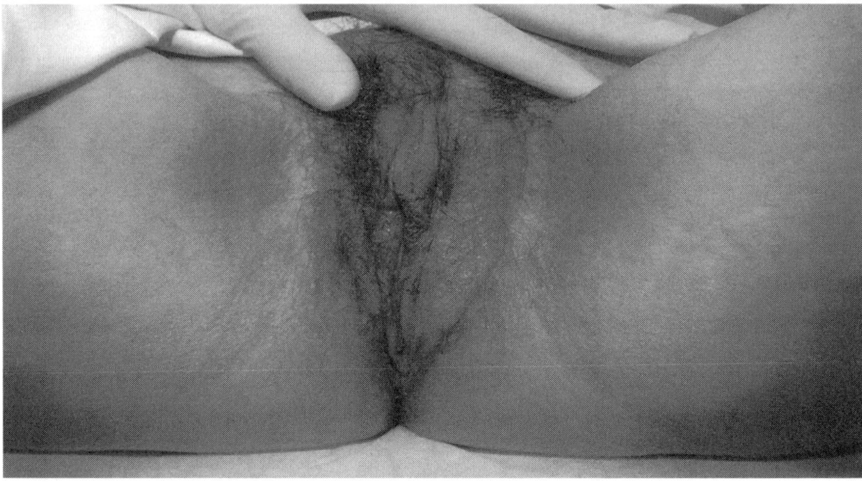

Figure 8 Lichen simplex: hyperkeratosis and erythema of the left labia majora. (*See color insert pp. 4 and 5.*)

the vulvar area in her sleep or be awakened by intense vulvar itching. Many times, a partner identifies that the woman is scratching without awakening.

The etiology of LSC of the vulva tends to be mechanical in nature. Whenever there is irritation that occurs long enough for the itch-scratch cycle to develop, the epidermis and stratum corneum of the vulva thicken (15). The skin of the vulva appears lichenified, with or without the presence of excoriations. The vulvar skin can appear white and crinkled, red, or even take on a violaceous hue. The skin changes are localized to the area of the itch (Figs. 8 and 9).

Treatment for LSC requires breaking the itch-scratch cycle. Topical low-to-moderate-potency steroid ointments are helpful. Occasionally, in severe cases, a high-potency steroid may be required. For women who are scratching during their sleep, the short-term use of amitriptyline 10 to 25 mg at bedtime will help the patient sleep through the itch sensation. It is also important for the patient to adhere to vulvar skin hygiene guidelines, as well as to use a daily skin protectant. A low-talc powder to help control moisture and perspiration is helpful. Zinc oxide ointment provides an effective moisture barrier that also has a slight drying effect, which is especially useful in warm climates. Lukewarm water with baking soda or colloidal oatmeal also provides symptomatic relief. If the skin is severely lichenified and macerated, an aluminum acetate 1:40 solution soak or compress (Domeboro Astringent Solution, Bayer, Morristown, NJ, U.S.A.) can assist with comfort and healing.

Lichen Sclerosus

Lichen sclerosus et atrophicus (LSA) is a cutaneous disease that has an affinity for the anogenital region. The exact etiology is unknown but there is evidence that it

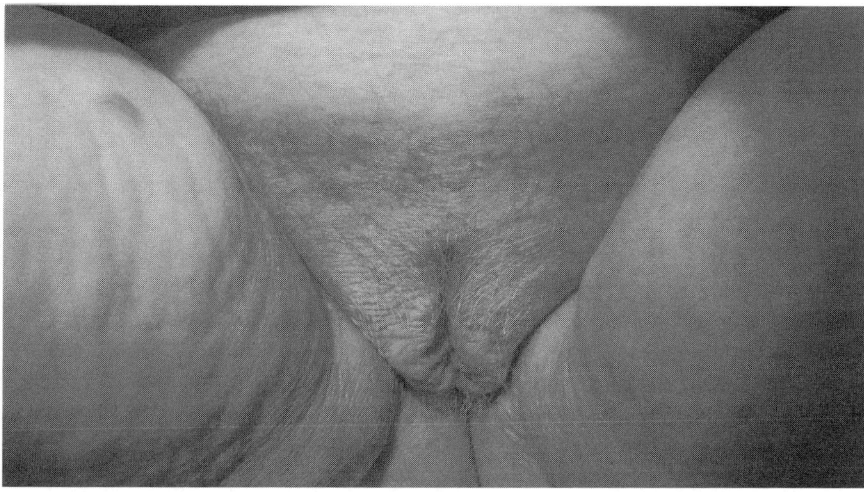

Figure 9 Lichen simplex: hyperkeratosis extending from the base of mons pubis to the labia majora bilaterally. (*See color insert pp. 4 and 5.*)

is autoimmune in nature. There might also be a genetic component, as it can be found in mother-daughter pairs. LSA can occur at anytime through the lifespan. LSA is an intensely pruritic disease, and sleep disturbance is a common complaint with anogenital LSA.

Vulvar appearance with LSA varies depending on the severity and length of time the patient has had the condition. The disease process disrupts the normal vulvar anatomy; typical changes include phimosis of the clitoral hood, involution of the labia minora, and scarring of the introitus.

The affected skin can have a thin, white, parchment paper-like appearance, it can be thin and red, or it can be thickened and white (16). All three of these skin variations can appear on the vulvar anogenital region together. There may be an "hourglass" pattern seen over the anogenital region, which can extend into the genitocrural folds. A vulvar biopsy may be useful in diagnosing LSA (Figs. 10–13).

Treatment for LSA is aimed at alleviating symptoms and preventing disease progression. Low-to-moderate-potency steroid ointments are useful. There is evidence that 0.1% tacrolimus ointment (Protopic®, Astellas Pharma U.S., Inc., Deerfield, IL, U.S.A.) is useful in the treatment of LSA (17,18). Symptom management strategies include following strict vulvar skin care and hygiene guidelines, using lukewarm water baking soda or colloidal oatmeal soaks, and applying an occlusive skin protectant daily to prevent urine and vaginal discharge from contacting affected skin.

Candida albicans

C. albicans vulvovaginitis is a common infection, which some authors estimate precipitates to 10 million office visits annually (19). In addition, many women

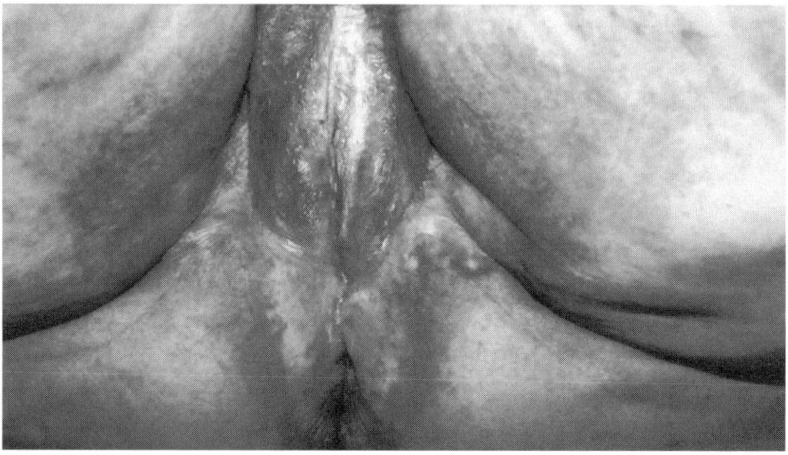

Figure 10 Lichen sclerosus: classic changes of lichen sclerosus of the vulva and perianal area in a postmenopausal woman, with areas of thin erythematous skin, white parchment paper-like skin in the perianal area, and thickened white skin. (*See color insert pp. 4 and 5.*)

self-diagnose a vulvovaginal yeast infection and treat with over-the-counter products without seeking medical assistance. It is estimated that 40% to 50% of women will have more than one episode and 10% to 20% will have complicated vulvovaginal candidiasis (20).

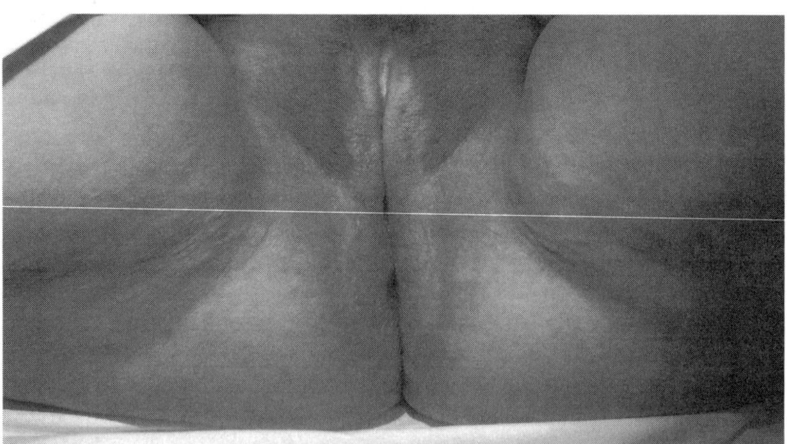

Figure 11 Lichen sclerosus: vulvar and perianal changes of lichen sclerosus in a young woman. (*See color insert pp. 4 and 5.*)

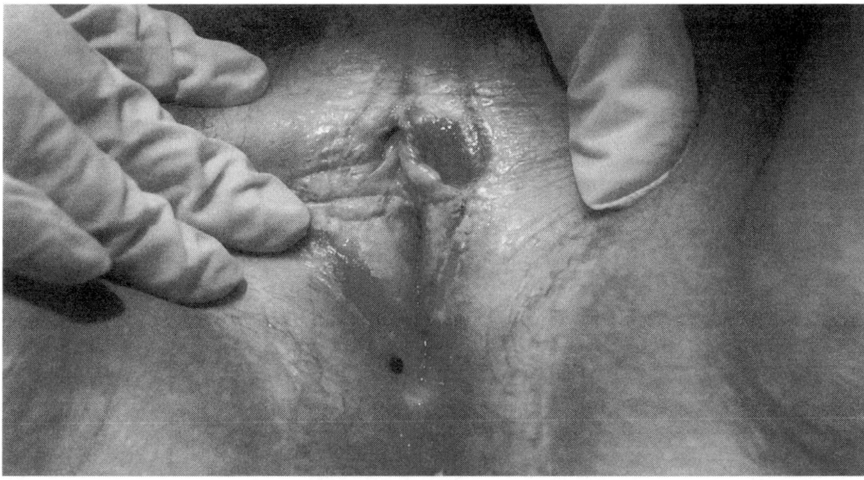

Figure 12 Lichen sclerosus: vulvar examination of the same patient as in Figure 10, with thin, erythematous skin and white hyperkeratotic skin. (*See color insert pp. 4 and 5.*)

C. albicans is the most common strain of *Candida* to cause infection in the vulvovaginal area (8). Women complain of vulvar itching and/or vaginal discharge. On examination, the vulvar skin and associated affected skin have an irregular or asymmetrical pattern, mild to intense erythema, edema of the

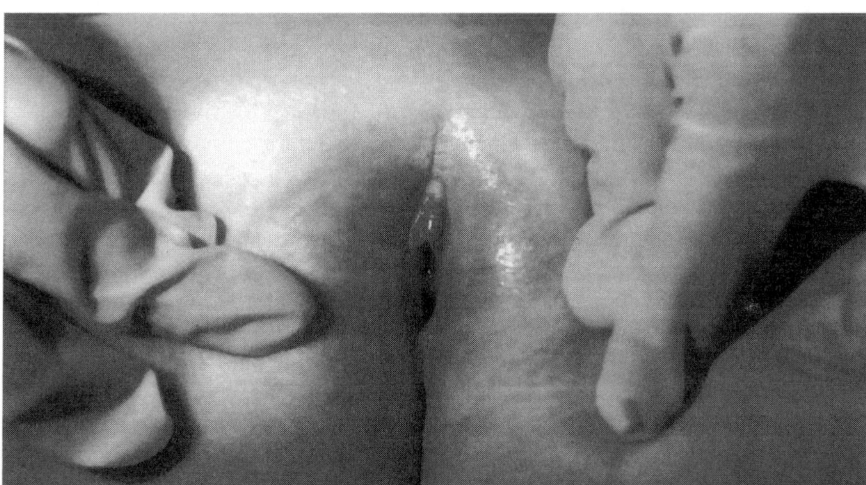

Figure 13 Lichen sclerosus: changes of lichen sclerosus in the periclitoral area and medial aspects of the labia majora in a three-year-old girl. (*See color insert pp. 4 and 5.*)

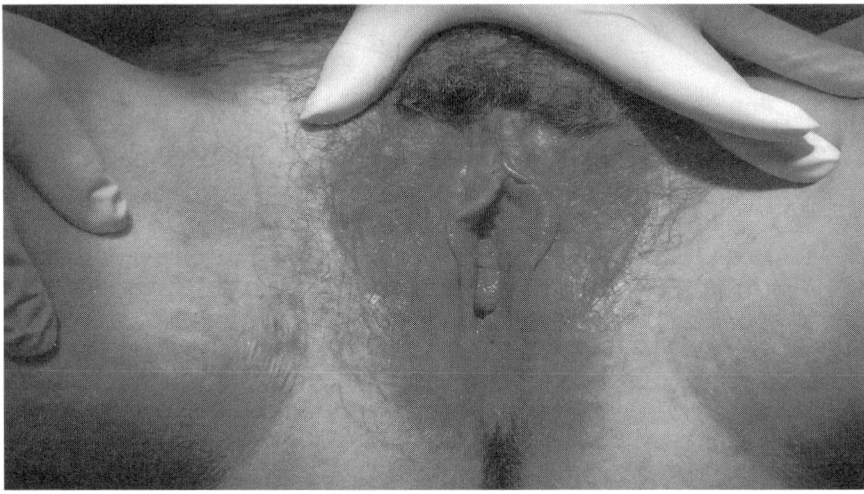

Figure 14 Yeast vulvovaginitis: irregular border of erythema, edema of the labia minora, satellite lesions extending to the right thigh and the perianal area. (*See color insert p. 5.*)

labia minora (usually), and edema of the labia majora (possibly). If the *C. albicans* infection spreads to the adjacent skin in the genitocrural folds, as well as to the perianal area, satellite pustules occur frequently in these skin areas as well. Excoriations can be present and there may or may not be vaginal discharge. Vaginal discharge can be scant to heavy, thin and milky, clumpy and curdy, or "cottage cheese-like." In addition, the woman may describe a foul, sweet, or strong odor associated with the discharge. Microscopic evaluation of the vaginal discharge usually documents the presence of hyphae and budding yeast. If the concentration of yeast is low, a yeast culture is useful to document the infection (Fig. 14).

Usually, *C. albicans* is treated with one of the imidazoles, either with one of the many topical vaginal preparations or with an oral antifungal preparation. Many of the intravaginal preparations can cause burning with application. For symptomatic relief, an antifungal-steroid combination ointment such as nystatin-triamcinolone to decrease the inflammation associated with vulvovaginal Candida infections. Lukewarm water soaks, as mentioned before, are soothing, as well.

Additional Diseases

Less frequently, pruritic vulvitis can be caused by senile atrophy, psoriasis, syringomas, pediculosis, and scabies. Trichomonas, which is also pruritic, is discussed later in this chapter.

DISEASES THAT CAUSE VULVAR PAIN

Vulvar Vestibulitis

Vulvar pain was documented as early as 1888, by Dr. Alexander J.C. Skene in his textbook *Treatise on the Disease of Women*, in which he identified "hyperesthesia of the vulva" (21). Vulvar vestibulitis syndrome (VVS) was first described by Woodruff and Parmley in 1983 (22). The criteria for the diagnosis were described by Eduard Friedrich in 1987. His three subjective and objective criteria are (23):

1. Severe pain on vestibular touch or attempted vaginal entry
2. Tenderness to pressure localized within the vulvar vestibule
3. Physical findings confined to vestibule erythema of various degrees.

Women with VVS experience substantial pain with tampon insertion, insertion of a speculum, or with sexual activity. When the insertional pain is associated with sexual activity, women usually experience relationship difficulties with their partners. When this occurs, lowered self-esteem is common and some women can experience substantial depression (1,24,25). In the more severe cases, women can experience pain and burning on a day-to-day basis when walking, sitting, wearing clothing that comes in contact with the vulva, after exercise, and wiping after urination. If the inflammatory process includes the periurethral ducts of the vestibule, women may complain of urgency and frequency in the absence of a urinary tract infection. Symptoms can also be totally unpredictable and unprovoked.

Vestibulitis is often undiagnosed and these patients may see multiple physicians prior to receiving an accurate diagnosis. It is imperative to identify the Bartholin's duct ostia on every examination and to evaluate for inflammation of the lesser vestibular glands (Figs. 15–17). Erythema is limited to the vulvar vestibule and there is a disproportionate pain-to-touch ratio when a cotton-tipped swab is pressed into the erythematous area.

Treatment strategies include applying a low-to-moderate-potency topical steroid ointment to decrease the inflammatory response. In addition, following strict vulvar skin care hygiene practices and using lukewarm water soaks of either baking soda or colloidal oatmeal help decrease inflammation and provide symptom relief. For some patients, the addition of oral calcium citrate daily in conjunction with a low-oxalate diet has proven helpful (26). Other nonsteroidal options to help decrease the inflammatory response and T-cell function include an immune suppressor such as tacrolimus ointment, but the efficacy has not been documented. Numerous other topical medications have been used, such as estrogen cream and lidocaine gel, and other treatment modalities such as surgery and laser ablation have been employed for treatment as well (27). It is the authors' experience that vulvar vestibulitis disease is self-limiting and, thus, conservative management best serves the patient.

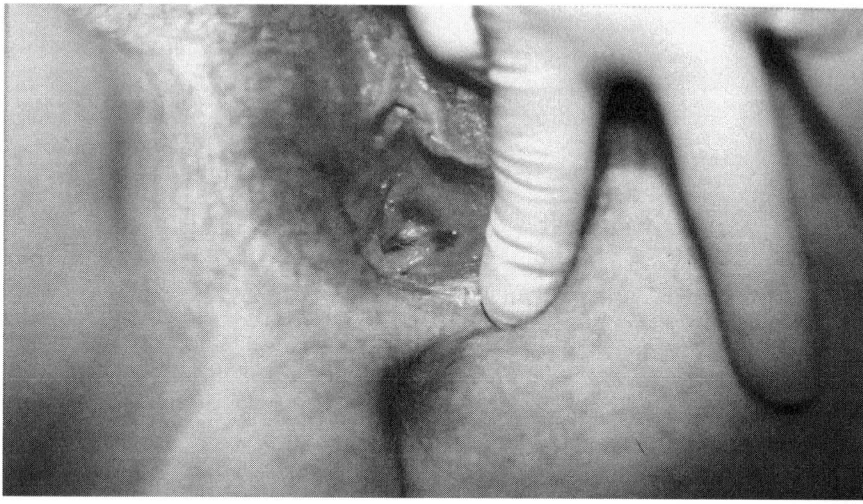

Figure 15 Vestibulitis: localized erythema in the left vestibule. (*See color insert p. 5.*)

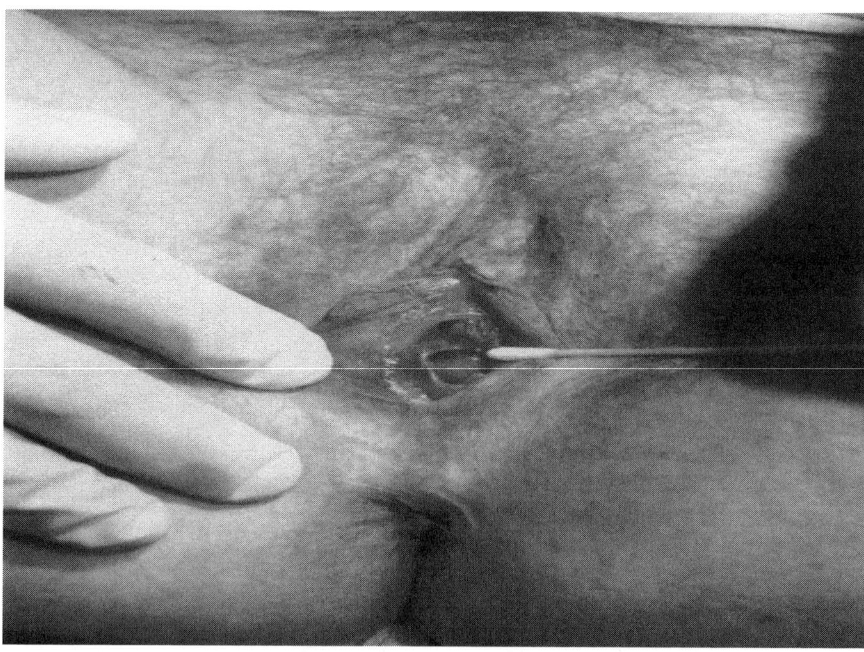

Figure 16 Vestibulitis: localized erythema in the right vestibule. (*See color insert p. 5.*)

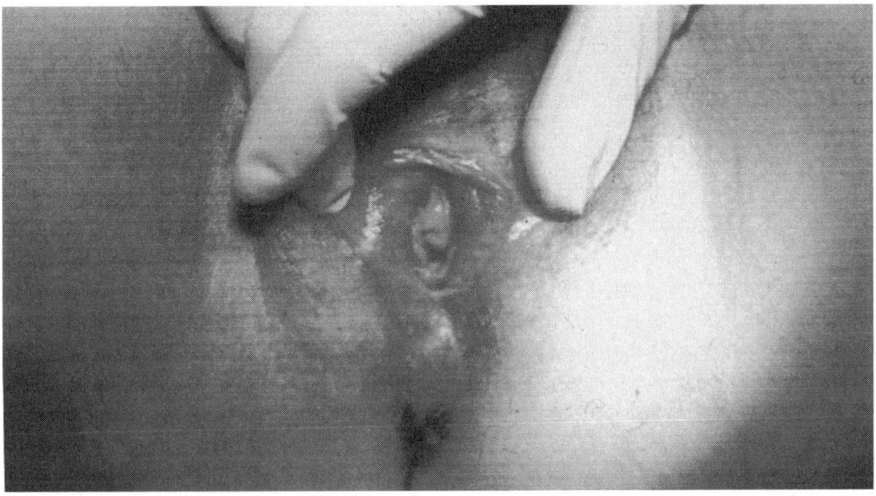

Figure 17 Vestibulitis: localized erythema in the right periurethral area. (*See color insert p. 5.*)

Erosive Lichen Planus

Lichen planus is an autoimmune disease that can occur anywhere on the body. When it occurs in mucous membranes, such as the oral mucosa and the vulvovaginal area, it tends to be erosive in nature (Fig. 18) (28). These erosions are quite painful during urination and daily activities, as well as with coital activity. There is usually a profuse white to yellow to greenish discharge present that patients often describe as "sticky." Examination of the mucous membranes of the mouth, vulva, and vagina demonstrate erythematous erosions. A lacy white pattern, known as Wickham's striae, can be present on the mucosal surfaces.

Treatments for lichen planus include removing contact irritants and following the vulvar skin care hygiene guidelines thoroughly. Low-to-high-potency steroid ointments applied to the vulva and vaginal creams/suppositories have been proven effective (29). In addition, recent case reports have shown that 0.1% tacrolimus (Protopic®, Astellas Pharma U.S., Inc., Deerfield, IL, U.S.A.) or 0.1% pimecrolimus (Elidel®, Allergan, Inc., Irvine, CA, U.S.A.) are also effective (30,31).

Ulcers

Ulcers of the vulvar vaginal area also cause pain. However, it is beyond the scope of this chapter to discuss genital ulcers adequately. One of the most common causes of genital ulcers is herpes simplex virus (HSV), which presents with exquisite pain and a vesicular rash on an erythematous base. HSV lesions are self-limiting, but with rapid identification, lesions can be treated with one of the antivirals, such as acyclovir, to limit the length of the outbreak.

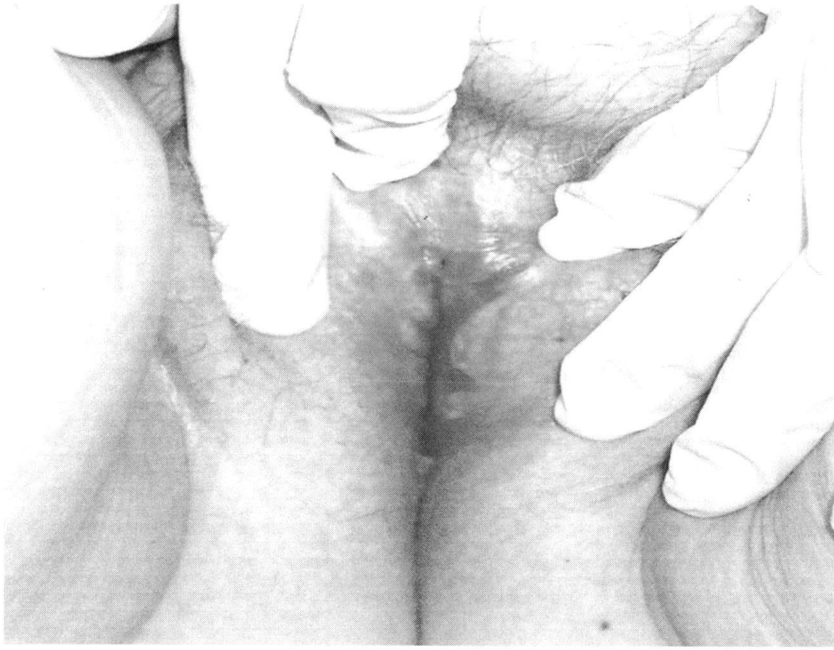

Figure 18 Erosive lichen planus: erosive changes of the introitus. (*See color insert p. 5.*)

Genital ulcerations can result from other infective organisms such as syphilis and Coxsackie virus. Ulcerations can occur from dermatoses, such as aphthous ulcers, Behçet's syndrome, severe contact dermatitis, pyoderma gangrenosum, or benign familial pemphigus (Hailey-Hailey's disease). Vulvar ulcerations also can be caused by malignancy, such as with basal cell carcinoma or squamous cell carcinomas of the vulva, and can arise in relation to systemic diseases processes, such as Crohn's disease. Finally, vulvovaginal ulcerations may result from traumatic causes such as immobility, with the development of decubitus ulcers, or from foreign bodies, such as a pessary used to treat pelvic organ prolapse and incontinence.

Additional Causes

Additional causes of pain include abscesses, Bartholin's duct cysts, Skene's duct cysts, and periurethral duct cysts.

DISEASES THAT CAUSE VAGINAL DISCHARGE

Bacterial Vaginosis

Bacterial vaginosis (BV) is an overgrowth of various anaerobic bacteria found normally in the vaginal ecosystem. Organisms include *Gardnerella vaginalis*,

Mobiluncus species, and Bacteroides species. Women describe a foul, usually "fishy" odor and a thin to milky discharge commonly (32). This odor comes from the release of trimethylamine in the alkaline environment of the vagina (33). Diagnosis is made microscopically by the presence of clue cells and the absence of Lactobacilli. The vaginal pH is elevated to 5 or higher. BV can be treated with either systemic antibiotics or chemotherapeutics, usually metronidazole, or intravaginal clindamycin or metronidazole (20).

Trichomoniasis Vaginalis

Trichomoniasis is a flagellated protozoan that can infect the vagina, causing a thin, watery, foamy discharge that is extremely pruritic. Diagnosis of a trichomonas infection can be made when microscopic evaluation of the vaginal discharge identifies the presence of the protozoan. Treatment for trichomonas includes metronidazole or tinidazole; patients with persistent recurrent infections should be referred to a medical specialist (20,33).

Additional Diseases

Additional causes of vaginal discharge include lichen planus and *C. albicans* yeast infection, which have been discussed earlier in this chapter.

CONCLUSION

A woman can experience irritation of the vulva at any time during her life. Some common irritative conditions are self-limiting, while others require a physician's treatment. Vulvovaginal irritative conditions can disrupt a woman's activities of daily living and sexual activities and, in some cases, result in problems with self-esteem leading to depression. Clinicians must rely on their skills in gynecology, dermatology, infectious disease, and psychology in order to diagnose and treat vulvovaginal irritative conditions effectively.

ACKNOWLEDGMENTS

We would like to acknowledge the effort and support of Cathy Fell and Cyndy Bohnenkamp in preparation of this manuscript.

REFERENCES

1. Gates EL, Galask RP. Psychological and sexual functioning in women with vulvar vestibulitis. J Psychosom Obstet Gynecol 2001; 22:221.
2. Jensen JT et al. Quality of life and sexual function after evaluation and treatment at a referral center for vulvovaginal disorders. Am J Obstet Gynecol 2003; 188:1629.
3. Bradley CB. Female sexual dysfunction. Postgrad Obstet Gynecol 2000; 20:1.
4. Lotery HE, Galask RP. Vulvar pain. Postgrad Obstet Gynecol 2002; 22:1.

5. Kennedy CM et al. Vulvar disease: a pelvic floor pain disorder? Am J Obstet Gynecol 2005; 192:1829.
6. Lotery HE. An Epidemiological Study of Women With Vulvar Burning Belfast: Faculty of Medicine and Health Sciences, Ireland, Queen University, 2004.
7. Kaufman RH, Faro S. Intraepithelial neoplasias of vulva and vagina. In: Manning, Mosby, eds. Benign Diseases of the Vulva, 4th ed., Mosby, St. Louis, 1994, chap. 7.
8. Fidel PL, Vazquez JA, Sobel JD. *Candida glabrata*: review of epidemiology, pathogenesis, and clinical disease with comparison to *C. Albicans*. Clin Rev 1999; 12:80.
9. Sobel JD. Vulvovaginitis due to *Candida glabrata*; an emergency problem. Mycoses 1998; 41:18.
10. Redondo-Lopez V et al. *Torulopsis glabrata* vaginitis: clinical aspects and susceptibility to antifungal agents. J Obstet Gynecol 1990; 76:651.
11. Sobel JP, Chaim W. Treatment of *Torulopsis glabrata* vaginitis: retrospective review of boric acid therapy. Clin Infect Dis 1997; 24:649.
12. White DJ et al. Combined topical flucytosine and amphotericin B for refractory vaginal *Candida glabrata* infection. Sex Transm Infect 2001; 77:212.
13. Sobel JD et al. Treatment of vaginitis caused by *Candida glabrata*: use of boric acid and flucytosine. Am J Obstet Gynecol 2003; 189:1297.
14. Baum SE, Morris JT. Amphotericin B douche for highly resistant *Candida* (*Torulopsis*) *glabrata* vaginitis. Infect Med 2001; 18:114.
15. Lynch PJ. Lichen simplex chronicus (atopic/neurodermatitis) of the anogenital region. Dermatol Ther 2004; 17:8.
16. Powell JJ, Wojnarowska FK. Lichen sclerosus. Lancet 1999; 353:22.
17. Kunstfeld R et al. Successful treatment of vulvar lichen sclerosus with topical tacrolimus. Arch Dermatol 2003;139:850.
18. Bohm M et al. Successful treatment of anogenital lichen sclerosus with topical tacrolimus. Arch Dermatol 2003; 139:922.
19. Kent HL. Epidemiology of vaginitis. Am J Obstet Gynecol 1991; 165:1168.
20. Centers for Disease Control and Prevention. Sexually transmitted diseases treatment guidelines 2002. MMWR Morb Mortal Wkly Rep 2002; 51:1.
21. Skene AJC. Treatise on the Disease of Women: For the Use of Students and Practitioners. New York: D. Appleton and Company, 1988.
22. Woodruff JD, Parmley TH. Infection of the minor vestibular gland. Obstet Gynecol 1983; 62:609.
23. Friedrich EG. Vulvar vestibulitis syndromes. J Reprod Med 1987; 32:110.
24. Schover LR, Youngs DD, Cannata R. Psychosexual aspects of the evaluation and management of vulvar vestibulitis. Am J Obstet Gynecol 1992; 167:630.
25. Sackett S et al. Psychosexual aspects of vulvar vestibulitis. J Reprod Med 2001; 46:593.
26. Solomons CC, Melmed MH, Heitler SM. Calcium citrate for vulvar vestibulitis: a case report. J Reprod Med 1991; 36:879.
27. Makela P, Sobel JD. Evaluation and management of vulvar vestibulitis syndrome: a poorly understood disorder. Postgrad Obstet Gynecol 2002; 22:1.
28. Eisen D. The vulvovaginal-gingival syndrome of lichen planus. Arch Dermatol 1994; 130:1379.
29. Anderson M, Kutznes S, Kaufman RH. Treatment of vulvovaginal lichen planus and vaginal hydrocortisone suppositories. Obstet Gynecol 2002; 11:359.

30. Lotery HE, Galask RP. Erosive lichen planus of the vulva and vagina. Obstet Gynecol 2003; 101:1121.
31. Jensen JT, Bird M, LeClair CM. Patient satisfaction after treatment of vulvovaginal erosive lichen planus with topical clobetazole and tacrolimus: a survey study. Am J Obstet Gynecol 2004; 190:1759.
32. Klebanoff MA et al. Vulvovaginal symptoms in women with bacterial vaginosis. Obstet Gynecol 2004; 104:267.
33. Brand JM, Galask RP. Trimethylamine: the substance mainly responsible for the fishy odor often associated with bacterial vaginosis. Obstet Gynecol 1986; 68:682.
34. Sobel JD, Nyirjesy P, Brown W. Tinidazole therapy for metronidazole-resistant vaginal trichomoniasis. Clin Infect Dis 2001; 33:1341.

7

Idiopathic Vulvodynia

Lauren D. Arnold
Douglass College, New Brunswick, New Jersey, U.S.A.

Gloria A. Bachmann
Robert Wood Johnson Medical School, University of Medicine and Dentistry of New Jersey, New Brunswick, New Jersey, U.S.A.

INTRODUCTION

Vulvodynia is a multifactorial chronic pain condition (1) that may affect up to 28% of women at some time during their lifetime (2). Prevalence figures for premenopausal women are as high as 12%. Characterized by symptoms of vulvar burning and pain (3), vulvodynia is an idiopathic condition that is not well understood. Historically, much of what was known about vulvodynia originated from case reports and studies conducted in clinical populations, resulting in controversy regarding its classification, diagnosis, and management. In the late 1990s, increased research funding, especially that awarded by the National Institutes of Health, provided support for structured scientific and clinical protocols designed to study the pathophysiology, treatment, and epidemiology of this condition. As more data emerge, it is beginning to appear that vulvodynia is not a highly localized pain disorder confined to the vulva; rather, vulvodynia may be indicative of a more generalized sensory abnormality in affected women.

Terminology and History

One of the earliest references to chronic vulvar pain in the medical literature is credited to T. Galliard Thomas, who described hyperesthesia of the vulva in *A Practical Treatise on the Diseases of Women* in 1891 (4). He noted an extreme sensitivity of the nerves supplying the vulva that was distinct from other gynecologic conditions, such as vaginismus. With the exception of redness, there were no physical abnormalities, and symptoms were triggered by friction, air, bathing, and/or pressure. Dyspareunia, or pain with intercourse, was cited as the most devastating symptom and often the reason a woman consulted a physician. Thomas attributed the origins of this vulvar pain to menopause or a "morbid mental state" (4). Because surgical removal of the labia minora and other vulvar tissues did not cure the patient, opium, chloroform, tannin, nitric acid, and local sedatives were recommended as potential treatments. Although this disorder was highlighted again by Skene in 1899 in *Treatise on the Diseases of Women* (5), there is little published literature until the late 1970s.

In 1975, the International Society for the Study for Vulvovaginal Disease (ISSVD) formally recognized a series of symptoms related to unexplained vulvar discomfort and termed the disorder "burning vulvar syndrome" (BVS). An ISSVD task force was established in 1982 to further investigate the condition. The findings were presented at the 1983 BVS Congress, where the term "vulvodynia" was coined (6) and defined as "chronic vulvar discomfort, especially that characterized by the woman's complaint of burning (and sometimes stinging, irritation, or rawness). Vulvodynia can have multiple etiologies, and use of this term for a patient's problem should prompt a thorough diagnostic evaluation" (6).

Just as there are many subsets of depression (7), not all vulvodynia is the same; duration, location, and nature of symptoms can vary greatly among patients. The past three decades have seen much controversy regarding the classification and description of this condition. In 1989, McKay proposed five categories of vulvodynia: vulvar vestibulitis, essential vulvodynia, vulvar dermatoses, cyclic vulvitis, and vulvar papillomatosis (8). Ten years later, the 1999 ISSVD World Congress encouraged clinicians to replace the term "vulvodynia" with "vulvar dysesthesia" and argued that the disorder be classified as "generalized" or "localized," based upon the location of symptoms. Within the localized forms of disease, there were three proposed subclassifications: vestibulodynia (formerly vulvar vestibulitis), clitoridynia, and "other" (9). A 2001 review by Graziottin, et al. (10) described seven subtypes of vulvodynia; the terminology and classification presented were not in agreement with the ISSVDs report.

When vulvodynia was revisited by the 2001 ISSVD World Congress, the terminology was again revised. "Vulvar dysesthesia" remained the preferred term, and two major categories—"provoked" and "spontaneous"—were recognized based upon the nature of pain stimulus; each of these was subdivided based upon the location of pain (generalized vs. localized) (11). Yet, this classification system was not accepted universally by clinicians and researchers. In April 2003, attendees of the National Institutes of Health Conference on Vulvodynia continued to debate the issue and resolved that two major subtypes of vulvodynia be recognized: dysesthetic vulvodynia and vulvar vestibulitis.

In early 2004, the National Vulvodynia Association supported this terminology and promoted it as follows (12):

- Dysesthetic Vulvodynia (generalized). Diffuse pain that is constant or intermittent; vestibular pressure does not always cause symptoms but may exacerbate existing symptoms.
- Vulvar Vestibulitis Syndrome (dysesthesia localized in the vestibule). Localized pain that occurs when pressure is applied to the vestibule; a burning sensation is the most common symptom.

In October 2003, the ISSVD World Congress reinstated the word "vulvodynia" to describe unexplained vulvar pain and recommended eliminating the term "vestibulitis." They again divided vulvodynia into two subtypes—generalized versus localized—as defined by symptom location; each of these is further classified into three categories—provoked, unprovoked, or mixed—based upon inciting factors. The 2003 ISSVD World Congress recommended universal acceptance and promotion of these terms, bringing uniformity and clarity to the way the disease is recognized, diagnosed, and discussed by health-care professionals (3).

SYMPTOMS

Currently, vulvodynia is defined as chronic vulvar discomfort characterized by soreness, rawness, burning, stinging, irritation, and/or stabbing pain (3,11,13–15). The definition of "chronic" is not specified, and researchers and clinicians describe a minimum symptomatic period of anywhere from three (2,16–18) to six months (1,19–23). The characteristics of discomfort are vague, in that it may be localized or diffuse, superficial or deep, and constant or provoked (3,13). Activities such as sexual intercourse (11,24), tampon insertion (24,25), exercise, and wearing snug clothing (24) incite and/or exacerbate symptoms. Because of the variation in the clinical presentation of vulvodynia, women may have difficulty describing their symptoms (26), and diagnosis is complicated.

ETIOLOGY

Several hypotheses have been proposed to identify etiological factors for vulvodynia. A high concentration of calcium oxalate crystals in the urine (27), allergies (28), hormonal relationships (29), history of abuse (30), genetics (25), psychological conditions (11), and recurrent infections (e.g., Candidiasis/yeast, human papilloma virus, and bacterial vaginosis) (20,31,32) have been thought to play a role in disease development. Yet, there is no agreement in the literature regarding these and other theories. Moreover, these issues have been described primarily in small, uncontrolled studies, and there is a lack of systematic, large-scale studies that explore them in greater depth (33).

PREVALENCE

It is estimated that as many as 200,000 women in the United States suffer from vulvodynia (13) and that up to 14 million U.S. women will experience chronic vulvar pain symptoms in their lifetime, 30% of whom will choose not to consult a clinician (16). Yet these numbers are only estimates, limited by a lack of population-based studies. The true extent of disease is unknown (Fig. 1; Ref. 34).

A national Gallup survey estimated that chronic gynecologic pain of at least six months' duration affects approximately 15% of U.S. women. While endometriosis, pelvic inflammatory disease, and yeast infections accounted for some of this pain, the majority of women surveyed had never received a diagnosis for their symptoms (35). A British health study reported that 13.3% ($n = 20$) of genitourinary clinic patients suffered from vulvar pain, but 75% of these cases were the result of an infectious agent (36). While these studies underscore the magnitude of general gynecologic and vulvar pain, they are not specific to vulvodynia and do not afford prevalence estimates in the general population.

In 1991, Goetsch reported that 15% ($n = 31$) of women screened in a gynecologic practice met diagnostic criteria for vulvar vestibulitis (25). However, these findings cannot be extrapolated to the general population, which includes women who do not seek care for their symptoms. Until recently, Goetsch had published the only prevalence data in the literature. In 2001, Harlow and colleagues performed the first population-based study to assess the prevalence of chronic vulvar pain and found that 18.5% ($n = 56$) of 303 women surveyed randomly in a Boston, Massachusetts community indicated a minimum three-month history of genital tract discomfort at some point in their life; 8.6% of the total population had symptoms at the time of the survey (17). A second Boston study found that of the 3,358 eligible women surveyed, 16% reported a lifetime history of burning, knife-like chronic vulvar pain of at least three months in duration, and 7% of participants experienced symptoms at the time of the study (16).

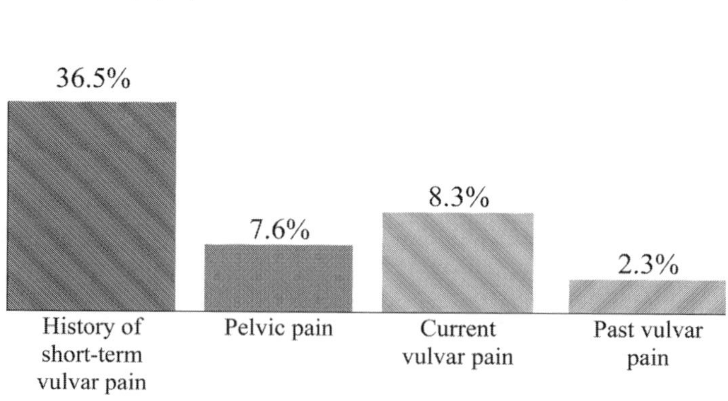

Figure 1 Prevalence of vulvodynia. *Source*: From Ref. 34.

Expanding on the work of Harlow et al., Reed (2) conducted a web-based survey with a national sample of 1,032 women and found a 27.9% lifetime prevalence of vestibular pain, with a 3% prevalence of symptoms lasting three months or longer. These two studies are important because, unlike earlier reports that focused on women seen in gynecological care settings, they were based on the general population. Yet, Reed's (2) national web-based survey yielded only a 23% response rate and, thus, additional studies with higher response rates are required to further explore prevalence and characteristics of vulvar pain at the national level.

DEMOGRAPHICS

A woman can develop vulvodynia at any time in her life, but studies report that the majority of afflicted women are of reproductive age. Sixty-five percent of Friedrich's patients (24) were between the ages of 20 and 40, and Harlow and Stewart's studies (16) indicate that cumulative incidence is greatest before age 25.

Historically, almost all women who sought care for unexplained vulvar pain were reported to be Caucasian (24,37,38). A case-control study by Dalton et al. (38) found that vulvodynia patients were more likely to be Caucasian relative to those without vulvodynia. It is thought that this heterogeneity is a function of the populations studied and not truly representative of those affected by the condition; population-based studies would address this concern. The initial work of Harlow et al. (17) in Boston failed to find racial disparities for chronic genital discomfort, but later study of Harlow and Stewart (16) suggests that vulvodynia is equally prevalent in Caucasians and African Americans, with Hispanics 80% as likely to experience symptoms.

To better understand vulvodynia in the African American community, Reed's web-based survey oversampled African American women. Consistent with the later findings of Harlow and Stewart (16), Reed et al. failed to identify Caucasian and African American racial disparities in the prevalence of vestibular pain and dyspareunia. Again, the low response rate obtained by Reed et al. justifies additional national studies to further examine and describe the ethnoracial composition of vulvodynia.

COMORBID CONDITIONS

Vulvodynia patients often have other medical complaints in addition to their vulvar symptoms. In a study of 301 vulvodynia patients at the University of British Columbia's Vulvar Disease Clinic, 55% indicated they had a suspected second chronic pain condition, including low-back pain, irritable bowel syndrome, migraine headaches, chronic fatigue syndrome, and fibromyalgia (39). That same study also reported a high proportion of patients with a history of yeast infections, a finding later supported by Harlow et al. (16). The

Reed et al. (2) web-based survey found that African American women with chronic vulvar pain were less likely than Caucasians to report a history of depression.

GYNECOLOGIC HISTORY

Past studies focused largely on the relationship between vulvar symptoms and gynecologic history. Although the preliminary findings of Harlow et al. (17) suggested that women who began menstruating at the age of 11 or younger are 2.4 times as likely to report chronic vulvar pain. The later work of Harlow and Stewart (16) suggested there is no risk associated with age at menarche. Pain and/or difficulty with first tampon use is associated with seven-fold greater odds of chronic vulvar pain (16). Women with vulvodynia are also 6.6 times as likely to have used oral contraceptives, an association that increases to 9.3 if oral contraceptive use began before the age of 16 (18).

PSYCHOSOCIAL AND SEXUAL ASPECTS

It was once proposed (and accepted) that psychological factors contributed to the development of vulvodynia (4). This concept has been debated widely and today vulvodynia is not considered to have psychogenic origins. However, it is accepted that the condition has a (noncausal) psychosomatic component and women with vulvodynia exhibit more somatic symptoms and harm-avoidance behavior than women without vulvodynia (1).

Similarly, the relationship between intercourse and vulvodynia is complex. Dyspareunia is one of the most common manifestations of pain, and nearly 75% of affected women experience painful intercourse (2,39). It has been demonstrated that women with vulvodynia are more likely to have had intercourse for the first time at age 18 or younger, to have had only one sexual partner, and to have a history of sexual problems (40). Women with vulvodynia are also more likely to have lost interest in sexual activity (40) and to rate intercourse as less important in their lives (41). To date, no relationship has been found between sexual victimization and vulvodynia (30,38,42).

DIAGNOSIS

In 1977, Friedrich and Dodson proposed guidelines for characterizing vulvodynia as follows:

1. Chronic symptoms
2. A lack of abnormal physical findings
3. Refraining from sexual intercourse because of symptoms
4. Emotional lability
5. Reluctance of the patient to acknowledge a psychological component to the condition (28).

Specific diagnostic criteria proposed by Friedrich in 1987 and still in use today include:

1. Vulvar erythema as the sole physical finding,
2. Pain upon vestibular touch or entry, and
3. Tenderness upon localized vestibular pressure (24).

In Friedrich's time, vulvodynia was thought to have psychosomatic origins and was diagnosed after all other causes were eliminated (28).

Today, vulvodynia remains a diagnosis of exclusion (26): pathologic findings are limited to erythema and causal agents cannot be isolated (28). Common presenting symptoms include vulvar burning, itching, aching, stinging, and stabbing pain (Fig. 2; Ref. 43). A comprehensive diagnostic work-up includes a symptom history, medical history, pelvic examination, vaginal cultures, and pain mapping. The pelvic examination should yield no physical abnormalities (6). Medical conditions that could cause symptoms, such as cysts, ulcers, tumors, spinal cord lesions, and dermatoses, must be ruled out, and vaginal cultures are needed to exclude urogenital infections (e.g., yeast infections, urinary tract infectious, herpes simplex, etc.) as the etiology of pain (26).

Pain mapping is an integral part of the diagnostic process. The traditional procedure for this is the cotton-swab test (10,26), in which the clinician applies

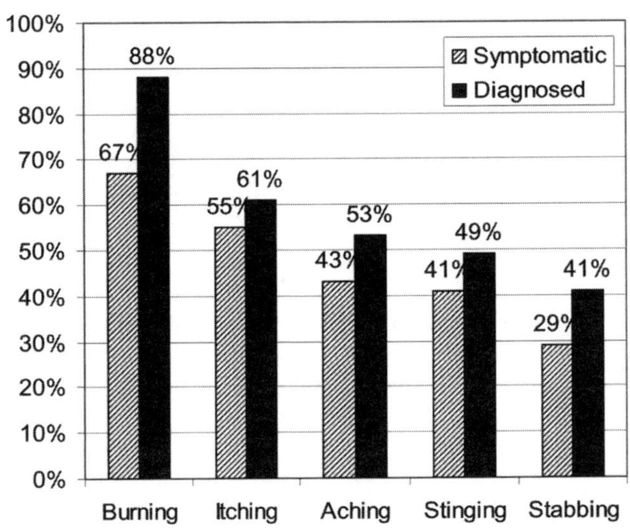

Figure 2 Self-reported vulvar pain descriptors obtained through University of Medicine and Dentistry of New Jersey survey data from a population of women with a clinically confirmed diagnosis of vulvodynia (DIAGNOSED) and a population of women who reported symptoms of vulvodynia via a telephone interview (SYMPTOMATIC). *Source*: From Ref. 43.

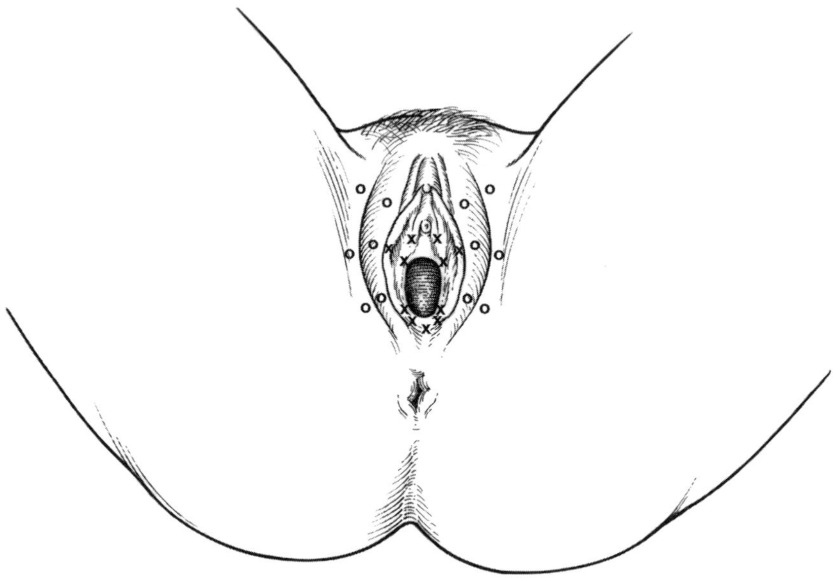

Figure 3 The cotton-swab test enables the clinician to map vulvar pain and allows the patient to rate pain sensation on a subjective scale.

pressure to designated areas of the vestibule using the swab (Fig. 3). The patient rates sensation on a scale of one (no pain) to five (maximum pain) (44). However, this test has limited reproducibility, because the outcome depends upon the clinician's subjective assessment of pain and the individual degree of pressure each practitioner exerts; the degree of pressure applied to the vulva varies from one clinician to another, and so this method lacks reliability.

An alternative to the cotton-swab test is the vulvalgesiometer, an instrument developed by investigators at McGill University in Montreal, Canada, specifically for the purpose of gathering standardized pain information from vulvodynia patients (45,46). The vulvalgesiometer consists of several syringes, each holding a spring calibrated to a preset tension. The clinician inserts a cotton-tipped swab into the end of the syringe and performs pain mapping. The spring standardizes the amount of pressure applied to each part of the vestibule and the patient indicates when pain is felt. As the degree of pressure applied is no longer dependent upon the clinician performing the examination, results should be consistent (45,46). Another method, a vulvar algesiometer designed by Curnow (47), utilizes a hand-held probe that is connected to a main control unit that runs an alternating current. Force delivered by the probe is increased until the patient reports pain. The maximum force utilized by this device is eight milli-newtons.

Although the diagnostic process can be complex and there is no common protocol used by clinicians, the critical point in making the diagnosis is to exclude all other pathologic entities that can be causing the vulvar pain (Fig. 4) (48).

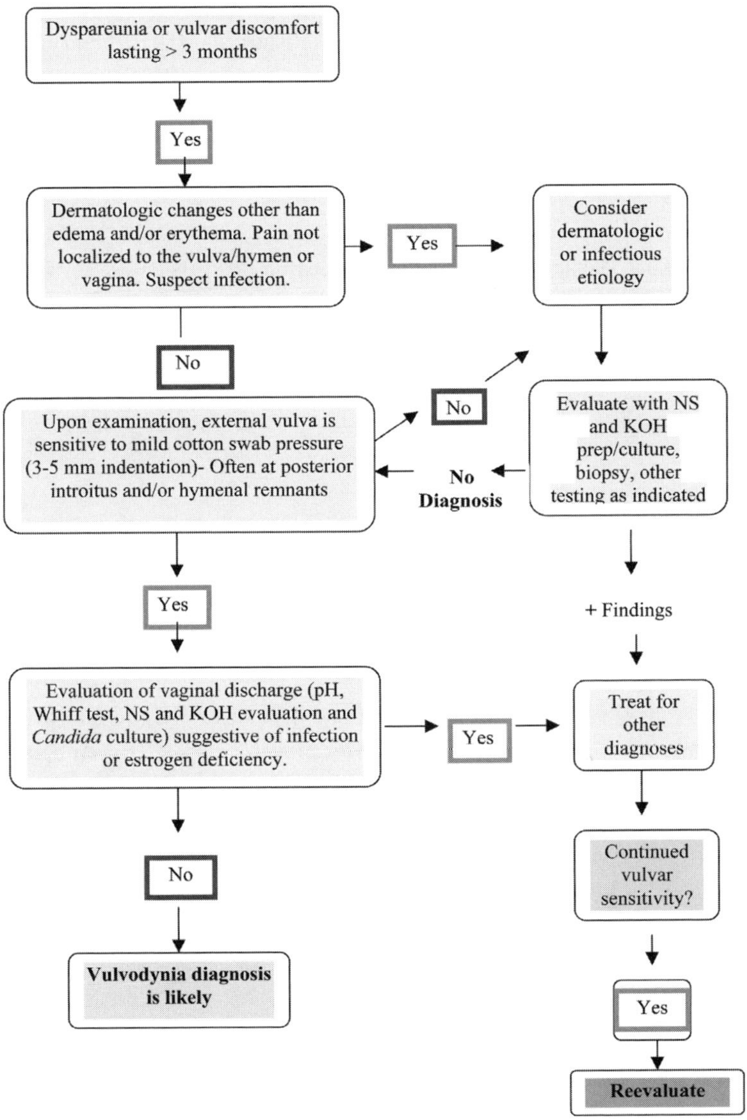

Figure 4 Diagnostic algorithm for vulvodynia. *Source*: From Ref. 47. (*See color insert p. 6.*)

TREATMENT

Not only is there no universal means of defining and diagnosing vulvodynia, there is no standard of care for treating this condition (13). Pharmacologic agents, such as tricyclic antidepressants (8,49) and corticosteroids (13), dietary changes, vitamin and mineral supplements (27), physical therapy (50), electromyographic biofeedback therapy (13,21,51,52), and surgery (21,24) have been used to treat vulvodynia with inconsistent success (Tables 1–3) (48).

Table 1 Topical Therapy Treatments for Vulvodynia

Treatment	Dosage/Regimen	Side effects	Basis for recommendation
Avoidance of topical irritants and allergens	Use mild soap or water for cleansing area, wear cotton underwear, and use fragrance-free sanitary products	None	Expert opinion
Estrogen (if estrogen deficiency is noted)	Vaginal cream used daily for 3 wk, then 2–3 times per wk as needed	Local: infrequent burning. Systemic: unclear	Expert opinion
Topical lidocaine, 5% gel or cream	Topically to the area of tenderness, prior to intercourse; or nightly, applying lidocaine gel to a cotton ball that is placed in the introitus and used overnight. Treatment duration is undetermined.	Occasional sensitivity/irritation	Expert opinion, study suggesting improvement in daily pain, the discomfort with intercourse
Cromolyn cream 4%	Apply 3 times to area of tenderness	Sensitivity to the agent or vehicle	Case report suggested improvement but randomized study did not

Source: Adapted from Ref. 48.

Table 2 Oral Therapy Treatments for Vulvodynia

Treatment	Dosage/regimen	Side effects	Basis for recommendation
Tricyclic anti-depressants	Amitriptyline, starting at 25 mg/day at bedtime for 10 days, increasing by 25 mg increments as tolerated to typical dosage of 50–100 mg/day (maximum dosage, 240 mg/day). Desipramine or imipramine at similar dosage. Nortriptyline at similar dosage, by to maximum or 100 mg/day	Oral dryness, constipation, weight gain (less common). Occasional neurological symptoms, cardiac arrhythmias, or urinary retention require discontinuation	Observational study and common usage
Paroxetine	10–20 mg/day, increasing as needed and tolerated to a maximum of 60 mg/day	Occasional restlessness, weight gain, fatigue, anorgasma	Expert opinion, case report
Venlafaxine	37.5 mg/day for 10 days, increasing to 75 mg/day, may increase to a maximum of 225 mg/day	Anorgasma, gastrointestinal problems, anxiety	Improvement noted for patients with diabetic neuropathy
Gabapentin	300 mg/day, increasing every 4 days by 300 mg/day (divided into 3 doses) to a maximum of 900 mg 3 times/day	Headache, nausea, vomiting fatigue, dizziness	Expert opinion, case reports
Calcium citrate (due to the citrate component)	2 tablets twice per day, increasing to 3–4 tablets twice per day	Tablets are large and difficult for some patients to swallow. Not indicated for women with a history of calcium-based renal stones	Common usage, case reports of use with low-oxalate diets

Source: Adapted from Ref. 48.

Table 3 Other Possible Treatments for Vulvodynia

Treatment	Dosage/regimen	Side effects	Basis for recommendation
Surgery (rare), perineoplasty or vestibulectomy (hypersensitive tissue is removed and replaced with vaginal mucosa advancement)	Surgical procedure confined to the posterior introitus; reserved for women who have not responded to other treatments	Discomfort, recovery time; rare reports of infection, bleeding, hematoma, wound separation, vaginismus, vaginal stenosis	Several case series, one study suggests 70% improvement
Pelvic floor muscle physical therapy and/or biofeedback	Performed by physical therapist who has undergone appropriate training	Discomfort, numerous visits, compliance with home exercises, possible high cost	Studies suggesting moderate effectiveness

Source: Adapted from Ref. 48.

Some women find nonmedical interventions such as bed rest, sitz baths, and ice packs helpful (11). One of the most widely used interventions is the low-oxalate diet, in which women are told to either totally avoid foods with high oxalate content or restrict their consumption of these foods. However, results with this type of diet are controversial. In addition, because adverse events resulting from this intervention are minimal, it is commonly used as an initial intervention on a "let's-see-what-happens" basis.

Another method of treatment that is gaining success is cognitive behavioral group therapy, in which women with vulvodynia meet as a group with a therapist over an 8- to 12-week period. The major problems with this type of intervention are poor compliance and the fact that most of the intervention focuses on dealing with pain rather than eliminating pain. Of the formal studies evaluating this type of interaction, a 30% improvement in pain is reported. While any of the aforementioned treatments may provide short-term relief, most do not provide a permanent solution.

CONCLUSION

Vulvodynia is a multifactorial, chronic painful condition that may affect nearly one-third of women at some time during their lives. Although identified as early as the 1800s, little published research exists prior to the late 1970s.

Vulvodynia is difficult to diagnose and currently remains a diagnosis of exclusion. Although there is no cure for vulvodynia, making the appropriate diagnosis and systematically treating the patient with interventions that have shown efficacy are priorities in delivering optimal patient care for this condition. It will only be through continued, multicenter, randomized, prospective, placebo-controlled trials that the etiology (or etiologies) and optimal treatment(s) that are evidenced based and safe will emerge.

REFERENCES

1. Danielsson I et al. Vulvar vestibulitis: a multi-factorial condition. BJOG 2001; 108:456.
2. Reed BD et al. Pain at the vulvar vestibule: a web-based survey. J Low Genit Tract Dis 2004; 8:48.
3. Moyal-Barracco M, Lynch PJ. 2003 ISSVD terminology and classification of vulvodynia: a historical perspective. J Reprod Med 2004; 49:772.
4. Thomas TG, Mundâe PF. A Practical Treatise on the Diseases of Women. 6th ed. Philadelphia: Lea Brothers & Co., 1891.
5. Skene AJC. Treatise on the Diseases of Women. For the Use of Students and Practitioners. 3rd ed. New York: D. Appleton and Company, 1898.
6. Burning vulva syndrome. Report of the ISVD task force. J Reprod Med 1984; 29:457.
7. American Psychiatric Association. Task Force on DSM-IV. Diagnostic and Statistical Manual of Mental Disorders: DSM-IV-TR. 4th ed. Washington, DC: American Psychiatric Association, 2000.
8. McKay M. Vulvodynia. A multifactorial clinical problem. Arch Dermatol 1989; 125: 256.
9. Edwards L, Lynch PJ. The terminology and classification of vulvodynia: past, present, and future. International Society for the Study of Vulvovaginal Disorders Newsletter, Summer, 3, 2000.
10. Graziottin A et al. Vulvodynia: the challenge of "unexplained" genital pain. J Sex Marital Ther 2001; 27:503.
11. Lynch PJ. Vulvodynia: a syndrome of unexplained vulvar pain, psychologic disability and sexual dysfunction. J Reprod Med 1986; 31:773.
12. About vulvodynia: what is vulvodynia? National Vulvodynia Association Website, Available at: http://www.nva.org/about_vulvodynia/what_is_vulvodynia.html. Accessed May 14, 2003.
13. Masheb RM et al. Vulvodynia: an introduction and critical review of a chronic pain condition. Pain 2000; 86:3.
14. McKay M et al. Vulvar vestibulitis and vestibular papillomatosis. Report of the ISSVD committee on vulvodynia. J Reprod Med 1991; 36:413.
15. Edwards L. Subsets of vulvodynia: overlapping characteristics. J Reprod Med 2004; 49:883.
16. Harlow BL, Stewart EG. A population-based assessment of chronic unexplained vulvar pain: have we underestimated the prevalence of vulvodynia? J Am Med Womens Assoc 2003; 58:82.
17. Harlow BL, Wise LA, Stewart EG. Prevalence and predictors of chronic lower genital tract discomfort. Am J Obstet Gynecol 2001; 185:545.

18. Bouchard C et al. Use of oral contraceptive pills and vulvar vestibulitis: a case-control study. Am J Epidemiol 2002; 156:254.
19. de Jong JM et al. Focal vulvitis: a psychosexual problem for which surgery is not the answer. J Psychosom Obstet Gynaecol 1995; 16:85.
20. Marinoff SC, Turner ML. Vulvar vestibulitis syndrome. Dermatol Clin 1992; 10:435.
21. Bergeron S et al. A randomized comparison of group cognitive–behavioral therapy, surface electromyographic biofeedback, and vestibulectomy in the treatment of dyspareunia resulting from vulvar vestibulitis. Pain 2001; 91:297.
22. Bergeron S et al. Vulvar vestibulitis syndrome: reliability of diagnosis and evaluation of current diagnostic criteria. Obstet Gynecol 2001; 98:45.
23. Witkin SS, Gerber S, Ledger WJ. Differential characterization of women with vulvar vestibulitis syndrome. Am J Obstet Gynecol 2002; 187:589.
24. Friedrich EG, Jr. Vulvar vestibulitis syndrome. J Reprod Med 1987; 32:110.
25. Goetsch MF. Vulvar vestibulitis: prevalence and historic features in a general gynecologic practice population. Am J Obstet Gynecol 1991; 164:1609.
26. Stewart EG. Developments in vulvovaginal care. Curr Opin Obstet Gynecol 2002; 14:483.
27. Solomons CC, Melmed MH, Heitler SM. Calcium citrate for vulvar vestibulitis. A case report. J Reprod Med 1991; 36:879.
28. Dodson MG, Friedrich EG, Jr. Psychosomatic vulvovaginitis. Obstet Gynecol 1978; 51:23s.
29. Bazin S et al. Vulvar vestibulitis syndrome: an exploratory case-control study. Obstet Gynecol 1994; 83:47.
30. Edwards L et al. Childhood sexual and physical abuse. Incidence in patients with vulvodynia. J Reprod Med 1997; 42:135.
31. Turner ML, Marinoff SC. Association of human papillomavirus with vulvodynia and the vulvar vestibulitis syndrome. J Reprod Med 1998; 33:533.
32. di Paola GR, Rueda NG. Deceptive vulvar papillomavirus infection. A possible explanation for certain cases of vulvodynia. J Reprod Med 1986; 31:966.
33. Bergeron S et al. Vulvar vestibulitis syndrome: a critical review. Clin J Pain 1997; 13:27.
34. Reed BD. Unpublished data, 2004.
35. Mathias SD et al. Chronic pelvic pain: prevalence, health-related quality of life, and economic correlates. Obstet Gynecol 1996; 87:321.
36. Denbow ML, Byrne MA. Prevalence, causes and outcome of vulval pain in a genitourinary medicine clinic population. Int J STD AIDS 1998; 9:88.
37. Gordon AS et al. Characteristics of women with vulvar pain disorders: responses to a Web-based survey. J Sex Marital Ther 2003; 29:45.
38. Dalton VK et al. Victimization in patients with vulvar dysesthesia/vestibulodynia. Is there an increased prevalence? J Reprod Med 2002; 47:829.
39. Sadownik LA. Clinical profile of vulvodynia patients. A prospective study of 300 patients. J Reprod Med 2000; 45:679.
40. Lamont J et al. Psychosexual and social profiles of women with vulvodynia. J Sex Marital Ther 2001; 27:551.
41. Reed BD et al. Sexual activities and attitudes of women with vulvar dysesthesia. Obstet Gynecol 2003; 102:325.

42. Reed BD et al. Psychosocial and sexual functioning in women with vulvodynia and chronic pelvic pain. A comparative evaluation. J Reprod Med 2000; 45:624.
43. Bachmann GA, Rosen R, Kelly SW, Rhoads GG. Vulvodynia: characteristics and associations with comorbidities and quality of life. Obstet Gynecol 2006; 10:617.
44. Spadt S. Suffering in silence: managing vulvar pain patients. Contemp Nurse Practitioner 1995; 1:32.
45. Pukall CF et al. Pain measurement in vulvodynia. J Sex Marital Ther 2003; 29:111.
46. Pukall CF, Binik YM, Khalife S. A new instrument for pain assessment in vulvar vestibulitis syndrome. J Sex Marital Ther 2004; 30:69.
47. Curnow JS, Barron I, Morrison G. Vulval algesiometer. Med Biol Eng Comput 1996; 34:266.
48. Reed BD. Vulvodynia. Female Patient 2005; 30:48.
49. Stolar AG, Stewart JT. Nortriptyline for depression and vulvodynia. Am J Psychiatry 2002; 159:316.
50. Bergeron S et al. Physical therapy for vulvar vestibulitis syndrome: a retrospective study. J Sex Marital Ther 2002; 28:183.
51. Glazer HI. Dysesthetic vulvodynia. Long-term follow-up after treatment with surface electromyography-assisted pelvic floor muscle rehabilitation. J Reprod Med 2000; 45:798.
52. Glazer HI et al. Electromyographic comparisons of the pelvic floor in women with dysesthetic vulvodynia and asymptomatic women. J Reprod Med 1998; 43:959.

8

Vulvar Vestibulitis Syndrome

Miranda A. Farage

Feminine Care Clinical Sciences, The Procter & Gamble Company, Cincinnati, Ohio, U.S.A.

Rudolph P. Galask

Department of Obstetrics and Gynecology, Vulvar Vaginal Diseases Clinic, University of Iowa Hospitals and Clinics, Roy J. and Lucille A. Carver College of Medicine, Iowa City, Iowa, U.S.A.

INTRODUCTION

Vulvar vestibulitis syndrome (VVS) is a perplexing disease involving pain limited to the vulvar vestibule without objective clinical findings to explain the symptoms. The condition impairs sexual function and creates substantial psychological distress. Its cause is unknown and there are few randomized studies evaluating the efficacy of interventions. This chapter reviews disease characteristics, possible etiologies, and approaches to management.

DEFINITION AND DISEASE CHARACTERISTICS

VVS is characterized by pain confined to the vulvar vestibule that occurs upon vestibular touch or attempted introital entry (e.g., intercourse, tampon insertion),

---

Reprinted from Farage MA, Galask RP. Vulvar vestibulitis syndrome: a review. European Journal of Obstetric & Gynecology and Reproductive Biology 2005; 123(1):9–16, with permission from Elsevier.

with minimal associated clinical findings. In 1987, Friedrich proposed three diagnostic criteria that define VVS (1):

1. Severe pain with vestibular touch or attempted vaginal entry
2. Tenderness in response to pressure on the vulvar vestibule
3. Physical findings limited to varying degrees of vestibular erythema

Because spontaneous remissions have been reported (1–3), the persistence of symptoms for more than six consecutive months is another often-used criterion.

Introital dyspareunia, the intensity of which may inhibit or prevent intercourse, is often the presenting symptom. Pain can occur in other situations that exert pressure upon the vestibule, such as tampon insertion and removal, bicycle and horseback riding, tight clothing, and prolonged periods of sitting.

Clinicians can assess the vestibular tenderness by applying a cotton-tipped swab to the vulvar vestibule in a clock-face pattern (1). Gentle touch provokes either hyperesthesia, a heightened intensity relative to the degree of applied pressure, or allodynia, the perception of a different sensation to that applied (i.e., pain rather than gentle touch). Thresholds to pain provoked by pressure are markedly lower in VVS patients (4). Reportedly, the areas most often affected are the mucosa around the openings of the Bartholin's gland ducts (4 o'clock and 8 o'clock positions) and the posterior aspect of the vestibule. However, studies using a randomized order of palpation challenge this as an artifact of increasing subjective pain with each successive clockwise or counterclockwise palpation (4).

Newer techniques have been proposed to standardize the measurement of induced vestibular pain. An assessment of various forms of thermal, tactile, and pressure stimuli demonstrated that a simple spring-pressure device (a manually operated 10 mL syringe with a spring inserted between the piston and the syringe cavity) was highly accurate in differentiating the VVS cases from controls and in distinguishing the most severe cases (5). A variation on this technique employs a vulvalgesiometer, which consists of a series of cylindrical syringe-like devices attached to a standard cotton-swab tip and springs of different compression rates for incremental pressure application (4). Though not available commercially, such tools may help refine diagnostic criteria by standardizing elicitation of the pain response.

Vestibular erythema is the most subjective and least specific of Friedrich's criteria: erythema is also present in normal subjects and determining its presence and severity depends upon clinical judgment. A recent evaluation of Friedrich's diagnostic criteria found that tenderness to vestibular pressure most reliably distinguished patients with and without VVS who had a history of dyspareunia; erythema was not a reliable criterion (6).

Some investigators distinguish between primary and secondary VVS. Primary VVS is distinguished by a history of introital dyspareunia from the first episode of sexual intercourse. Secondary VVS is preceded by symptom-free intercourse. It is unclear whether these are different entities or represent different onsets of the same disease process. Characteristically, women with primary VVS are younger, more likely to be nulliparous, and less likely to have involvement of the whole vestibule; but they do not differ in other demographic, social, or medical variables (7,8). An elevated systemic pain response to the thermal stimulus of the forearm has been associated with primary VVS (9), yet patients with primary or secondary VVS report similar symptoms and perceived symptom severity (8).

Some patients experience pain confined to the posterior vestibule (including the fourchette and the Bartholin's glands) and others have pain in the posterior and in the anterior vestibule (10). The latter type is thought to be more recalcitrant to treatment. As noted earlier, however, localized distinctions in pain have been challenged as an artifact of the order of palpation.

PREVALENCE AND PATIENT DEMOGRAPHICS

The prevalence of VVS in the general population is unknown. The prevalence of women diagnosed with VVS was 20% over a four-year period among the cohort of women presenting to a referral center for vulvovaginal disorders (11), 15% among patients seen over a six-month period in a gynecology clinic (12), and 1.3% among 24 walk-in patients in a genitourinary clinic (13). Patients ranged in age from 20 to 40 and were predominantly Caucasian. Case-control studies from North America suggest that VVS is more common in white women of reproductive age than in African American women (14). A global web-based survey initiated by highly educated, internet-savvy women with complaints of vulvar pain found that 90% of the 428 respondents were Caucasian women of reproductive age (15). The reported prevalence of VVS and dysesthetic vulvodynia in this survey was 55% and 43%, respectively; however, the reported diagnoses lacked independent confirmation and more than one diagnosis could be chosen by respondents.

Available demographic statistics may be skewed by cultural differences in the likelihood of seeking intervention as well as by diagnostic delays. The only available population-based survey, which comprised 4915 women aged 18 to 64 from ethnically diverse communities in the Boston, Massachusetts (U.S.) area, found that 40% of women with vulvar pain sought no treatment, while 60% of those who did so consulted three or more health-care providers over several years before obtaining a diagnosis (16). About 16% of respondents reported histories of chronic burning or knife-like vulvar pain or pain on vulvar contact experienced over a period of at least three months; 12.4% complained specifically of pain on vulvar contact (16). Caucasian and African American women reported a similar lifetime prevalence but Latino women were 80% more likely to have experienced vulvar pain than the other two groups. Women with a history of vulvar pain were almost eight times more likely to have experienced difficulty or pain with first tampon use (16,17). The survey suggests that vulvar pain syndromes are more widespread among various ethnic groups than previously thought, but does not fully distinguish between women whose pain is elicited by vestibular contact VVS and those who have chronic or unremitting vulvar pain in the absence of stimulation (dysesthetic vulvodynia).

DIFFERENTIAL DIAGNOSIS

The differential diagnosis can be difficult, which often leads to diagnostic delays. The hallmark characteristics of VVS are the character of the pain (raw, burning pain or sharp, knife-like pain) (6), its localization (confined to the vulvar vestibule), and its elicitation (in response to touch or pressure). Thus, VVS differs from dysesthetic vulvodynia, which involves chronic, often nonlocalized vulvar pain that occurs with or without stimulation. These two vulvar pain syndromes are distinguished from contact dermatitis, the vulvar dermatoses, and acute vulvovaginal infection by minimal clinical findings (i.e., visual, microscopic, and/or histopathologic), other than the symptom of pain with an unexplained cause.

Other organic causes of vulvar pain must be ruled out before establishing the diagnosis of VVS. Itch is not a symptom; hence, the absence of vulvar itch is a distinguishing characteristic from acute vulvovaginal candidiasis, allergic contact dermatitis, lichen simplex chronicus, lichen sclerosus, and lichen planus. The absence of skin or mucosal lesions, or of visual signs of inflammation other than mild vestibular erythema also distinguish VVS (and dysesthetic vulvodynia) from contact dermatitis, lichen simplex chronicus, lichen sclerosus, erosive lichen planus, and genital herpes simplex.

Microscopic findings help to exclude infectious vulvitis. Patch testing with standard allergens is not recommended unless allergic contact dermatitis (delayed contact hypersensitivity) is suspected in the differential diagnosis; no relevant reactions either to standard allergens or to a series pertinent to perianal or vulvar disorders were found in VVS patients (18). However, a subset of women with VVS exhibited immediate-type (or Type I) hypersensitivity to seminal fluid, as assessed by their plasma antibody titers to pooled semen samples. A majority of these patients reported that their symptoms began with an episode of sexual intercourse and that they experienced symptoms only during and after intercourse. Hence, allergy to a component of seminal fluid may be an unrecognized contributing or exacerbating factor in some cases of VVS.

Traditionally, histopathology has been of little value except to exclude other conditions. The inflammatory nature of this syndrome is the subject of debate; a nonspecific inflammatory infiltrate is observed in the tissue surrounding the vestibular glands, but this is also seen in normal tissue (19). Recently, computerized image analysis of immunostained biopsy samples has demonstrated that the number of degranulated mast cells localized to the minor vestibular glands and the overall heightened innervation of the tissue are distinguishing factors in patients with severe VVS (20).

ETIOLOGY

The etiology of VVS is unknown. A perplexing array of variables has been associated with the condition, suggesting a multifactorial pathogenesis.

Neuropathy Secondary to Inflammation

The prevailing theory is that VVS is a neuropathic disorder involving abnormal pain perception, postulated to result from sensitization of the vestibular nerve fibers and the establishment of a sympathetically maintained pain loop. In this theory, unidentified trigger events (presumably some form of chronic inflammation) activate and cause prolonged firing of the sympathetic Type C nerve fibers responsible for transmitting noxious chemical or thermal stimuli to the brain; this, in turn, causes the wide dynamic range neurons in the brain to respond abnormally, such that mild stimuli are perceived as pain. The process has been suggested first to result in the localized pain of VVS, then to progress to the chronic, generalized vulvar pain of dysesthetic vulvodynia (21).

Several lines of investigation support a neuropathic etiology for VVS. Consistent with other neuropathic pain syndromes, thresholds to thermal and mechanical stimuli are lowered in VVS patients (4,5,22). The affected tissue is hyperalgesic to thermal, tactile, and pressure stimuli, sometimes involving a hyperpathic "after pain" that lasts for minutes after removal of the stimulus (5). Neuronal hyperplasia is observed in the most afflicted areas of the vestibular tissue (20,23,24). Neurochemical characterization of these free nerve endings indicates that they are nociceptors responsible for transmitting noxious stimuli to the brain (25). Doppler perfusion imaging has revealed heightened erythema and increased superficial blood flow in the posterior vestibule of VVS patients, which suggests either the presence of classic inflammation or neurogenically induced vasodilation (26).

Recent evidence highlights a potential genetic predisposition to chronic inflammation among VVS-afflicted women. Proinflammatory variants of the polymorphic *interleukin-1* receptor antagonist gene and the *melanocortin-1* receptor gene are substantially more prevalent in VVS patients (27,28). The risk of VVS rises additively in women who carry proinflammatory variants of both genes (28). Homozygosity for allele 2 of the *interleukin-1* receptor antagonist gene leads to a reduced capacity to terminate an inflammatory response. Notably, markedly reduced induction of *interleukin-1* receptor antagonist was observed in the blood of VVS patients compared to controls (29).

Separately, a deficiency in interferon-α production, unrelated to these genotypes, may contribute to the chronic vestibular inflammation in a subset of VVS patients by reducing their ability to combat intracellular infection (30). Some VVS patients have impaired natural killer cell function, which is involved in tumor surveillance and antiviral immune activity (31). Studies have also demonstrated significantly reduced estrogen receptor expression in localized regions of the vestibular mucosa from VVS patients (32). Because estrogen both stimulates the antibody response and inhibits T-cell mediated inflammation, localized insensitivity to circulating estrogen may increase vulvar susceptibility to inflammation caused by infectious agents.

Although these lines of evidence support a pathogenic role for inflammation, they do not establish a causative relationship to nociceptor sensitization and hyperproliferation. Associations between an altered pattern of innervation of the posterior vestibule and local tissue inflammation (33) and between hyperinnervation of the vestibular epithelium and the number of degranulated mast cells around the vestibular glands are suggestive (20). Conversely, other researchers have found no evidence for active tissue inflammation in VVS patients, as assessed by inflammatory markers (cyclo-oxygenase-2 and inducible nitric oxide synthase) that are usually upregulated during the inflammatory process. A complicating factor in identifying possible inflammatory triggers is the delay between first onset of symptoms and first diagnosis; inflammation associated with an initiating event either may subside by the time patients are evaluated or may persist only in the most severe cases.

Infection

A history of genital infections is a risk factor for VVS (34). Early etiologic hypotheses focused on epidemiologic links to vulvovaginal candidiasis and genital human papilloma virus (HPV) infection. One study reported a history of recurrent candidiasis in 80% of VVS cases (35); others found the prevalence of Candida infection to be within the range found in normal subjects (36). The diagnosis of candidiasis in the aforementioned studies was often presumptive; hence, early misdiagnosis of VVS as candidiasis could have contributed to the observed statistical linkage. More recent investigations, which corroborated referring physicians' statements or prior laboratory results with patient reports, found VVS risk to be associated with a history of bacterial vaginosis, *Candida albicans*, pelvic inflammatory disease, trichomoniasis, and vulvar dysplasia (34).

The epidemiological association with HPV has been controversial. Studies investigating this hypothesis (most of which examined a limited number of viral subtypes) have produced mixed but mostly negative results (37,38). Laser or cryogenic treatment for prior HPV also has been suggested as a possible precipitating factor for VVS. Recent case-control studies utilizing physician-reported diagnoses found no increased risk associated with prior HPV infection, genital warts, chlamydia, genital herpes, or gonorrhea (34). Emerging data on host factors, such as reduced immune cell function (30–32) and genetic susceptibility to chronic inflammation (27–29), support the hypothesis that either bacterial or viral infections, or other potential inflammatory triggers (exposure to noxious chemicals, laser treatment, semen allergy), may play a role in VVS pathogenesis.

Physical Causes

Dysfunction of pelvic floor muscles may be a component of VVS (39). The variables of pelvic floor muscle instability at rest, elevated resting baseline electromyographic response, and poor muscle recovery after contraction differentiated VVS-afflicted women from controls. Such studies do not distinguish whether these variations of pelvic floor muscular responses are predisposing or causative factors, or consequences of the syndrome.

Diet

Urinary excretion of oxalates, which causes burning and itching of the urethra, was proposed as a contributing factor based on a case report of symptom relief in a single patient whose symptoms were associated with hyperoxaluria and elevated urine pH (40). This etiologic theory was bolstered by the association of VVS and interstitial cystitis (41–43); both the vulvar vestibule and the urinary bladder are derived from the same embryologic cells and innervated by branches of the same nerves, suggesting the potential for a shared pathogenesis. However, a prospective study of low oxalate diets in 130 patients and 23 controls failed to confirm therapeutic efficacy (44).

Psychosexual Dysfunction

Multiple studies have examined the potential etiologic role of psychosexual factors (45–51). Women with VVS experience greater psychological distress and sexual dissatisfaction than healthy controls (46). Although some investigators propose that the syndrome has a purely psychogenic origin (52), others dispute this, pointing to evidence of pain relief by surgical excision of affected portions of the vestibule (53). Studies of the prevalence of psychological distress fail to distinguish whether such impairment is predisposing, precipitating, perpetuating, or simply the result of having an unmitigated pain syndrome. Qualitative research, which examines patients' commentary as an adjunct to standardized psychological profiling, suggests that sexual dysfunction and psychological distress are the consequences of, rather than the cause of, VVS. For example, when asked about the impact of the disease, VVS sufferers reported dramatic negative effects on sexuality, intimate relationships, and psychological well-being, which bore no correlation with how they rated such factors prior to symptom onset (49). Changes associated with disease onset included reduced sexual interest, satisfaction, and willingness to engage in sexual or noncoital intimacy, along with high levels of frustration and increased symptoms of clinical depression. Therefore, optimal treatments must address both physical and psychological sequelae of VVS.

MANAGEMENT

No accepted curative therapy for VVS exists and current approaches to management lack clear etiologic foundations. A dearth of rigorous, randomized prospective trials exists for most therapies; evidence for their efficacy derives largely from single case studies or case series, in which each patient was her own control. Studies also differed in the definition of success criteria, including the endpoints assessed (e.g., pain, dyspareunia, sexual function), the extent of recovery (e.g., partial or significant improvement, complete remission), and the duration of follow-up.

Interventions include symptom relief, biofeedback, pharmacologic treatment of putative infectious causes, psychosocial and supportive therapies, and surgery to remove afflicted vestibular tissue.

Symptom Relief

Applying topical anesthetic to the vestibule about 10 to 15 minutes prior to intercourse may relieve dyspareunia (54). A case report of a single patient described pain relief for 12 months after treatment with a 6-week course of the submucosal infiltrations of betamethasone and lidocaine (55). Favorable results in 15 of 22 patients (either remission or marked improvement at 12 or 24 months of follow-up) were obtained with submucosal infiltrations of lidocaine and methylprednisone (56). Presumably, such treatments combine immediate anesthetic effects as well as immediate and depot anti-inflammatory or immunomodulating effects of the steroid.

Low-dose tricyclic antidepressants have been employed on the basis of their effectiveness in treating dysesthetic vulvodynia. These agents are indicated for efficacious pain reduction rather than for their effects on mood. In a series of 230 VVS patients, a three- to six-month course of low-dose amitriptyline resulted in a 60% positive response rate after five years of follow-up (3).

Biofeedback

Biofeedback is a good conservative first choice in treatment. Two independent studies demonstrated the effectiveness of electromyographic biofeedback of the pelvic floor musculature in VVS patients with severe, chronic, introital dyspareunia (57,58). The therapy involves a program of in-home, biofeedback-assisted, pelvic floor muscle rehabilitation exercises using portable equipment. Using resumption of intercourse as a measure of treatment efficacy, success rates in the two studies were 78% and 89%, respectively.

Antifungal and Antiviral Agents

Historically, clinicians prescribed oral fluconazole as a treatment, despite little evidence of efficacy, based on a presumptive association with Candida infection (59,60). In one of the few long-term, follow-up studies of this approach, maintenance antifungal therapy resulted in a 71% cure rate among women who had positive Candida cultures at initial diagnosis (3).

Injectable interferon-β and interferon-α have been investigated with mixed results on the basis of the presumptive association of VVS with HPV infection (61–64). Treatment appeared to be more effective in HPV-associated cases. Recent reports of a genetic deficiency in interferon-α production among some VVS patients (30) have led to a resurgence of interest in therapy with exogenous interferon-α targeted at the appropriate subset of afflicted women (65).

Supportive and Multimodal Approaches

The comprehensive treatment of VVS should include some form of supportive therapy. VVS disrupts intimate relationships and causes great distress. Because of the intimate nature of their pain, many women delay seeking treatment; those who do are often frustrated and demoralized after appointments with multiple clinicians or after trying numerous interventions without success (15). Because of the significant impact of VVS on intimate relationships and psychological well-being, optimal treatment must address both the psychosexual and physical aspects of the disease. Clinicians must be willing to probe emotional and sexual concerns with sensitivity and be able to make referrals to mental health professionals if necessary (46,49). Supportive psychosocial approaches (such as cognitive-behavioral sex therapy) can serve as primary or adjunctive therapy. Some clinicians advocate integrated treatment programs consisting of physical therapy (including biofeedback), pain management, and psychosexual support as the principal forms of intervention (66).

Surgery

Surgery is generally reserved for the most refractive cases of VVS. The efficacy of surgical excision of painful vestibular tissue has been reviewed extensively elsewhere (67). Case series indicate that surgery is an effective form of therapy, with symptom relief in 60% to 90% of cases (35,53,68–70). It should be noted that the definition of a successful outcome (pain reduction, resumption of intercourse, etc.) varies among these studies and that most women served as their own control.

The most conservative surgical technique, vestibuloplasty, involves vertical excision of the posterior vaginal introitus without vaginal advancement. In partial vestibulectomy, the posterior portion of the vulvar vestibule is removed, with advancement of the vaginal epithelium to cover the excised portion. Perineoplasty, the most aggressive intervention, extends from just below the urethra to the fourchette; the vaginal epithelium is advanced laterally to the labia minora and posteriorly to the perineal body.

A comparative study involving 21 women found that vestibuloplasty failed to relieve symptoms in 10 patients, while perineoplasty resulted in complete remission in 9 of 11 patients (71). Removal of only the posterior vestibule, coupled with interferon treatment of the remaining anterior vestibule, was as effective as total perineoplasty and had fewer surgical complications (72).

A 10-year retrospective chart review at the Mayo Clinic provided substantial evidence for the effectiveness of vestibulectomy, lending further support for this more conservative approach (70).

A partially randomized and nonrandomized study involving 48 women comparing cognitive behavioral therapy (CBT) and CBT preceded by vestibulectomy found both treatments to be equally effective (73). Notably, although the study was to have been a randomized trial of CBT and surgery, it became difficult to continue assigning patients to surgery once it became apparent that the two treatments were equally effective; therefore, some patients were given the option of choosing surgical intervention prior to CBT. Because of the small group sizes (only 14 women participated in the randomized portion), the power of the statistical analysis and the study conclusions have been criticized (74). A later comparison of CBT, electromyographic biofeedback, and vestibulectomy found that all treatments resulted in improvements in pain perception and sexual function at a six-month follow-up, although vestibulectomy was significantly more successful (75). After two years, vestibulectomy remained superior in its impact on vestibular pain perception, but was no different to CBT, specifically with regard to coital pain (76). It is unclear whether the duration of the physical and psychosocial interventions (12 weeks) was sufficient for an effective comparison of these alternative measures.

It should be noted that the data supporting the efficacy of surgery are not accepted universally. Some investigators have challenged study methodologies and the assumptions involved in measuring success rates; they believe that the psychosocial aspects of the syndrome are underappreciated and view surgery as unwarranted for a condition that has no clearly defined etiology (52,77).

CONCLUSION

VVS is a debilitating syndrome involving unexplained, localized vestibular pain on contact accompanied by minimal objective clinical findings. The etiology is unknown and possibly is multifactorial. The prevailing theory postulates that the syndrome is a neuropathic disorder of abnormal pain perception triggered by some form of chronic inflammation. Possible triggers include infectious agents, excessive use of irritating topical products or medications, prior laser or cryogenic treatments for HPV infection, and Type I hypersensitivity to seminal fluid. Mounting evidence suggests that VVS-afflicted women are predisposed genetically to chronic inflammatory responses or may have impaired immune defenses against infectious agents. Evidence also exists for physical (pelvic musculature dysfunction, vaginismus) and psychological contributing factors. Rigorous randomized prospective trials evaluating alternative therapeutic approaches are lacking. Conservative interventions with some evidence for efficacy are anesthetic symptom relief, pain modulation with low-dose tricyclic antidepressants, and electromyographic biofeedback. Antifungal or interferon therapy may be beneficial for selected subsets of patients. Surgical excision of afflicted portions of the vestibule produces relief but is reserved for chronic, recalcitrant cases when other treatments have failed. Patients with VVS benefit from supportive therapy; a multimodal treatment approach may be optimal to address both the physical symptoms and the psychological sequelae. More research is required to elucidate etiologic mechanisms and produce effective, evidence-based treatments for this complex disease.

REFERENCES

1. Friedrich EG Jr. Vulvar vestibulitis syndrome. J Reprod Med 1987; 32:110.
2. Marinoff SC, Turner ML. Vulvar vestibulitis syndrome: an overview. Am J Obstet Gynecol 1991; 65:1228.
3. Pagano R. Vulvar vestibulitis syndrome: an often unrecognized cause of dyspareunia. Aust N Z J Obstet Gynaecol 1999; 39:79.
4. Pukall CF, Binik YM, Khalife S. A new instrument for pain assessment in vulvar vestibulitis syndrome, J Sex Marital Ther 2004; 30:69.
5. Lowenstein L et al. Vulvar vestibulitis severity—assessment by sensory and pain testing modalities. Pain 2004; 107:47.
6. Bergeron S et al. Vulvar vestibulitis syndrome: reliability of diagnosis and evaluation of current diagnostic criteria. Obstet Gynecol 2001; 98:45.
7. Bornstein J, Mamanm M, Abramovici H. "Primary" versus "secondary" vulvar vestibulitis: one disease, two variants. Am J Obstet Gynecol 2001; 184:28.
8. Witkin SS, Gerber S, Ledger WJ. Differential characterization of women with vulvar vestibulitis syndrome. Am J Obstet Gynecol 2002; 187:589.
9. Granot M et al. Primary and secondary vulvar vestibulitis syndrome: systemic pain perception and psychophysical characteristics. Am J Obstet Gynecol 2004; 191:138.
10. Bornstein J et al. Severe vulvar vestibulitis. Relation to HPV infection. J Reprod Med 1997; 42:514.
11. Hansen A, Carr K, Jensen JT. Characteristics and initial diagnoses in women presenting to a referral center for vulvovaginal disorders in 1996–2000. J Reprod Med 2002; 47:854.
12. Furlonge CB et al. Vulvar vestibulitis syndrome: a clinico-pathological study. Br J Obstet Gynaecol 1991; 98:703.
13. Denbow ML, Byrne MA. Prevalence, causes and outcome of vulval pain in a genitourinary medicine clinic population. Int J STD AIDS 1998; 9:88.
14. Foster DC, Woodruff JD. Case-control study of vulvar vestibulitis syndrome, J Womens' Health 1995; 4:677.
15. Gordon AS et al. Characteristics of women with vulvar pain disorders: responses to a Web-based survey. J Sex Marital Ther 2003; 29(suppl):1, 45.
16. Harlow BL, Stewart EG. A population-based assessment of chronic unexplained vulvar pain: have we underestimated the prevalence of vulvodynia? J Am Med Women's Assoc 2003; 58:82.
17. Harlow BL, Wise LA, Stewart EG. Prevalence and predictors of chronic lower genital tract discomfort. Am J Obstet Gynecol 2001; 185:545.
18. Nunns D et al. Is patch testing necessary in vulval vestibulitis? Contact Dermatitis 1997; 37:87.

19. Lundqvist EN et al. Is vulvar vestibulitis an inflammatory condition? A comparison of histological findings in affected and healthy women. Acta Derm Venereol 1997; 77:319.
20. Bornstein J, Goldschmid N, Sabo E. Hyperinnervation and mast cell activation may be used as histopathologic diagnostic criteria for vulvar vestibulitis. Gynecol Obstet Invest 2004; 58:171.
21. Cox JT. Deconstructing vulval pain. Lancet 1995; 345:53.
22. Bohm-Starke N et al. Psychophysical evidence of nociceptor sensitization in vulvar vestibulitis syndrome. Pain 2001; 94:177.
23. Bohm-Starke N et al. Increased intraepithelial innervation in women with vulvar vestibulitis syndrome. Gynecol Obstet Invest 1998; 46:256.
24. Tympanidis P, Terenghi G, Dowd P. Increased innervation of the vulval vestibule in patients with vulvodynia. Br J Dermatol 2003; 148:1021.
25. Bohm-Starke N et al. Neurochemical characterization of the vestibular nerves in women with vulvar vestibulitis syndrome. Gynecol Obstet Invest 1999; 48:270.
26. Bohm-Starke N et al. Increased blood flow and erythema in the posterior vestibular mucosa in vulvar vestibulitis(1). Obstet Gynecol 2001; 98:1067.
27. Jeremias J, Ledger WJ, Witkin SS. Interleukin 1 receptor antagonist gene polymorphism in women with vulvar vestibulitis. Am J Obstet Gynecol 2000; 182:283.
28. Foster DC, Sazenski TM, Stodgell CJ. Impact of genetic variation in interleukin-1 receptor antagonist and melanocortin-1 receptor genes on vulvar vestibulitis syndrome. J Reprod Med 2004; 49:503.
29. Gerber S et al. Defective regulation of the proinflammatory immune response in women with vulvar vestibulitis syndrome. Am J Obstet Gynecol 2002; 186:696.
30. Gerber S et al. A deficiency in interferon-alpha production in women with vulvar vestibulitis. Am J Obstet Gynecol 2002; 186:361.
31. Masterson BJ, Galask RP, Ballas ZK. Natural killer cell function in women with vestibulitis. J Reprod Med 1996; 41:562.
32. Eva LJ et al. Estrogen receptor expression in vulvar vestibulitis syndrome. Am J Obstet Gynecol 2003; 189:458.
33. Westrom LV, Willen R. Vestibular nerve fiber proliferation in vulvar vestibulitis syndrome. Obstet Gynecol 1998; 91:572.
34. Smith EM et al. Case-control study of vulvar vestibulitis risk associated with genital infections. Infect Dis Obstet Gynecol 2002; 10:193.
35. Mann MS et al. Vulvar vestibulitis: significant clinical variables and treatment outcome. Obstet Gynecol 1992; 79:122.
36. Bazin S et al. Vulvar vestibulitis syndrome: an exploratory case-control study. Obstet Gynecol 1994; 83:47.
37. Wilkinson EJ et al. Vulvar vestibulitis is rarely associated with human papillomavirus infection types 6, 11, 16, or 18. Int J Gynecol Pathol 1993; 12:344.
38. Bergeron C et al. Vulvar vestibulitis. Lack of evidence for a human papillomavirus etiology. J Reprod Med 1994; 39:936.
39. White G, Jantos M, Glazer H. Establishing the diagnosis of vulvar vestibulitis. J Reprod. Med 1997; 42:157.
40. Solomons CC, Melmed MH, Heitler SM. Calcium citrate for vulvar vestibulitis. A case report. J Reprod Med 1991; 36:879.

41. Fitzpatrick CC et al. Vulvar vestibulitis and interstitial cystitis: a disorder of urogenital sinus-derived epithelium? Obstet Gynecol 1993; 81:860.
42. Stewart EG, Berger BM. Parallel pathologies? Vulvar vestibulitis and interstitial cystitis. J Reprod Med 1997; 42:131.
43. Tarr G, Selo-Ojeme DO, Onwude JL. Coexistence of vulvar vestibulitis and interstitial cystitis. Acta Obstet Gynecol Scand 2003; 82:969.
44. Baggish MS, Sze EH, Johnson R. Urinary oxalate excretion and its role in vulvar pain syndrome. Am J Obstet Gynecol 1997; 177:507.
45. Brotto LA, Basson R, Gehring D. Psychological profiles among women with vulvar vestibulitis syndrome: a chart review. J Psychosom Obstet Gynaecol 2003; 24:195.
46. Gates EA, Galask RP. Psychological and sexual functioning in women with vulvar vestibulitis. J Psychosom Obstet Gynaecol 2001; 22:221.
47. Green J et al. A review of physical and psychological factors in vulvar vestibulitis syndrome. Int J STD AIDS 2001; 12:705.
48. Jantos M, White G. The vestibulitis syndrome. Medical and psychosexual assessment of a cohort of patients. J Reprod Med 1997; 42:145.
49. Sackett S et al. Psychosexual aspects of vulvar vestibulitis. J Reprod Med 2001; 46:593.
50. Schover LR, Youngs DD, Cannata R. Psychosexual aspects of the evaluation and management of vulvar vestibulitis. Am J Obstet Gynecol 1992; 167:630.
51. Van Lankveld JJ, Weijenborg PT, ter Kuile MM. Psychologic profiles of and sexual function in women with vulvar vestibulitis and their partners. Obstet Gynecol 1996; 88:65.
52. de Jong JM et al. Focal vulvitis: a psychosexual problem for which surgery is not the answer. J Psychosom Obstet Gynaecol 1995; 16:85.
53. Bornstein J et al. Vulvar vestibulitis: physical or psychosexual problem? Obstet Gynecol 1999; 93:876.
54. Gibbons JM. Vulvar vestibulitis. In: Steeg JS, Metzger DH, Levy BS, eds. Chronic Pelvic Pain. Philadelphia: W.B. Saunders, 1998:181.
55. Segal D, Tifheret H, Lazer S. Submucous infiltration of betamethasone and lidocaine in the treatment of vulvar vestibulitis. Eur J Obstet Gynecol Reprod Biol 2003; 107:105.
56. Murina F et al. Treatment of vulvar vestibulitis with submucous infiltrations of methylprednisolone and lidocaine. An alternative approach. J Reprod Med 2001; 46:713.
57. Glazer HI et al. Treatment of vulvar vestibulitis syndrome with electromyographic biofeedback of pelvic floor musculature. J Reprod Med 1995; 40:283.
58. McKay E et al. Treating vulvar vestibulitis with electromyographic biofeedback of pelvic floor musculature. J Reprod Med 2001; 46:337.
59. Ashman RB, Ott AK. Autoimmunity as a factor in recurrent vaginal candidosis and the minor vestibular gland syndrome. J Reprod Med 1989; 34:264.
60. Marinoff SC, Turner ML. Hypersensitivity to vaginal candidiasis or treatment vehicles in the pathogenesis of minor vestibular gland syndrome. J Reprod Med 1986; 31:796.
61. Bornstein J, Pascal B, Abramovici H. Treatment of a patient with vulvar vestibulitis by intramuscular interferon beta; a case report. Eur J Obstet Gynecol Reprod Biol 1991; 42:237.

62. Bornstein J, Pascal B, Abramovici H. Intramuscular beta-interferon treatment for severe vulvar vestibulitis. J Reprod Med 1993; 38:117.
63. Umpierre SA et al. Human papillomavirus DNA in tissue biopsy specimens of vulvar vestibulitis patients treated with interferon. Obstet Gynecol 1991; 78:693.
64. Marinoff SC et al. Intralesional alpha interferon. Cost-effective therapy for vulvar vestibulitis syndrome. J Reprod Med 1993; 38:19.
65. Hofmann RG. Alferon and vulvar vestibulitis. J Am Med Women's Assoc 2003; 58:131.
66. Graziottin A, Brotto LA. Vulvar vestibulitis syndrome: a clinical approach. J Sex Marital Ther 2004; 30:125.
67. Haefner HK. Critique of new gynecologic surgical procedures: surgery for vulvar vestibulitis. Clin Obstet Gynecol 2000; 43:689.
68. Bergeron S et al. The surgical treatment of vulvar vestibulitis syndrome: a follow-up study. J Sex Marital Ther 1997; 23:317.
69. McCormack WM, Spence MR. Evaluation of the surgical treatment of vulvar vestibulitis. Eur J Obstet Gynecol Reprod Biol 1999; 86:135.
70. Gaunt G, Good A, Stanhope CR, Vestibulectomy for vulvar vestibulitis. J Reprod Med 2003; 48:591.
71. Bornstein J et al. Perineoplasty compared with vestibuloplasty for severe vulvar vestibulitis Br J Obstet Gynaecol 1995; 102:652.
72. Bornstein J, Abramovici H. Combination of subtotal perineoplasty and interferon for the treatment of vulvar vestibulitis. Gynecol Obstet Invest 1997; 44:53.
73. Weijmar Schultz WC et al. Behavioral approach with or without surgical intervention to the vulvar vestibulitis syndrome: a prospective randomized and non-randomized study. J Psychosom Obstet Gynaecol 1996; 17:143.
74. van der Werf-Eldering MJ, Batstra L. To cut or not to cut: treatment of vulvar vestibulitis syndrome. J Psychosom Obstet Gynaecol 2004; 25:77.
75. Bergeron S et al. A randomized comparison of group cognitive—behavioral therapy, surface electromyographic biofeedback, and vestibulectomy in the treatment of dyspareunia resulting from vulvar vestibulitis. Pain 2001; 91:297.
76. Bergeron S, Binik YM, Khalife S, In favor of an integrated pain-relief treatment approach for vulvar vestibulitis syndrome. J Psychosom Obstet Gynaecol 2002; 23:7.
77. Marin G. Vestibulectomy as treatment for vestibulitis. J Reprod Med 2001; 46:1078.

9

Vulvar Therapies: Evidence Vs. Testimony

Natalie Moulton-Levy
Jefferson Medical College, Philadelphia, Pennsylvania, U.S.A.

Howard I. Maibach
Department of Dermatology, University of California School of Medicine, San Francisco, California, U.S.A.

INTRODUCTION

Management of vulvar conditions requires special consideration, as there are unique emotional, psychological, and physiologic components that clinicians must address. Thus, currently accepted therapeutic techniques for vulvar disease are specific, reflecting the necessary modifications of treatments for standard dermatologic diseases. This chapter describes the vulvar lesions encountered most commonly and discusses their evidence-based therapies. Unfortunately, the number of published randomized clinical trials (RCTs) for management of vulvar disease is limited.

VULVODYNIA

The cause of vulvodynia is multifactorial. As such, most effective treatments are interdisciplinary and highly patient specific. There are few clinical trials (with inadequate numbers of participants) demonstrating the efficacy of therapies to treat this disorder; placebo-controlled studies are yet to be performed.

Vulvar pain syndromes can be emotionally devastating. It has been suggested that there is a psychological component to vulvodynia; however, many patients are reluctant to seek psychological help. It is of utmost importance for the caregiver to provide emotional support and education about the disorder (1). Patients may also benefit from support group participation.

Medical therapy for patients with all subtypes of vulvodynia consists of treatments generally used for treating neuropathic pain. Several reports, including a noncontrolled retrospective study (2), suggest that oral tricyclic antidepressants, specifically 100–150 mg of amitriptyline or desipramine, may be effective in reducing pain. The retrospective study showed that 58% of patients "responded well" to treatment and 20% were "cured" after six months. As some patients do not wish to take a psychiatric drug, it is important to explain that the medication is being used for its neuromodulating effect. (Though tricyclic antidepressants are used commonly to treat neuropathic pain, the FDA has not cleared these agents for pain indications.) In order to minimize potential adverse side effects, clinicians often prescribe tricyclic antidepressants at an initial dose of 5–10 mg daily, with the dose increasing gradually to 150 mg per day, as tolerated by the patient, or until the symptoms have been controlled. The average time required for effective treatment is seven months, after which the treatment can be discontinued or tapered. Side effects of tricyclic medications include drowsiness, fatigue, mouth and eye dryness, constipation, increased appetite, and urinary retention. Within the tricyclic antidepressant class, desipramine has one of the best side-effect profiles: it is less sedating, has lower anticholinergic effects, and leads to less weight gain. This agent, however, is more likely than amitriptyline to produce tremulousness. Desipramine can be prescribed in the same dosages as amitriptyline, but should be taken at night. In addition, there have been reports of the efficacy of treating this condition with nontricyclic antidepressants, such as selective serotonin re-uptake inhibitors and venlaxafine (2).

For women who cannot tolerate tricyclics or whose pain does not improve, gabapentin may be an acceptable alternative (2). Patients can start with low doses and increase the dose gradually to 900–3600 mg per day, divided into three or four dosages. Limited noncontrolled case reports demonstrate gabapentin's efficacy in treating vulvodynia; however, many clinicians report successful treatment with gabapentin. Side effects include drowsiness, fatigue, dizziness, nausea, vomiting, and ataxia.

Lidocaine (5% ointment) is the topical therapy used most commonly. Long-term overnight topical treatment may minimize pain (3). Lidocaine ointment may cause erythema and numbness. Other topical treatments that might be beneficial include 2% amitriptyline with 2% baclofen (4), applied one to three times daily; side efects include contact dermatitis, dry mouth, drowsiness, and constipation. Additional topical treatments include estradiol cream (4) (0.01%, twice a day for a minimum of 4 to 8 weeks), capsaicin (4), and cytokines (5). Of note, estradiol may cause vaginal bleeding.

Neuromuscular dysfunction can contribute to pain. Pelvic floor muscle rehabilitation combined with biofeedback has been beneficial in relieving pain by up to 40% to 60% in several noncontrolled clinical trials (2). If pelvic floor abnormalities are identified by surface electromyography, regularly exercising the muscles twice daily for 8 to 12 months has been shown to be beneficial, with improvement noted after several months (6). Unfortunately, therapists and physiatrists skilled in this type of training are not widely available.

Trigger-point injections of 0.2 to 0.3 mL of 3 mg/mL triamcinolone acetonide may be of great benefit in treating patients with localized pain (5). An additional injection after four to six months may provide permanent pain relief. Intralesional interferon-α (IFN-α) injections have been reported to be beneficial (7). Treatment consists of one million units of IFN-α injected three times per week for four weeks circumferentially at the vestibule periphery. Side effects such as fever, malaise, and myalgias can be reduced by pretreatment with acetaminophen or ibuprofen. Patients also sometimes experience pain at the site of injection, which may be minimized by pretreatment with a topical anesthetic. Improvement one year after the therapy is variable.

Some researchers believe that the pathophysiology involves an adverse reaction to *Candida*. Therefore, treatment for this subtype can include antifungal medication, even in patients with negative cultures. This treatment regimen proved beneficial in an RCT (8). The most common regimen is fluconazole, 150 mg orally once weekly for two months and then once every other week for two to four months (8).

Severe or refractory vulvar vestibulitis, which has failed medical treatment for six months, can be treated surgically with vulvar vestibulectomy (9). Many surgeons remove all areas of the vestibule, including areas that do not exhibit pain, because vestibulectomy failures result in recurrences in remaining vestibule tissue. Surgical excision has been curative or produced significant improvement of symptoms in 66% to 85% of patients (9). However, hematoma, wound dehiscence, poor healing, symptom recurrence, or worsening of pain can occur after vestibulectomy. Flashlamp-excited dye laser treatment has been somewhat successful in reducing the need for resective surgery (4).

High oxalate levels may cause vulvar irritation, contributing to the pain of vulvodynia. A low-oxalate diet with calcium citrate supplementation to inhibit absorption of oxalate can reduce pain symptoms (10). However, other studies have failed to detect increased oxalate levels in patients with vulvodynia, and have shown no correlation between oxalate levels and symptom improvement (4).

ECZEMATOUS AND PAPULOSQUAMOUS VULVAR DERMATOSES

Contact Dermatitis (Irritant and/or Allergic)

Contact dermatitis can be either irritant (nonimmunologic) and/or allergic (immunologic). Lesions occur on areas of the vulva that contact environmental irritants or antigens. It is essential to restore the normal skin barrier and protect the skin from additional injury. Treatment begins with identification and withdrawal of the offending substance. To prevent recurrence, careful documentation of possible irritants or allergens is necessary. Women with vulvar dermatoses should be patch tested to define or rule out disease-causing agents (11).

After irritant withdrawal, symptoms of nonimmunologic contact dermatitis should disappear rapidly. However, if the lesions are of allergic etiology, signs and symptoms can persist for days after the discontinuation of the allergen. Though clinical improvement is apparent and supported by clinical trials, there has been no RCT evaluating treatment for contact dermatitis of the vulva.

Common habits can cause mucocutaneous irritation, and behavior modifications are necessary to reduce risk of vulvar irritation and ensure successful management. Modifications include, but are not limited to, use of cotton underwear, lubrication with sexual contact, washing with mild soap, keeping the vulva clean and dry, and avoidance of cosmetics, perfumes, or other caustic substances in this sensitive area. Aluminum acetate in water (e.g., Burow's solution), topical creams (such as Sorbolene or aqueous cream), sitz baths with mild soap, and lubricants (such as petroleum jelly) are helpful in some cases. Secondary bacterial or *Candida* infections require specific treatment.

Antipruritic medications, such as antihistamines, are not of great therapeutic benefit except as soporific agents. Drugs with antihistamine and sedative properties, such as doxepin (10–20 mg at night), can be helpful in controlling nocturnal scratching (12).

Topical corticosteroids can be helpful in cases of irritant contact dermatitis that are unresponsive to conservative therapy. These agents may reduce inflammation in allergic contact dermatitis, but typically are not used for the long-term treatment. Ointments are preferred to creams or lotions, which can be dry and irritating. Topical corticoids are most effective when applied and covered with a barrier, such as plastic wrap, a gauze dressing, cotton gloves, or petroleum jelly.

Pharmacologic treatment consists of mid- to high-potency topical corticosteroids, such as triamcinolone, betamethasone, and fluocinolone (2), usually for 14 days or until symptoms have resolved. At this point, a weaker corticosteroid, such as 1% hydrocortisone, can be continued for an additional two to three months. This cycle can be repeated if disease activity flares. In cases of mild disease, low-potency steroids are safer and are preferred, typically. Use low-potency topical steroids, such as hydrocortisone 2.5%, on thinner skin and for patients who prefer to use a topical preparation regularly. Alternatives include intralesional triamclinone injections every three to six months. Brief courses of systemic corticosteroids are reserved for severe or recalcitrant dermatitis. Adequate dosage and an adequate taper length are important points to consider. Treatment with topical corticosteroids should be limited, as long-term use may induce telangiectasias, skin friability, striae formation, and easy bruising. Caution must also be taken to avoid rebound inflammation upon withdrawal from long-term, high-potency corticosteroids. See Chapter 12 for a more thorough discussion of contact dermatitis of the vulva.

Atopic Dermatitis

Endogenous atopic dermatitis is not curable but, typically, is readily treatable. Though there are clinically effective treatment options, no randomized or controlled trials have been performed. Primary treatment is aimed at avoiding exacerbating factors, which, in limited cases, can control symptoms effectively.

Moisturizers can be helpful in rehydrating the skin and helping to relieve symptoms. Symptomatic benefit may be obtained from wet Burow's solution compresses applied for 30 minutes several times daily. Mild topical corticosteroids such as 0.5% to 1% hydrocortisone cream applied several times daily can further aid healing and alleviate irritation in mild to moderate atopic dermatitis (13). Strong topical corticosteroids may be needed to control severe acute disease. To prevent side effects, highly potent corticosteroids should be used for only short periods. Oral corticosteroids are used occasionally to treat chronic atopic dermatitis, but should not be used regularly.

Topical tacrolimus (14) and pimecrolimus (15) have been shown to be more effective than placebo in treatment of generalized atopic dermatitis. Tacrolimus is a macrolide immunosuppressant with multiple immune-modulating effects, including suppression of proliferating T lymphocytes, and inhibition of interleukin-2. Because of the limited side effects of local burning, this drug may be particularly useful in sensitive areas, such as the vulva. These topical agents have been found in clinical experience to be an effective new therapeutic regimen for vulvar disease, but data specific to the vulvar area are lacking.

The immunosuppressant azathioprine is a purine analog that has been shown by double-blind, placebo-controlled clinical trials to be effective as monotherapy for generalized atopic dermatitis (16). It is thought to act through the inhibition of DNA and RNA synthesis (17). For severe or refractory vulvar disease, azathioprine is used typically as a corticoid-sparing adjunct. Side effects include gastrointestinal discomfort. Rare but severe complications include renal impairment, liver disease, and bone marrow suppression; clinicians should monitor the patient's complete blood count every two weeks and it is advisable to check liver and renal function tests periodically. This drug should not be prescribed to pregnant women, as both the drug and its metabolites cross the placenta and are potential teratogens. Azathioprine has not been studied for specific use in the vulvar region and should be used with caution.

Psoriasis

Treatment of psoriasis is aimed at symptom relief and minimizing Koebner's phenomenon. After PUVA—psoralen (P) and long-wave ultraviolet radiation (UVA)—treatment for extensive, generalized disease, psoriatic vulvar plaques may remain due to inadequate phototherapy in this region (18). Thus, vulvar psoriasis may require separate treatment. This disorder often requires more aggressive and prolonged treatment than dermatitis.

For cases of limited disease, clinicians can attempt initial treatment with a low-potency topical corticosteroid, such as 1% hydrocortisone cream. However, when used as monotherapy, such drugs are seldom effective for disease control. Many cases can be treated successfully with a 14-day course of mid- to high-potency topical corticosteroid. Intralesional corticosteroids may be an alternative (13). Systemic steroids often produce a rebound flare-up of the disease and should be avoided.

Randomized, placebo-controlled studies have proven both topical tacrolimus and pimecrolimus successful for treating generalized disease but not for vulvar psoriasis. Clinically, tacrolimus has been effective in treating psoriasis of the vulva.

Tazarotene, a retinoid, and calcipotreine, a topical vitamin D_3 analog, are used to treat generalized psoriasis without the adverse effects of steroid treatment. These have not been studied specifically for use in vulvar disease.

Weak tar preparations, such as 3% liquor picis carbonis in aqueous cream, are possible alternatives. Generally, however, tar preparations are irritating to the vulvar skin and should be avoided.

Seborrheic Dermatitis

Treatment is similar to that for contact dermatitis. Exacerbating factors, such as excessive sweating, emotional distress, and tight clothing should be minimized. Hydrocortisone cream is the most effective medical therapy (18). Acute episodes may be treated with sitz baths or topical aluminum acetate solution. Antibiotics should be administered for secondary infection.

Lichen Sclerosus

Effective treatment of lichen sclerosus will control symptoms, minimize scarring, and allow for early detection of malignant change. As a result of compelling data from clinical trials, treatment recommendations have changed recently. The current recommended and accepted treatment for all forms of lichen sclerosus is the potent topical corticosteroid ointment, clobetasol propionate (19,20). One RCT comparing clobetasol, testosterone, progesterone, and petroleum jelly showed higher rates of symptom control with clobetasol (75%) (21). Clobetasol 0.05% gel or cream provides rapid symptomatic improvement in over 90% of women treated. It also reverses some of the histological changes and is effective in long-term disease control. The medication should be applied once daily (22), and treatment typically lasts two to three months. The dose should be tapered gradually and then used only when symptoms recur, typically fewer than once or twice per week. There is some evidence that lichen sclerosus of the vulva may be treated with long-term maintenance therapy (23). The patient should be advised that this therapy is not curative and recurrence is likely.

If lesions recur, re-treatment may be necessary. Potential side effects include cutaneous atrophy or adrenal suppression but, in practice, these complications are rare. There is anectodal suggestion that intralesional injections of triamclinone every three to six months may be appropriate alternative therapy (24).

In the past, androgens and progesterones have been used widely. Androgenic side effects are common and include clitoral enlargement, hirsutism, amenorrhoea, increased libido, and voice changes (25). Side effects of progesterone include changes in vaginal discharge. Placebo-controlled trials have demonstrated that testosterone (26) is no more effective in the treatment of lichen sclerosus. Clinical trials have also indicated that prednisolone is not an effective treatment (27).

Surgical therapies, such as excision followed by skin grafting, vaginoplasty, and vulvectomy, have been used for treatment of lichen sclerosus; however, there are no data proving their effectiveness. Surgical treatments are associated with a recurrence rate and surgery is not currently recommended in the absence of vulvar intraepithelial neoplasia (VIN) or malignancy (27). In contrast, surgical intervention is always necessary in the case of lichen sclerosus complicated by malignant disease. In severe cases, with extensive fissuring and scar formation, surgical correction may be considered. Topical steroids postoperatively may help prevent recurrence. Other ablation techniques include cryotherapy (28) and laser therapy (29). These have not been investigated, recurrence rates are high, and there can be significant post-procedural discomfort, resulting in limited use of these therapeutic modalities.

Photodynamic therapy (PDT) with topical 5-aminolaevulinic acid and argon laser light has been reported to result in clinical improvement (30).

Several studies (31,32), including a placebo-controlled trial (31), showed some efficacy of systemic retinoids for treatment of lichen sclerosus; however, there are many intolerable and potentially harmful side effects. There is no evidence demonstrating the effectiveness of topical retinoids and clinical use is unlikely because these drugs cause severe skin irritation.

Case studies have demonstrated the efficacy of treating anogenital lichen sclerosus with low-dose PUVA (33), as well as with PUVA cream photochemotherapy (34). It has been postulated that radiation suppresses collagen synthesis and induces collagenase activity, leading to softening of sclerotic skin plaques.

Tacrolimus is also a promising agent for treating lichen sclerosus. There have been multiple RCTs indicating the efficacy of this drug in generalized disease. Case reports demonstrate treatment success specifically with genital lesions (35,36); however, further investigation is necessary at this time.

Lifetime risk of developing squamous cell carcinoma in the affected area is approximately 4% (37). At the minimum, patients should have yearly follow-up to monitor for malignancy. Clinicians should advise patients to return sooner if they notice any growth or ulceration. Any erosions, ulcers, and hyperkeratotic or erythematous areas should be evaluated with biopsy.

There is debate as to whether asymptomatic patients should be treated and this decision should be based on each individual case. Treatment may prevent disease progression and, possibly, malignant transformation. This, however, must be considered in the context of the multiple disadvantages to long-term therapy. Regardless of treatment decision, all patients should have long-term follow-up.

Lichen Planus

Little data support the efficacy of any specific therapy for vulvar lichen planus. Typically, vulvar lesions of lichen planus are treated with a potent topical corticoid cream such as clobetasone. Intralesional corticosteroids are used for refractory disease. Antihistamines are also helpful in treating pruritis. Generally, systemic steroids are reserved for severely symptomatic disease (38); upon discontinuation, oral steroid dosages must be tapered.

There have been reports indicating the value of vaginal suppositories in treatment of this disease (39); 25 mg hydrocortisone suppositories intravaginally twice daily for two months resulted in improvement in 16 of 17 women in one series.

Oral and topical retinoids have proven effective for generalized disease and there have been some reports of success of these agents with vulvar disease (40). However, data are too few to make any conclusive recommendations regarding use of these agents. Additionally, topical retinoids cause significant irritation and may worsen lesions.

Griseofulvin has been reported in one case series to be efficient in managing patients with vulvar disease. However, subsequent study failed to reproduce these results (38). Small studies have shown cyclosporin to be effective in treatment of severe disease (38). Cyclosporine acts by suppressing proliferating T cells and inhibiting lymphokine production. Side effects of this powerful drug can be severe, and include nephrotoxicity. It is essential to monitor the renal function of patients taking this drug every two weeks (16).

Oral or topical dapsone may be effective in chronic, recalcitrant cases. An uncontrolled case series demonstrated the efficacy of the drug, particularly when used in conjunction with oral corticosteroids. The exact mechanism of action is unknown but is believed to be anti-inflammatory, possibly through alterations of neutrophil function (16). Rarely, dapsone has been associated with hemolytic anemia or agranulocytosis. During therapy, complete blood count (CBC) should be measured regularly; most advise monitoring liver and renal function, as well. Before initiating the therapy, a glucose-6-phosphate dehydrogenase (G-6-PD) screen is recommended, as G-6-PD deficiency is a contraindication to drug use.

Recent studies have also shown topical tacrolimus 0.1% ointment to be effective in treating erosive vulvar lichen sclerosus (41). A more recent retrospective series investigating topical tacrolimus therapy demonstrated symptom control and clinical improvement in 94% of patients (42).

There have also been case studies demonstrating the use of PUVA cream phototherapy in genital lichen planus (36). At present, however, data are limited.

Surgical methods of treatment include excision, cryotherapy, and carbon dioxide laser. Blunt dissection may be performed with addition of potent topical steroids in the postoperative period (38).

As with lichen sclerosus, these patients should be monitored regularly because of an increased risk of developing vulvar malignancy (38).

Lichen Simplex Chronicus

Treatment is similar to that for chronic eczematous inflammation. Mainstays of the therapy are avoidance of known irritants or allergens and the use of topical mid- to high-potency corticosteroids. There is some evidence supporting intralesional triamclinone injections (5–10 mg/mL) every three to six months. Antihistamines are often used as antipruritics and those with sedative properties provide additional benefit as soporific agents (13).

BENIGN VULVAR NODULES OR TUMORS

In most cases, excision of solid lesions is diagnostic as well as therapeutic. Pigmented vulvar lesions include lentigo and nevi. Approximately 2% to 5% of melanomas, but only 0.1% of nevi, are located on the vulva, leading theories that vulvar nevi are at increased risk for malignant transformation (43). As such, detection and careful evaluation of vulvar nevi are critical. The benign lesions of seborrheic keratosis do not require treatment. However, excision can be performed at the patient's request, often for cosmesis.

In the case of acrochordons (fibroepithelial polyps) and hidradenomas, simple excision is curative. These is no evidence that patients with these lesions are at increased risk for malignancy (43). Achrocondon is usually asymptomatic, but repeated trauma and irritation can cause it to become ulcerated. If the lesion is in a troublesome location, such as the panty line or groin fold, it can be removed in an outpatient setting with local anesthesia and simple electrocautery or scissor excision.

Fibroma and related fibromyoma should be removed for diagnostic purposes to exclude a rare leiomyosarcoma or sarcoma. Lipomas usually do not require surgical excision unless they become painful or are cosmetically unacceptable to the patient. Painless, firm, Bartholin's masses, especially postmenopausal, should be excised to rule out Bartholin's gland malignancy (13).

INFECTIOUS DISEASES

Bacterial

Abscesses and Cellulitis

Vulvar sites often affected by abscesses or cellulitis include the hair follicle, apocrine glands, Skene's glands, and, most commonly, Bartholin's glands.

The infection is usually polymicrobial in nature, with both aerobic and anaerobic (*Bacteroides* species and other colonic and vaginal bacteria) flora. *C. trachomatis* and *N. gonorrhoeae* are encountered frequently.

The treatment of Bartholin's glands infections depends on the patient's symptoms. Asymptomatic women less than 40 years of age do not need treatment. Therapy for symptomatic cellulitis, with or without an abscess, consists of broad-spectrum antibiotics and warm sitz baths. In the case of isolated abscesses without evidence of cellulitis, antibiotics are not necessary (44). Spontaneous rupture and drainage of an abscess sometime occurs, but recurrence is likely. Definitive treatment involves surgical drainage with a Word catheter, marsupialization, or excision. The former two treatments are office-based procedures and can be performed using local anesthesia.

The treatment of choice for a symptomatic abscess is a Word catheter, which provides a convenient and highly successful method of creating a fistula from the duct of the gland to the vestibule. Most cases resolve after a few days of drainage and the catheter often falls out within a week. Ideally, the catheter should remain in place for four to six weeks, during which time an epithelial sinus will form. Sitz baths two to three times daily after the procedure may help with discomfort, keep the area clean, and hasten the healing process. Coitus may be resumed after catheter insertion.

If the abscess is too deep, Word catheter placement is impractical, and other options must be considered. Simple incision and drainage is an easy procedure but is discouraged because of the high risk of abscess recurrence, which has been reported as high as 13% (44). Also, incision and drainage may complicate later attempts at Word catheter placement or marsupialization. Nonetheless, if a Word catheter proves ineffective, incision and drainage is an acceptable option before proceeding to surgical excision. The incision for abscess drainage should be made on the mucosal, rather than the cutaneous surface. If the abscess recurs, more definitive therapy in the form of marsupialization or complete excision of the gland may be required, but these procedures are not the initial treatment of choice.

Marsupialization is a more complex procedure, involving incision and drainage followed by suturing the walls of the cyst to the skin. As with Word catheters, postoperative sitz baths can be beneficial. The recurrence rate following marsupialization is approximately 5% to 15% (44). Complications include dyspareunia, hematoma, and infection. There is a report of sepsis after marsupialization of a Bartholin's gland abscess in a gravida (45) and pregnant women should be considered high risk and managed accordingly.

Excision of Bartholin's gland and duct is another option. Though some clinicians routinely suggest excisional surgery following the first infection, more commonly surgery is reserved for the patient with persistent infection or multiple abscess recurrences. Some experts advocate for excision and biopsy for gland enlargement in women more than 40 years of age in order to evaluate for possible Bartholin's gland adenocarcinoma (13). Excision should be performed only in the absence of active infection. This is not an office procedure, as regional block or general anesthesia is necessary. Associated complications include intraoperative hemorrhage, hematomas, scarring, and dyspareunia.

Necrotizing Fasciitis

The presence of cellulitis, deteriorating vital signs, and a deep, spreading, painful erythema, especially in the postpartum or postoperative patient, should raise concern for necrotizing fasciitis. Necrotizing fasciitis is a rapidly progressive infection commonly caused by mixed aerobic–anaerobic bacteria. Unfortunately, antibiotic treatment usually proves ineffective. Necrotizing fasciitis is a surgical emergency requiring immediate and extensive surgical debridement of the necrotic fascia to prevent septic shock and fatal complications. Patients may require several debridements and skin grafts are often needed to repair large defects. Due to the emergent nature of this condition, women presenting with vulvar cellulitis, with risk factors for necrotizing fasciitis (obesity, diabetes mellitus, corticosteroid use, or immunosuppressed states) should be hospitalized for treatment with intravenous broad-spectrum antibiotics, including a penicillin and surgical treatment (46).

Treponema pallidum (Syphilis)

For over 50 years, administration of penicillin G to patients with syphilis has resulted in resolution of lesions and decreased transmission rates, and has prevented sequelae of the disease effectively. On the basis of the clinical results, penicillin is accepted as the treatment of choice for syphilis. No comparative trials have been conducted to determine the optimal dose, preparation, or length of therapy. The efficacy of most treatment recommendations is based on experience with the disease supported by case studies, clinical trials, and clinical experience. Data are not reinforced by results from RCTs, but at this time, conducting such a trial would most likely be of little additional benefit.

Parenteral penicillin G is the preferred drug for the treatment of all stages of syphilis (47) (treatment for tertiary syphilis will not be discussed further). For primary and secondary syphilis, the recommended treatment regimen is a single dose of benzathine penicillin G, 2.4 million U intramuscularly. If within six months of treatment, nontreponemal titers do not decrease four-fold, the patient should be retreated with benzathine penicillin G, 2.4 million U intramuscularly weekly for three weeks.

Treatment alternatives for penicillin-allergic patients include doxycycline (100 mg twice daily for 14 days), tetracycline (500 mg 4 times daily for 14 days), erythromycin (30–40 g given in divided doses over a period of 10–15 days), or penicillin desensitization. Tetracycline can cause gastrointestinal side effects; the other agents may increase the patient's compliance.

Some data demonstrate the efficacy of ceftriaxone for the treatment of early syphilis. However, the optimal dose and duration of therapy have not been defined clearly. The current recommendation is 1 g daily either intramuscularly or intravenously for 8 to 10 days.

Small studies, including one randomized comparative pilot study, indicate that azithromycin, as a single oral dose of 2 g or two doses one week apart, may be effective in treating early primary syphilis (48). This treatment is an attractive future alternative because it is administered orally. Recent reports have documented strains of *T. pallidum* with functional resistance to azithromycin (49).

Because they currently lack recommendation by the Center for Disease Control (CDC), and their efficacy are supported by limited data, clinicians must follow patients receiving ceftriazone and azithromycin closely.

Regardless of the drug used for treatment, patients treated for syphilis may develop the Jarisch-Herxheimer reaction, an acute febrile reaction starting within 24 hours of treatment initiation. This condition is characterized by fever, headache, and myalgias. Patients should be informed about this possible adverse reaction.

Parenteral penicillin G is the only documented efficacious treatment for syphilis during pregnancy. Thus, penicillin-allergic pregnant women with syphilis in any stage should be desensitized and treated with penicillin. Tetracycline and doxycycline should not be used during pregnancy. Erythromycin should not be used because it does not cure the infected fetus reliably. The Jarisch-Herxheimer reaction may induce early labor or cause fetal distress; however, this concern should not delay or prevent therapy.

Haemophilus ducreyi (Chancroid)

Successful treatment for chancroid cures the infection, resolves the clinical symptoms, and prevents transmission to others. Recently, *H. ducreyi* has shown resistance to many pharmacologic agents, such as trimethoprim-sulfametrole, penicillin, and tetracycline, some of which have been used traditionally for its treatment. Worldwide, there have been reports of isolates with intermediate resistance to ciprofloxacin, ceftriaxone, and erythromycin. Current regimens accepted by the World Health Organization (WHO) and CDC are as follows: oral erythromycin (500 mg three or four times a day for seven days), oral azithromycin (1 g single dose), intramuscular ceftriaxone (250 mg single dose), oral ciprofloxacin (500 mg twice a day for three days), oral ciprofloxacin (500 mg single dose), and spectinomycin (2 g single dose, intramuscularly) (47,50).

Intramuscular azithromycin and ceftriaxone allow for one-dose therapy. For ciprofloxacin, there is some debate concerning the duration of therapy; the WHO recommends a single 500 mg oral dose and the CDC recommends 500 mg daily for three days. A recent double-blind, RCT showed comparable cure rates (51). The WHO and CDC also differ in their recommendations of the frequency of dosing of erythromycin. The WHO recommends 500 mg treatment four times per day, whereas the CDC recommends the same dose three times per day. Both regimens appear effective.

With treatment, buboes smaller than 5 cm typically resolve in one to two weeks. Larger buboes, as well as fluctuant buboes, should be aspirated or incised, and drained for symptomatic relief and to avoid spontaneous rupture, chronic ulceration, and tissue loss. Partners should be examined and treated and sexual contact should be avoided until treatment is complete and lesions have resolved. Pregnant women should be treated with either erythromycin or ceftriaxone regimens.

Patients with HIV infection have reduced healing and persistent infection and, therefore, should have careful follow-up.

Donovanosis (*Granouloma inguinale, Calymmatobacterium granulomatis*)

Few trials report appropriate antibiotic choice or duration of therapy for treatment of Donovanosis. However, current CDC recommendations are as follows (47): oral trimethoprim-sulfamethoxazole 800 mg/160 mg twice daily or oral doxycycline 100 mg twice daily. Alternatives include ciprofloxacin 750 mg twice daily, erythromycin base 500 mg four times a day, and azithromycin 1 g once per week. Regardless of antibiotic choice, treatment should be continued for at least three weeks or until the lesions have healed. Larger lesions may require longer periods of treatment. Some clinicians recommend adding an aminoglycoside, such as gentamicin 1 mg/kg intravenously every eight hours, if improvement is not apparent within the first few days of therapy.

Patients should be seen regularly until symptoms resolve. Follow-up is essential, as patients may relapse 6 to 18 months after seemingly effective treatment.

Pregnant and lactating women should be treated with erythromycin, with consideration given to the addition of gentamicin. Azithromycin may prove efficacious in this population, but there currently are no published data.

Lymphogranuloma venereum (*Chlamydia trachomatis* strain)

Oral doxycycline (100 mg, twice a day for three weeks) is the drug of choice for this genital infection. Oral erythromycin (500 mg four times a day for 21 days) is an appropriate alternative (47). Azithromycin (1 g once weekly for three weeks) appears effective, although there are no supporting clinical data. Successful treatment provides symptomatic relief, cures the infection, and prevents continued tissue damage. Scarring, which results from tissue reaction, is unaffected by antibiotic treatment. Buboes can persist, as they are not affected by antibiotic therapy. Persistent buboes may require aspiration or incision and drainage.

Patients should be followed clinically until signs and symptoms have resolved. Pregnant and lactating women should be treated with erythromycin.

Fungal

Candidiasis

Multiple double-blind, randomized studies have proven the efficacy of both oral and topical antifungals for the treatment of candidiasis. Administration route is largely dependant on patient preference. Topical antifungals include butoconazole, clotrimazole, miconazole, nystatin, terconazole, and tioconazole. Table 1 summarizes topical treatments tested in RCTs. Cure rates are over 80%, with

Table 1 RCT-Supported Topical Medications Proven Beneficial for Uncomplicated Vulvovaginal Candidiasis

Treatment	Placebo controlled?	Comment	Reference
Butoconazole 2% cream 5 g for 3 days	Yes	Also compared to clotrimazole and miconazole	(52)
Butoconazole 2% cream 5 g, 1 time	No	Compared to miconazole	(53)
Clotrimazole 1% cream 5 g for 7–14 days	No	Compared to terconazole	(54)
Clotrimazole 100 mg vaginal tablet for 7 days	No	Compared to clotrimazole 14 days and miconazole, also to oral fluconazole	(55–57)
Clotrimazole 100 mg vaginal tablet, 2 tablets for 3 days	No	Compared to tiaconazole, itraconazole, and oral fluconazole	(58–60)
Clotrimazole 500 mg tablet, 1 time	Yes	Also compared to oral fluconazole	(60–65)
Miconazole 2% cream 5 g for 7 days	Yes	Also compared with terconazole	(66)
Nystatin 100,000 unit table for 14 days	Yes	Has also been compared to intravaginal imidazoles	(67)
Tioconazole 6.5% ointment 5 g, 1 time	No	Compared to terconazole	(68)
Teraconazole 0.4% cream 5 g for 7 days	No	Compared to clotrimazole	(69)
Teraconazole 0.8% cream 5 g for 3 days	No	Compared to tioconazole	(68)
Teraconazole 80 mg suppository for 3 days	Yes	Also compared to miconazole, and oral fluconazole	(66,70)

Abbreviation: RCT, randomized clinical trial.

symptomatic resolution in 48–72 hours and mycological cure within four to seven days (71). Oral azoles (fluconazole, itraconazole, ketoconazole) also achieve high cure rates; however, fluconazole is currently the only FDA-approved agent (72). Itraconazole has been found to be as effective. Both methods of administration are available in prescription and over-the-counter forms. Oral agents may be preferable because of convenience and avoidance of skin sensitization, which has been associated with topical antifungals. Side effects of fluconazole are mild and infrequent, but include gastrointestinal intolerance, headache, and rash (71). There is increased hepatotoxicity with concomitant use of fluconazole with other hepatotoxic drugs, most notably statins. Oral azoles should not be used during pregnancy. One RCT has shown boric acid to be as effective in treatment as nystatin; however, this agent can cause skin irritation, is toxic if ingested, and should not be first-line therapy (73).

Candidia vulvitis can be classified into complicated and uncomplicated forms (51). Uncomplicated infection, which affects 90% of patients, is caused typically by *Candida albicans* and responds to a short-course oral or topical antifungal. There are currently many effective single-dose oral regimens, such as one-time dose of fluconazole, 150 mg. The rare infection with azole-resistant *C. albicans* requires higher doses of fluconazole. Ketoconazole is effective in treating uncomplicated candidiasis; however, hepatitis is a rare but serious side effect and the risks outweigh the benefits of its use in treating candidiasis.

Complicated candidiasis, seen in approximately 10% of the cases, requires antimycotic therapy for 10–14 days (72). Microbial infections with Candida species other than *C. albicans*, particularly *C. glabrata*, are less susceptible to azoles and azole therapy is unreliable. *C. glabrata* and the other non-*albicans* infections frequently respond to topical boric acid, 600 mg/d for 14 days or to topical flucytosine.

Recurrent vulvitis, defined as four or more episodes per year, is usually due to azole-susceptible *C. albicans* (72). Clinicians should assess patients for possible risk factors, such as uncontrolled diabetes mellitus, immunosuppression, or chronic antibiotic therapy. Multiple studies have demonstrated the effectiveness of a six-month antifungal maintenance suppressive therapy after an initial two-week induction regimen, resulting in negative cultures. Typically, induction is achieved with an oral azole. Acceptable maintenance therapies include oral fluconazole (150–200 mg weekly), oral ketoconazole (100 mg daily), oral itraconazole (100 mg every other day), or daily therapy with any topical azole (47). Two small RCTs provide insufficient evidence about regular prophylaxis with intravaginal imidazoles (74,75).

Viral

Herpes Simplex Virus

Randomized trials (76,77), including one placebo-controlled trial for acyclovir (78), show effective clinical management of disease with three oral antivirals: acyclovir, famciclovir, and valacyclovir, each of which is an acyclic nucleoside analog. These drugs result in clinical improvement, but do not eradicate latent virus nor do they affect the frequency or severity of recurrences after discontinuation. Topical antivirals offer little benefit and are not recommended.

Effective treatment will decrease shedding, as well as length and severity of symptoms of initial episodes of genital herpes, with both types 1 and 2. According to the Sexually Transmitted Diseases Guidelines, primary infection should be treated with acyclovir, 400 mg tid, acyclovir 200 mg five times daily, famciclovir 250 mg tid, or valacyclovir, 1 g bid (47). Treatment should last for 7 to 10 days. Following the course of medication, treatment is extended if healing is incomplete. Studies comparing these agents have shown equal efficacy.

Antiviral therapy for recurrent genital herpes can be administered either episodically or continously for disease suppression. Effective episodic treatment of recurrent herpes is most effective if initiated within one day of lesion onset, or during the prodrome, if possible (47). Episodic treatment decreases the time to active disease resolution and duration of shedding by one to two days (79). Each of the recommended drugs has been shown in RCTs to be effective (80–82). Recommended regimens include acyclovir (400 mg three times a day for five days or 800 mg bid for five days), famciclovir 125 mg bid for five days), or valacyclovir (500 mg bid for 3 to 5 days or 1 g daily for 5 days) (47). An RCT indicated that a 3-day course of valacyclovir 500 mg twice daily is as effective as a 5-day course (83). Though these drugs are equally efficacious, acyclovir is the least expensive and cost should be considered when choosing agents for prolonged therapy. Clinicians should counsel patients about how to identify recurrences and should provide a supply of antiviral medication for future use.

Herpes simplex virus suppression indicated in patients with more than six outbreaks per year (47). Recommended treatment options include acyclovir (400 mg twice daily), valacyclovir (500–1000 mg once daily), or famciclovir (250 mg twice daily) (47). Valacyclovir 500 mg once a day might be less effective than other dosing regimens in patients with more than 10 episodes per year (47). Daily suppressive therapy decreases symptomatic recurrence by up to 70% to 80%, increases quality of life, and decreases transmission to uninfected partners (79). Therapy with 500 mg of valacyclovir once daily for eight months can reduce disease transmission by up to 48% (79). Nonetheless, clinicians should advise patients that suppressive therapy reduces, but does not eliminate, viral shedding (84). There has been no increase in side effects noted with long-term therapy. Safety has been documented with daily acyclovir therapy for as long as six years and for one year with valacyclovir or famciclovir (79). For many patients, the frequency of recurrences diminishes with time. Because of this fact, periodic discussion regarding discontinuation of suppressive treatment is advised.

It is critical for clinicians to provide education and counseling to infected individuals and their partners. Education should include an explanation of the natural course of the disease, asymptomatic viral shedding, sexual and perinatal transmission, and methods to reduce transmission. Counseling may help, because some patients are troubled more by the psychological manifestations of the disease than the physical symptoms. Initial counseling can be provided at the first visit; the patient may benefit from direction to websites or printed materials for further support.

For HIV-positive patients, lesions may be larger, more painful, with longer healing time and more recurrences. Higher medication dose and longer treatment times may be necessary. Episodic or suppressive antiviral therapy should be considered (47).

Genital Warts (*Condyloma acuminata* Caused by Human Papilloma Virus)

Sixty percent of *Condyloma acuminata* is estimated to resolve spontaneously within two years; nonetheless, patients frequently request treatment (47) for various reasons, including cosmesis and symptom relief. Despite the fact that there is such a high rate of spontaneous resolution, the natural course of the disease varies; the condition may remain unchanged or warts may increase in size or number. Counsel patients that although the lesions may not be present, the virus may always be present in the genital tract, and that recurrences are common, generally in six months after treatment (85). It is unknown whether treatment reduces transmission, as there is no established laboratory marker of infectivity. Existing data indicate that currently available therapies for genital warts may reduce but probably do not eradicate infectivity (86).

There is a variety of treatment options that have been proven in RCTs to be safe and effective. Some treatments have been used for a long time and have shown promising in years of clinical practice. There are other new treatment options the efficacy of which is supported by research data, but that the long-term safety and efficacy have not been demonstrated in practice.

Treatment options may be either physician or patient applied. In the case of patient-applied treatment, if possible, the health-care provider should apply the initial treatment to demonstrate correct application techniques. The two recommended patient-applied treatments are podofilox and imiquimod, the efficacy of which has been supported by data from RCTs.

Podofilox is a purified podophyllin resin available in a 0.5% solution. The medication should be applied to visible warts twice daily for three days, followed by four days without therapy, a cycle that can be repeated as necessary, up to four times (47). There are eight randomized, placebo-controlled trials and many more RCTs supporting the use of podophyllotoxin that report clearance rates of up to 77% within six weeks of treatment (85). Recurrences have been reported for up to 34% of patients followed in clinical trials (87). The safety of podofilox during pregnancy has not been established.

Imiquimod is an immunomodulator with a mechanism of action that is not understood completely, but studies indicate that the chemical induces cytokines, such as IFN-α, thus activating antiviral activity. The 5% cream should be applied at bedtime, three times a week for up to 16 weeks. Six to 10 hours after application, the treatment area should be washed with soap (47). Imiquimod has been studied in a number of clinical trials, including five which were placebo controlled (88,89). Imiquimod is currently FDA-approved treatment for genital warts and has up to 70% clearance rate (85) without recurrence in up to 37% (89). Most studies indicate that this drug is less effective in men than in women (85). Side effects include skin irritation and erythema.

Four recommended provider-administered treatments include cryotherapy, podophyllin resin, acetic acid, or surgical removal. Cryotherapy with liquid nitrogen or cryoprobe can be repeated every 1 to 2 weeks (47). Nonplacebo-controlled clinical trials show efficacy similar to that of bi- and tri-chloroacetic acid, better treatment success than with podophyllin, and possibly less efficacy than electrosurgery (90). The practitioner should attempt to freeze the lesion itself, avoiding the surrounding skin. Complications include burning and ulceration, which usually resolve in 7 to 10 days with little or no scarring. Recurrences rates may be 40% to 75% (85).

This regimen has not been investigated in a placebo-controlled trial; however there are many data comparing podophyllin to the various other treatment options, and there is consensus that efficacy in clearing lesions is similar (86). However, the recurrence rate can be as high as 60%. Provider-administered podophyllin resin is most effective for lesions that are 2 cm or less in diameter (47). A 10% to 25% solution can be applied to visible warts weekly, as necessary. If regression is not achieved after four applications, an alternative therapy should be considered. Transmucosal systemic absorption does occur and this solution should not be applied intravaginally. Complications include a subjective burning sensation or actual ulceration, which can affect as many as 30% of patients (86). Washing the area one to four hours after treatment will minimize severe irritation associated with prolonged exposure. Neurologic, hematologic, febrile complications, and death have been associated with topical podophyllin. Podophyllin is cytotoxic and is contraindicated during pregnancy.

An 80% to 90% solution of bi- or tri-chloroacetic acid is an effective treatment for small lesions, as shown by two RCTs comparing it with cryotherapy (86). Treatment may be repeated weekly, for up to four weeks. Some recommend applying petrolatum ointment, talcum powder, or bicarbonate soda to skin in contact with the treatment area to avoid extensive irritation. The solution can be washed off six to eight hours after treatment and a sitz bath with baking soda may relieve some discomfort. Overall, this regimen has a better side effect profile than podophyllin and can be used safely by pregnant women.

Genital warts can be excised by tangential scissor, shave excision curettage, or punch biopsy, and treatment can be repeated as necessary. RCTs demonstrate no difference in the results achieved by laser and surgical excision, or between the clearance rates as compared with podophyllin. However, surgical excision is more effective in preventing recurrence than is podophyllin (86).

Alternative surgical techniques include loop electrosurgical excision procedures (LEEP) and laser surgery with CO_2 laser. Electrosurgery uses thermal coagulation to destroy genital warts. Randomized trials showed a slightly greater efficacy of electrotherapy compared with cryotherapy, but this difference did not persist after three to five months of follow-up. One placebo-controlled trial found electrosurgery to be only slightly more effective in clearing lesions than placebo (86).

Laser therapy uses focused, infrared light energy to vaporize genital warts. In general, laser is reserved for larger lesions and the lesions must be destroyed down to the base to minimize recurrence rates. Some authors suggest that the clearance of warts is better when laser therapy is performed under colposcopic examination. Recurrence rates in a randomized controlled design ranged from 60% to 80% (91).

Several other promising treatment options exist for genital warts. Topical IFN can be used to treat recurrent or resistant genital warts. Treatment efficacy has been supported by three placebo-controlled clinical trials and a trial with podophyllotoxin, which showed wart clearance to be increased substantially. IFN-α and -β can be used as adjuvants to surgery (92,93). Side effects are generally limited to burning and itching. Systemic IFN has been studied in RCTs with inconsistent results. This drug causes immunosuppression and its risks outweigh the benefits for use as treatment for the treatment of genital warts.

The antiviral cidofovir has been reported effective in limited case series. One study has shown a 65% response rate (85). Typically, this drug is used as a 1% gel applied for five days straight, followed by one week rest, for up to six cycles. Four hours after application, the area must be washed. In a placebo-controlled trial, 47% of cidofovir-treated patient achieved complete remission compared with none of the placebo controls (94). Another placebo-controlled trial in HIV-positive patients showed similar results (95). In HIV-infected patients, one randomized (but not placebo controlled) study showed the efficacy of cidofovir combined with electrosurgery, with a significant reduction of recurrences in patients treated with both cidofovir and electrosurgery in comparison to patients treated by surgery alone (96). These data are based on few subjects and further investigation is necessary; however cidofovir remains a promising option for the future.

Another clinically effective, patient-applied treatment is 5-fluorouracil (5-FU) 5% cream. Small clinical trials support its efficacy as monotherapy (97) and 5-FU with adreneline gel has been tried and proven effective by a randomized, double-blind, placebo-controlled study (98). Associated side effects include erythema, edema, and skin ulceration. Though initial studies produced positive results, with the limited available data and with the potential toxic effects of the drug, this is not currently considered first-line therapy.

Molluscum Contagiosum

Lesions of molloscum contagiusum often involute spontaneously, without scarring. Despite this, the lesions are often treated to prevent patient's discomfort, as well as autoinocculation and transmission.

Mechanical treatments, such as curettage, cryotherapy, and electrosurgery achieve moderate to high initial success rates with variable recurrence rates (99), but can result in pain and mild scarring. Case reports show that CO_2 laser therapy may be an effective alternative (100), although keloid formation is possible after treatment (101). Curettage allows for the added benefit of confirmatory diagnosis. However, the success of physical ablation treaments has not been evaluated adequately and placebo-controlled studies are lacking.

Chemical therapies include trichloroacetic acid, 5-FU, bleomycin (99), canthridin, phenol, salicylic acid, lactic acid, and strong saline solution (102). Tretinoin cream may be useful as adjuvant therapy (102). Randomized controlled trials have proven the success of podophyllotoxin as treatment for molluscum contagiosum; however, these results are yet to be reproduced in a study with female participants (103). Local use of cytotoxic agents may result in skin reactions, pain, or adverse systemic effects (99).

Immunomodulators may be of benefit in treating molluscum contagiosum, especially in severe or treatment-resistant cases. In the past, IFN was used to treat molluscum contagiosum; however, results for genital lesions are variable (99). Imiquimod is used currently to treat genital molluscum contagiosum and its efficacy is supported by multiple studies (104,105), which show total clearance rates of 53%, with additional subjects showing substantial reduction in lesion size. Recurrence rates were as low as 7% after 12 months (104). Treatment typically lasts from 4 to 16 weeks. Advantages include ease of application. There are few local side effects, including erythema, pruritis, and erosion; typically, tissue damage is less than damage resulting from ablation.

Currently, cidofovir is being used for treating molluscum contagiosum (106), as are other poxviridae (107). Studies show promising results of treating HIV-infected patients with advanced molluscum contagiosum with topical and intravenous cidofovir (108). Any added benefit in this population may be due to antiviral effects.

Patients should be educated that after treatment, the condition may recur due to re-inoculation from sexual partners.

Ectoparasitic Infections

Scabies (*Sarcoptes scabiei*)

The CDC-recommended treatment regimens for scabies include permetrin, lindane, and ivermectin (47). Effective alternatives include crotamiton, precipitated sulfur, and possibly benzyl benzoate (109). Even if they are asymptomatic, household contacts and sex partners from the previous month should be treated, as well. Bedding and clothing must be decontaminated and sexual contact should be avoided until partners are cured (47). A few small studies have shown permethrin to be more effective compared with lindane and crotamiton in clinical, parasitic, and subjective cure (109). One larger trial showed no difference between permethrin and lindane (110). Despite conflicting data, permethrin is

Table 2 RCT-Supported Treatment Options for Scabies

Treatment	Placebo controlled?	Comments	Reference
Permethrin	No	More effective when compared with crotamiton, lindane; larger study showed no difference when compared to lindane	(111–115) (112, largest, 476 subjects)
Crotamiton	No	Comparison with lindane showed no difference, see comments for permethrin	(111,112)
Lindane	No	See comments for permethrin and crotamiton	(111,113–117)
Ivermectin (the only oral agent)	Yes	Showed no difference when compared with benzyl benzoate or lindane	(117)
Sulfur	No	More effective when compared with benzyl benzoate	(118)
Benzyl benzoate	No	See comments for sulfur	(118)

Abbreviation: RCT, randomized clinical trial.

first-line treatment for scabies in adults and children over two months of age (47), a recommendation most likely based on clinical practice and reviews. Table 2 summarizes RCT-supported treatments for scabies.

Permethrin 5% cream should be applied once to affected areas and washed off 8 to 14 hours later (47). Advantages include a limited side-effect profile and safety for use by pregnant women and children. Adverse reactions include burning, stinging, and exacerbation of recurrence of pruritis (119). Permethrin is more expensive than lindane and crotamiton, and cost should be considered in choosing therapy. There have been a few documented cases of permethrin-resistant scabies (120) and the number may be much higher.

Lindane 1% should be applied one time and washed off six to eight hours later; some clinicians recommend a second application one week later. Generally, lindane is an appropriate alternative treatment for scabies; however, there have been reports of possible resistance (47) and there are multiple possible adverse side effects. Convulsions may occur if applied after a bath or in patients with extensive dermatitis (121). Lindane has also been associated with the development of aplastic anemia (122,123) and brain tumors in children (120), though data are few. Accidental ingestion can lead to lindane-induced central nervous system toxicity, manifested by headache, nausea, vomiting, tremors, convulsions, respiratory failure, coma, and death (124). It is possible that toxic side effects are due to overexposure or improper use. Lindane should not be used by patients with seizures or neurologic disease (119), pregnant or lactating women, or by children under two years of age (47). Exercise caution when prescribing this drug for any child weighing less than 50 kg (110 lbs.) (125). Because of the multiple and potentially lethal side effects, the FDA in 2003 issued a public health advisory concerning the use of topical lindane for the treatment of scabies and lice (125). Despite this advisory, due to its low cost, ease of administration, and high efficacy, the use of lindane will likely continue. Thus, to reduce the incidence of toxicity, clinicians must warn against overuse and educate patients about proper product application techniques.

Crotamiton 10% lotion/cream should be applied once, and reapplied 24 hours later, without washing between applications. The patient may bathe 48 hours after the final application (47). Some health-care providers suggest a five-day application (119,126). In nonrandomized trials, cure rates have been as high as 70% (127), although the only RCT studying crotamiton found it to be no more effective than lindane (111). Some health-care providers do not recommend using crotamiton because of the lack of toxicity data (127). There have been cases of crotamiton resistance (128).

Ivermectin, the only oral scabies treatment (100–200 mg/kg, and repeated in two weeks) is very useful for severe infection (47). Studies have shown cure after single dose, even for immunocompromised patients (129). A review of published clinical trials showed no consensus regarding most effective dosing regimens (130). Although one small randomized, placebo-controlled trial demonstrated the effectiveness of this drug (131), subsequent RCTs have shown that ivermectin is more beneficial than benzyl benzoate or lindane (109).

Epidemics occurring in nursing homes or hospitals must be controlled by treating the entire population at risk. In such epidemics, if topical agents fail, ivermectin may be considered (132). Tolerance is typically good; however one study demonstrated increased mortality with ivermectin treatment among elderly, debilitated persons (133); however, the authors failed to address the effect of confounding factors on the results. Therefore, the validity of this study is questionable (109). Case reports suggest usefulness in severe infection, although a single oral dose might be inadequate in this scenario (120,134). Anecdotally, topical ivermectin has been used with success (127). Common side effects include headache, abdominal pain, and vomiting. Of note, ivermectin is not recommended for pregnant or lactating patients and its safety for children less than 15 kg (33 lbs) has not been determined (47).

Sulfur is the oldest known treatment for scabies. Currently, a 6% ointment of precipitated sulfur applied for three consecutive nights is used as alternative treatment for pregnant women and children under two months of age (47), or in situations in which other options are intolerable. This drug was shown to be more effective than benzyl benzoate in one RCT (135). Its advantages include low cost, but it is difficult to apply and can cause skin irritation.

Benzyl benzoate, 10% to 25% in a lotion, is applied for 24 hours on three to five consecutive days to treat scabies (120). Though it has been used for decades, its effectiveness has not been proven. Studies show it to be less effective than sulfur (135) and it has not been compared with permethrin (109). However, according to recent reports, benzyl benzoate may be helpful in certain cases of crusted scabies or in recurrent disease (127). Disadvantages include skin irritation and high treatment failure, possibly due to incorrect application. It should not be used by pregnant and lactating women, infants, and young children less than two years of age. Because of the lack of supporting data, and the ease, effectiveness, and availability of other options, this treatment is used rarely.

Malathion, an organophosphate acetylcholinesterase inhibitor, was once used to treat scabies. This agent has not been investigated in RCTs (109). Lack of data, bad odor, and the need for a long treatment period have caused this drug to fall out of favor.

As rash and pruritis may persist for up to two weeks after treatment, clinicians should re-evaluate patients with scabies after two weeks. Some health-care providers recommend retreatment after two weeks for patients who remain symptomatic, whereas others advocate for retreatment only if live mites are seen. Patients with initial treatment failure should be retreated with an alternative therapy (47).

Pediculosis Pubis (*Phthirus pubis*)

Currently, the CDC recommends treatment with permethrin, lindane, and pyrethins with piperonyl butoxide. Other options include malathion and, possibly, ivermectin. Most of these preparations were discussed in the previous section and will be described only briefly here.

Permethrin 1% cream should be applied to the affected areas and rinsed off after 10 minutes (47). Higher cure rates are reported after a sccond application one week after the first (120). Permethrin is usually the first line of treatment, although resistance increases, which may present a problem (120).

Lindane 1% shampoo is also used topically, applied to the affected area, and washed off after four minutes. Lindane may have neurologic and hematologic side effects and should not be used by children and pregnant and lactating women (47).

Another effective treatment is natural pyrethrins with piperonyl butoxide, applied to the affected area and washed off after 10 minutes (47). A second application one week later increases the cure rate (120). There are various vehicles available, including liquids, gels, and foams. Pyrethrin can provoke in respiratory distress in patients allergic to ragweed (120).

Malathion, a 0.5% lotion, should be applied and left in place for 8 to 12 hours, then washed off (85). As stated previously, malathion is not used frequently.

Oral ivermectin has been used in trials (126,136) but is not currently recommended for lice. A 0.8% ivermectin lotion was successfully applied to 25 patients with head lice. As with scabies, recent household contacts and sex partners must be treated, bedding and clothing must be decontaminated, and sexual contact should be avoided. If lice are seen at follow-up in one to two weeks, the patient should be retreated.

VULVAR NEOPLASM

Vulvar Intraepithelial Neoplasia

Surgical treatment for frankly invasive vulvar carcinoma is indicated clearly; however, no commonly accepted treatment for VIN exists. The goal of treatment is to minimize symptoms and halt progression to invasive cancer, while attempting to preserve anatomy and sexual function. Options include topical agents, wide local excision, laser therapy, and skinning vulvectomy. Management is individualized based upon biopsy, extent of disease, and symptoms. Table 3 summarizes vulvar neoplasm treatments supported by nonRCTs.

Table 3 Nonrandomized Trial-Supported Treatment for Vulvar Neoplasm

Stage	Primary treatment	Additional therapies
VIN	Local excision (137), skinning vulvectomy (139), laser (138), LEEP (138)	Promising topicals: imiquimod (21,137), 5-FU (139), IFN-α (143), PDT (144)
Stage I	If <1 mm: Local excision with wide or radical margins (140) If >1 mm: Add lymphadenectomy (141)	Laser/LEEP (138)
Stage II	3-Incision conservative or radical vulvectomy with bilateral inguinofemoral lymphadenectomy (141)	Laser/LEEP (138)
Stage III	3-Incision radical vulvectomy with bilateral inguinofemoral lymphadenectomy (141) If >1 node positive, add postoperative groin and pelvic irradiation (142)	Primary chemoradiation therapy (145), preoperative chemoradiation (146), preoperative radiation (147)
Stage IV	Radical or en bloc vulvectomy and lympadenectomy, remove metastases (141) If >1 positive node, add postoperative groin and pelvic irradiation (142)	Primary chemoradiation therapy (145), preoperative chemoradiation (146), preoperative radiation (147)

Abbreviations: VIN, vulvar intraepithelial neoplasia; 5-FU, 5-fluorouracil; IFN-α, interferon-α; LEEP, loop electrosurgical excision procedures; PDT, photodynamic therapy.

Lower grade VIN may be managed best with a conservative, nonsurgical treatments that preserve vulvar anatomy. Several chemotherapeutic agents appear promising, but are yet to be proven by RCTs.

Imiquimod is currently FDA approved for treatment of genital warts is being used currently to treat human papillomavirus-associated VIN. In a few small noncontrolled studies, topical 5% imiquimod cream three times weekly was found to clear VIN II/III (137,148). Studies have shown at least 75% overall response (148). Efficacy, however, may be limited when dysplasia extends into ducts of glands or into hair follicles (138). Invasive carcinoma must be ruled out prior to therapy, as invasive disease has been found after treatment with imiquimod. Further studies investigating efficacy are warranted.

In a case series, topical 5% 5-FU showed response rates of 50% to 60% (139). 5-FU, however, causes chemical desquamation that can result in significant discomfort, inflammation, and painful ulcerations. There has been one case report of successful treatment of extensive VIN III with topical 1% cidofovir. Further investigation is necessary to determine the role of these drugs in the treatment of VIN.

One small randomized, double-blind, crossover study evaluated topical IFN-α in 18 patients with VIN III. The study compared IFN-α versus IFN-α with nonoxyl-9 and showed 67% response rate in all patients, independent of the addition of nonoxyl-9 (143). Although the results appear promising, the efficacy cannot be determined until a placebo-controlled trial with more participants is performed.

For the low-grade VIN, surgery may be unnecessary. However, untreated VIN III lesions have a high incidence of conversion to invasive squamous cell carcinoma; typically, surgery is the best management (137). Surgical excision can be diagnostic as well as therapeutic, offering an advantage over ablative or medical management options. This is important because of the frequency of undetected coexisting invasive squamous cell carcinoma. In a case series of patients treated with excision, more than 20% had underlying invasive disease, the majority of which was more than 1 mm (137,149). Local excision with 5 mm margins is sufficient treatment in unifocal disease with disease-free biopsy margins and no evidence of stromal invasion (137). Although excision through the depth of the epidermis is satisfactory, removing some underlying dermis may be of added benefit to rule out invasive disease (139). Disfigurement is a disadvantage; however, excision and close follow-up reduce the chance of development of invasive cancer. Nonetheless, in a 15-year follow-up study of patients after surgical excision, recurrence or persistence occurred in 48%, and disease progressed to frankly invasive carcinoma in 7% (150). Despite the widespread use of surgical treatment, there are no systematic reviews or RCTs showing the effects of surgical treatment for VIN.

Several noncontrolled studies support the use of laser therapy (excision and vaporization) as alternative treatment for multiple, small lesions (138,139). Laser excision has a cure rate of up to 87% (136,150). The cure rate after one treatment with laser vaporization is up to 75% (137,138,151). Most other cases achieve disease control with a second or third treatment (138,139). Some patients who received additional treatment developed invasive squamous cell carcinoma subsequently (137). A retrospective cohort study showed a significant increase in disease recurrence or persistence with laser vaporization as compared to local excision (150); subsequent smaller uncontrolled studies have had varied results. It is essential to rule out invasive cancer before using laser vaporization, as this modality involves tissue ablation. Superficial laser treatment may be more appealing cosmetically than the other surgical techniques—for example, clitoral involvement—in which case precision minimizes deformity and sexual dysfunction (149). In areas with hair, dysplastic cells are deeper and superficial treatment is not appropriate; in this case, laser causes scarring and deformity. Recurrence is common in these regions; thus, standard surgical excision is preferable (140).

Skinning vulvectomy is recommended for more extensive lesions. Skin is removed subepidermally, allowing for preservation of subcutaneous tissue. Closure is either by reapproximation or with a skin graft (140).

Electrosurgery has been used with success and, when compared to laser, appears to be as efficacious in clearing disease, but further study is necessary (138,152). Though used in the past, cryosurgery can have up to 90% recurrence rate (153); however, data have been derived from studies with few participants. Because of the availability and better success of other options, electrosurgery is not recommended.

In uncomplicated cases, an alternative to standard therapy is PDT. Topical 5-aminolevulinic acid can be applied to the vulvar lesion and activated with light. Multiple noncontrolled studies show similar efficacy as conventional treatment options in clearing all grades of VIN. Advantages of PDT include short healing time and minimal disfiguration (144). However, PDT can be associated with significant patient discomfort, including burning sensations and pain; in addition, recurrence of VIN is common after this treatment (139) and response rates in multifocal lesions and lesions with increased pigmentation and hyperkeratosis are lower (144). Nonetheless, PDT deserves further investigation.

Invasive Vulvar Neoplasm

Several histologic types of invasive vulvar carcinoma include squamous cell carcinoma, Paget's disease, basal cell carcinoma, melanoma, Bartholin gland carcinoma, and sarcoma. Treatment for all these types is similar.

Surgery is the primary treatment for invasive vulvar cancer. Historically, en bloc vulvectomy was the standard of care. This procedure includes vulvectomy and inguinal and upper femoral node dissection. However, en bloc vulvectomy results in severe genital disfigurement and is accompanied by a high incidence of treatment-related complications, including 1% to 5% mortality rates (154). Currently, more conservative surgical techniques are preferred and are equally effective in limited, non-aggressive disease. Farias-Eisner, et al. (155) reported similar survival rates when comparing patients with Stage I and Stage II disease after treatment with conservative versus radical vulvectomy. Nonetheless, in advanced, aggressive disease, radical vulvectomy may be necessary.

Alternatives to surgery include radiotherapy and/or chemotherapy. Chemotherapy alone is of limited efficacy in vulvar cancer, but the combination of chemotherapy and radiotherapy appears effective (147). Radiation (142) and chemoradiation (146) can also be adjuvants to surgery. For patients with any stage of vulvar carcinoma who are unable to undergo surgery, radical radiation (147) alone may enhance survival.

Local surgical excision with wide or radical margins is treatment of choice for Stage I vulvar carcinoma (140,141). With less than 1 mm stromal invasion, fewer than 1% of cases are complicated by inguinofemoral lymph node metastases, and this procedure alone is adequate (139). Mohs microsurgery allows for complete removal of the primary lesion.

For more invasive Stage I lesions (>1 mm), the risk of nodal metastases is 8% and additional unilateral lymphadenectomy is suggested (147). Ansink, et al. (156) authored a systematic review of two nonrandomized case-controlled observational studies investigating the effect of surgical treatment in early squamous cell carcinoma of the vulva (cT1-2N0M0 tumors). With lateralized, node-negative disease, radical local excision with complete ipsilateral lymphadenectomy appears effective. Both studies reported similar recurrence rates in local excision as compared with radical vulvectomy (157,158). One nonrandomized case-controlled study supports that ipsilateral dissection is as effective as bilateral dissection (157). Alternatively, for central lesions, bilateral lymphadenectomy is indicated (139). When resecting nodes, it is imperative to take both iliac and femoral nodes; one study found that leaving the femoral nodes resulted in a 4% groin recurrences (146). Though not first-line treatment, LEEP and CO_2 laser may be acceptable alternatives to conventional surgery (138).

Three-incision conservative or radical vulvectomy with bilateral inguinofemoral lymphadenectomy is used to treat Stage II disease (139). Five-year survival rates are 80% to 90% (131). Survival and disease-free interval are similar for modified radical vulvectomy and en bloc radical vulvectomy (159). Both LEEP and CO_2 laser may be acceptable alternatives (138).

For Stage III vulvar cancer, radical vulvectomy with inguinal and femoral lymphadenectomy is the currently accepted first-line therapy (139). In a randomized trial, participants with two or more positive nodes who underwent radical vulvectomy and bilateral inguinal and femoral groin node dissections showed significantly better survival with postoperative groin and pelvic irradiation than with pelvic node dissection (142). Therefore, if nodes are positive, it is currently accepted practice to add pelvic and groin irradiation. A study investigating the role of radiation alone showed recurrence rates of 10% in patients with Stage III/IV disease (142), proving that radiation alone is an unacceptable alternative for surgery. It is, however, an appropriate therapy for patients who are unable to tolerate or are unsuitable candidates for surgery (142). Preoperative radiation therapy may improve operability and decrease the extent of surgery required (147). Chemoradiation as pretreatment before surgical excision may lessen tumor burden, allowing for more conservative excision. In a Phase II study by the Gynecologic Oncology Group, Moore et al. (146) over 97% of patients treated with combination therapy were free of disease. Alternatively, chemoradiation can be used as primary treatment for vulvar cancer (145). Trials have resulted in complete response rates of 53% to 89% and disease-free survival rates of 47% to 84%, with a median follow-up of 37 months (147).

Chemotherapeutic agents with demonstrated effectiveness in combination with radiation include 5-FU, cisplatin, mitomycin C, bleomycin, methotrexate (139). Disadvantages of combination therapies include multiple complications due to each individual intervention, as well as the risk for cumulative toxicity.

Surgical management of Stage IV vulvar cancer is radical or en block vulvectomy and lymphadenectomy and removal of metastases (139). With two or more positive nodes, surgery followed by radiation has better survival than postoperative pelvic node dissection (134). Preoperative radiation (147) or chemoradiation (146) may decrease the tumor size and the extent of surgery required. Chemoradiation (145) alone is an acceptable alternative to surgery. For those intolerable of or unsuitable for surgery or chemotherapy, radical radiation therapy alone may increase survival (147).

Close follow-up is necessary to detect recurrence. Without nodal involvement, the five-year survival rate after radical local excision is up to 75%. Inguinal recurrences may require vulvectomy. Radiation or chemoradiation may be used with or without surgery for palliation.

There is no standard treatment for metastatic disease. If distant metastases are present, salvage cytotoxic chemotherapy with cisplatin, methotrexate, bleomycin, mitomycin C, and cyclophosphamide may be appropriate (139). Prognosis is poor.

Verrucous carcinoma is a squamous cell carcinoma variant treated with wide local excision (160). If node positive, lymphadenectomy should be performed, as well. Radiation is contraindicated because it may induce anaplastic transformation and increase the likelihood of metastases (161).

CONCLUSION

The vulva is a physiologically unique area and requires unique therapeutic consideration. Therapies that are used to treat general disease may not have the same effect when used to treat the vulvar area. It is important to address the need for specific treatment options for this area.

This chapter reviews current therapies for common vulvar conditions. Though these disorders are encountered commonly in the population, there are few convincing data supporting therapeutic regimens. Most of the recommended treatment options are based on clinical experience and case reports, with few supportive clinical trials. There are alarmingly few RCTs proving treatment safety or efficacy, or determining optimal doses, preparations, or length of therapy. Existing studies have small participant populations and are methodologically imperfect. As a result, few conclusions can be made safely.

With women comprising over half of the U.S. population, it is essential that we gain understanding about the specific nature of the vulva, and how this affects the ways that we treat disease processes specific to this area. Further research is needed in order to appropriately elucidate safety, effectiveness, and physiologic mechanisms of available vulvar therapies.

REFERENCES

1. Edwards L. New concepts in vulvodynia. Am J Obstet Gynecol 2003; 189:S24.
2. McKay M. Dysesthetic ("essential") vulvodynia. Treatment with amitriptyline. J Reprod Med 1993; 38:9.
3. Zolnoun DA, Hartmann KE, Steege JF. Overnight 5% lidocaine ointment for treatment of vulvar vestibulitis. Obstet Gynecol 2003; 102:84.
4. Haefner HK et al. The vulvodynia guideline. J Low Genit Tract Dis 2005; 9:40.
5. Gerber S et al. Topical cytokine cream for vulvar vestibulitis. Poster presented at: Vulvodynia and Sexual Pain Disorders: a State of the Art Consensus Conference, Atlanta, GA, Oct 2004.
6. Bergeron S et al. Physical therapy for vulvar vestibulitis syndrome: a retrospective study. J Sex Marital Ther 2002; 28:183.
7. Marinoff SC et al. Intralesional alpha interferon. Cost-effective therapy for vulvar vestibulitis syndrome. J Reprod Med 1993; 38:19.
8. Bornstein J et al. A pure versus complicated vulvar vestibulitis: a randomized trial of fluconazole treatment. Gynecol Obstet Invest 2000; 50:194.
9. Haefner HK. Critique of new gynecologic surgical procedures: surgery for vulvar vestibulitis. Clin Obstet Gynecol 2000; 43:689.
10. Solomons CC, Melmed MH, Heitler SM. Calcium citrate for vulvar vestibulitis. A case report. J Reprod Med 1991; 36:879.
11. Farage MA, Maibach HI. The vulvar epithelium differs from the skin: implications for cutaneous testing to address topical vulvar exposures. Contact Dermatitis 2004; 51:201.
12. Welsh BM et al. Management of common vulval conditions. Med J Aust 2003; 178:391.
13. Foster D. Vulvar disease. Obstet Gynecol 2002; 100:145.
14. Cheer S, Plosker G. Tacrolimus ointment: a review of its therapeutic potential as a topical therapy in atopic dermatitis. Am J Clin Dermatol 2001; 2:389.
15. Meurer M et al. Pimecrolimus cream in the long-term management of atopic dermatitis in adults: a six-month study. Dermatology 2002; 205:271.
16. Wakelin S, Maibach HI. Handbook of Systemic Drug Treatment in Dermatology. London: Manson Publishing, Ltd., 2002.
17. Meggit S, Reynolds N. Azathioprine for atopic dermatitis. Clin Exp Dermatol 2001; 26:369.
18. McKay M. Vulvar manifestations of skin disorders. In: Black M, McKay M et al., eds. Obstetric and Gynecologic Dermatology. London: Mosby, 2002.

19. Dalziel K, Millard PR, Wojnarowska F. The treatment of vulvar lichen sclerosus with a very potent topical corticosteroid (clobetasol propionate 0.05%) cream. Br J Dermatol 1991; 124:4614.
20. Lorenz B, Kaufman RH, Kutzner SK. Lichen sclerosus. Therapy with clobetasol propionate. J Reprod Med 1998; 43:7904.
21. Bracco G et al. Clinical and histologic effects of topical treatments of vulval lichen sclerosus. J Reprod Med 1993; 38:40.
22. Lagos BR, Maibach HI. Frequency of application of topical corticosteroids: an overview. Br J Dermatol 1998; 139:7636.
23. Sinha P, Sorinola O, Luesley DM. Lichen sclerosus of the vulva. Long-term steroid maintenance therapy. J Reprod Med 1999; 44:621.
24. Mazdisnian F et al. Intralesional injection of triamcinolone in the treatment of lichen sclerosus. J Reprod Med 1999; 44:332.
25. Paslin D. Treatment of lichen sclerosus with topical dihydrotestosterone. Obstet Gynecol 1991; 78:1046.
26. Sideri M et al. Topical testosterone in the treatment of vulvar lichen sclerosus. Int J Gynecol Obstet 1994; 46:536.
27. Abramov Y et al. Surgical treatment of vulvar lichen sclerosus: a review. Obstet Gynecol Surv 1996; 51:193.
28. August PJ, Milward TM. Cryosurgery in the treatment of lichen sclerosus et atrophicus of the vulva. Br J Dermatol 1980; 103:667.
29. Kartamaa M, Reitamo S. Treatment of lichen sclerosus with carbon dioxide laser vaporization. Br J Dermatol 1997; 136:356.
30. Hillemans P et al. Photodynamic therapy of vulvar lichen sclerosus with 5-aminolevulinic acid. Obstet Gynecol 1999; 93:714.
31. Bousema MT et al. Acitretin in the treatment of lichen sclerosus et atrophicus of the vulva: a double-blind, placebo-controlled study. J Am Acad Dermatol 1994; 30:225.
32. Virgili A et al. Open study of topical 0.025% tretinoin in the treatment of vulval lichen sclerosus. One year of therapy. J Reprod Med 1995; 40:614.
33. Kreuter A et al. Low-dose ultraviolet-A1 phototherapy for lichen sclerosus et atrophicus. Clin Exp Dermatol 2001; 26:30.
34. Reichrath J, Reinhold U, Tilgen W. Treatment of genito-anal lesions in inflammatory skin diseases with PUVA cream photochemotherapy: an open pilot study in 12 patients. Dermatology 205:245.
35. Kunstfeld R et al. Successful treatment of vulvar lichen sclerosus with topical tacrolimus. Arch Dermatol 2003; 139:850.
36. Bohm M et al. Successful treatment of anogenital lichen sclerosus with topical tacrolimus. Arch Dermatol 2003; 139:922.
37. Wallace HJ. Lichen sclerosus et atrophicus. Trans Rep St. Johns Hosp Dermatol Soc 1971; 57:9.
38. Lewis F. Vulval lichen planus. Br J Dermatol 1998; 138:569.
39. Anderson M, Kutzner SM, Kaufman RH. Treatment of vulvovaginal lichen planus with vaginal hydrocortisone suppositories. Obstet Gynecol 2002; 100:359.
40. Edwards L. Vulvar lichen planus. Arch Dermatol 1989; 125:1677.
41. Lotery H, Galask R. Erosive lichen planus of the vulva and vagina. Obstet Gynecol 2003; 101:1121.

42. Byrd J, Davis M, Rogers R. Recalcitrant symptomatic vulvar lichen planus: response to topical tacrolimus. Arch Dermatol 2004; 140:715.
43. Larrabee R, Kylander D. Benign vulvar disorders. Identifying features, practical management of nonneoplastic conditions and tumors. Postgrad Med 2001; 109:151.
44. Omole F, Simmons BJ, Hacker Y. Management of Bartholin's duct cyst and gland abscess. Am Fam Physician 2003; 68:135.
45. Miller NR. Sepsis after Bartholin's duct abscess marsupialization in a gravida. J Reprod Med 2001; 46:913.
46. Gallup D et al. Necrotizing fasciitis in gynecologic and obstetric patients: a surgical emergency. Am J Obstet Gynecol 2002; 187:305.
47. Workowski KA et al. U.S. Centers for Disease Control and Prevention guidelines for the treatment of sexually transmitted diseases: an opportunity to unify clinical and public health practice. Ann Intern Med 2002; 137:255.
48. Hook EW et al. A randomized, comparative pilot study of azithromycin versus benzathine penicillin G for treatment of early syphilis. Sex Transm Dis 2002; 29:486.
49. Lukehart S et al. Macrolide resistance in treponema pallidum in the United States and Ireland. N Engl J Med 2004; 351:154.
50. World Health Organization. Guidelines for the management of sexually transmitted infections, 2003. Available at: http://whqlibdoc.who.int/publications/2003/9241546263.pdf. Accessed Sept 21, 2005.
51. Martin D et al. Comparison of azithromycin and ceftriaxone for the treatment of chancroid. Clin Infect Dis 1995; 21:409.
52. Brown D Jr et al. Butoconazole vaginal cream in the treatment of vulvovaginal candidiasis: comparison with miconazole nitrate and placebo. J Reprod Med 1986; 31:1045.
53. Brown D et al. Butoconazole nitrate 2% for vulvovaginal candidiasis. J Reprod Med 1999; 44:933.
54. Lebherz T et al. A comparison study of the efficacy of two vaginal creams for vulvovaginal candidiasis, and correlations with the presence of Candida species in the perianal area and oral contraceptive use. Clin Ther 1983; 5:409.
55. Franklin R. Seven-day clotrimazole therapy for vulvovaginal candidiasis. South Med J 1978; 71:141.
56. Sobel JD et al. The fluconazole vaginitis study group, single oral dose fluconazole compared with conventional clotrimazole topical therapy of Candida vaginitis. Am J Obstet Gynecol 1995; 172:1263.
57. Goode MA et al. Single dose fluconazole versus clotrimazole in the treatment of vaginal candidiasis. International Pharmaceutical Abstracts (ASHP Midyear Clinical Meeting) 1992; 27:61.
58. Stein GE et al. Single-dose tioconazole compared with 3-day clotrimazole treatment in vulvovaginal candidiasis. Antimicrob Agents Chemother 1986; 29:969.
59. Tobin JM, Loo P, Granger SE. Treatment of vaginal candidosis: a comparative study of the efficacy and acceptability of itraconazole and clotrimazole. Genitourin Med 1992; 68:36.
60. Woolley PD. Comparison of clotrimazole, fluconazole and itraconazole in vaginal candidiasis. Br J Clin Pract 1995; 49:65.
61. Fleury F, Hodgson C. Single-dose treatment of vulvovaginal candidiasis with a new 500 mg clotrimazole vaginal tablet. Adv Ther 1984; 1:349.

62. Guess EA, Hodgson C. Single-dose topical treatment of vulvovaginal candidiasis with a new 500 mg clotrimazole vaginal tablet. Adv Ther 1984; 1:137.
63. Adetoro OO. Comparative trial of a single dose of fluconazole (150 mg) and a single intravaginal tablet of clotrimazole (500 mg) in the treatment of vaginal candidiasis. Curr Ther Res 1990; 48:275.
64. Boag FC et al. Comparison of vaginal flora after treatment with a clotrimazole 500 mg vaginal pessary or a fluconazole 150 mg capsule for vaginal candidosis. Genitourin Med 1991; 67:232.
65. Van Heusden AM et al. A randomized, comparative study of a single oral dose of fluconazole versus a single topical dose of clotrimazole in the treatment of vaginal candidosis among general practitioners and gynaecologists. Eur J Obstet Gynaecol Reprod Biol 1994; 55:123.
66. Thomason JL et al. Terconazole for the treatment of vulvovaginal candidiasis. J Reprod Med 1990; 35:992.
67. Isaacs JH. Nystatin vaginal cream in monilial vaginitis. Illinois Med J 1973; 3:240.
68. Clark C et al. A multicenter comparison of one-dose tioconazole ointment with three-dose terconazole cream in vulvovaginal candidiasis. J Womens Hlth 1993; 2:189.
69. Palacio-Hernanz A, Sanz-Sanz F, Rodriquez-Noriega A. Double-blind investigation of R-42470 (terconazole cream 0.4%) and clotrimazole (cream 1%) for the topical treatment of mycotic vaginitis. Chemioterapia 1984; 3:192.
70. Slavin MB et al. Single dose oral fluconazole vs intravaginal terconazole in treatment of candida vaginitis. J Florida Med Assoc 1992; 79:693.
71. Sobel JD. Vaginitis. N Engl J Med 1997; 337:1896.
72. Sobel J et al. Vulvovaginal candidiasis: epidemiologic, diagnostic and therapeutic considerations. Am J Obstet Gynecol 1998; 178:203.
73. Spence D. Candidiasis (vulvovaginal). Clin Evid 2004; 12:2490.
74. Watson MC, Grimshaw JM, Bond CM et al. Oral versus intra-vaginal imidazole and triazole anti-fungal treatment of uncomplicated vulvovaginal candidiasis (thrush). Cochrane Database Syst Rev 2001; CD008245.
75. Stein GE, Mummaw N. Placebo-controlled trial of itraconazole for treatment of acute vaginal candidiasis. Antimicrob Agents Chemother 1993; 37:89.
76. Fife KH et al. Valaciclovir versus acyclovir in the treatment of first-episode genital herpes infection: results of an international, multicenter, double-blind randomized clinical trial. Sex Transm Dis 1997; 24:481.
77. Loveless M, Harris W, Sacks S. Treatment of first episode genital herpes with famciclovir, Programs and Abstracts of the 35th Interscience Conference on Anitmicrobial Agents and Chemotherapy, San Francisco, Sept 17–20, 1995, Abstract A12.
78. Mertz G et al. Double-blind placebo-controlled trial of oral acyclovir in the first episode genital herpes simplex virus infection. J Am Med Assoc 1984; 252:1147.
79. Jungmann E. Genital herpes. Clin Evid 2004; 11:2073.
80. Stone K, Whittington W. Treatment of genital herpes. Rev Infect Dis 1990; 12:610.
81. Wald A et al. Two-day regimen of acyclovir for treatment of recurrent genital herpes simplex virus type 2 infection. Clin Infect Dis 2002; 34:944.
82. Wald A. New therapies and prevention strategies for genital herpes. Clin Infect Dis 1999; 28:S4.

83. Strand A et al. Aborted genital herpes simplex virus lesions: findings from a randomised controlled trial with valaciclovir. Sex Transm Infect 2002; 78:435.
84. Wald A et al. Frequent genital herpes simplex virus 2 shedding in immunocompetent women: effect of acyclovir treatment. J Clin Invest 1997; 99:1092.
85. Dupin N. Treatment of genital warts. Clin Dermatol 2004; 22:48.
86. Buck H. Genital warts. Clin Evid 2004; 12:1.
87. Beutner K et al. Patient-applied podofilox for treatment of genital warts. Lancet 1989; 1:831.
88. Edwards L et al. Self-administered topical 5% imiquimod cream for external anogenital warts. Arch Dermatol 1998; 134:25.
89. Moore R et al. Imiquimod for the treatment of genital warts: a quantitative systematic review. BMC Infect Dis 2001; 1:3.
90. Stone KM et al. Treatment of external genital warts: a randomised clinical trial comparing podophyllin, cryotherapy, and electrodesiccation. Genitourin Med 1990; 66:16.
91. Duus B et al. Refractory condylomata acuminata: a controlled clinical trial of carbon dioxide laser versus conventional surgical treatment. Genitourin Med 1985; 61:59.
92. Gross G et al. Systemically administered interferon alfa-2a prevents recurrence of condylomata acuminata following CO2-laser ablation—influence of the cyclic low-close therapy regime. Genitourin Med 1996; 76:71.
93. Gross G et al. Recombinant interferon beta gel as an adjuvant in the treatment of recurrent genital warts: results of a placebo-controlled double blind study in 120 patients. Dermatology 1998; 196:330.
94. Snoeck R et al. Phase II double-blind, placebo-controlled study of the safety and efficacy of cidofovir topical gel for the treatment of patients with human papillomavirus infection. Clin Infect Dis 2001; 33:597.
95. Matteelli A. Efficacy and tolerability of topical 1% cidofovir cream for the treatment of external anogenital warts in HIV-infected persons. Sex Transm Dis 2001; 28:343.
96. Orlando G et al. Combined surgery and cidofovir is an effective treatment for genital warts in HIV-infected patients. AIDS 2002; 16:447.
97. Krebs HB. Treatment of extensive vulvar condylomata acuminata with topical 5-fluorouracil. South Med J 1990; 83:761.
98. Swinehart JM et al. Development of intralesional therapy with fluorouracil/adrenaline injectable gel for management of condylomata acuminata: two phase II clinical studies. Genitourin Med 1997; 73:481.
99. Ting P, Dytoc M. Therapy of external anogenital warts and molluscum contagiosum: a literature review. Dermatol Ther 2004; 17:68.
100. Amstey MS, Trombetta GC. Laser therapy for vulvar molluscum contagiosum infection. Am J Obstet Gynecol 1985; 153:800.
101. Friedman M, Gal D. Keloid scars as a result of CO_2 laser for molluscum contagiosum. Obstet Gynecol 1987; 70:394.
102. Brown T, Yen-Moore A, Tyring S. An overview of sexually transmitted diseases. Part II. J Am Acad Dermatol 2001; 357:661.
103. Syed TA, Lundin S, Ahmad M. Topical 0.3% and 0.5% podophyllotoxin cream for self-treatment of molluscum contagiosum in males. A placebo-controlled, double-blind study. Dermatol 1994; 189:65.

104. Hengge UR et al. Self-administered topical 5% imiquimod for the treatment of common warts and molluscum contagiosum. Br J Dermatol 2000; 143:1026.
105. Liota E et al. Imiquimod therapy for molluscum contagiosum. J Cutan Med Surg 2000; 4:76.
106. De Clercq E, Neyts J. Therapeutic potential of nucleoside/nucleotide analogues against poxvirus infections. Rev Med Virol 2004; 14:289.
107. Tuzun B et al. Anogenital lesions (viral diseases and ectoparasitic infestations): unapproved treatments. Clin Dermatol 2002; 20:668.
108. Zabawski EJ Jr, Cockerell CJ. Topical and intralesional cidofovir: a review of pharmacology and therapeutic effects. J Am Acad Dermatol 1998; 39:741.
109. Walker GJ, Johnstone PW. Interventions for treating scabies. Cochrane Database Syst Rev 2000; 2:CD000320.
110. Schultz MW et al. Comparative study of 5% permethrin cream and 1% lindane lotion for the treatment of scabies. Arch Dermatol 1990; 126:167.
111. Amer M, El-Gharib I. Permethrin versus crotamiton and lindane in the treatment of scabies. Int J Dermatol 1992; 31:357.
112. Taplin D et al. Comparison of crotamiton 10% cream (Eurax) and permethrin 5% cream (Elimite) for the treatment of scabies in children. Pediatr Dermatol 1990; 7:67.
113. Hansen RC, Remmers E, Menter MA. A controlled comparative trial of permethrin 5 per cent cream and 1 per cent lindane lotion for the treatment of scabies. Clin Res 1986; 34:160.
114. Schultz MW et al. Comparative study of 5% permethrin cream and 1% lindane lotion for the treatment of scabies. Arch Dermatol 1990; 126:167.
115. Taplin D et al. Permethrin 5% dermal cream: a new treatment for scabies. J Am Acad Dermatol 1986; 15:995.
116. Chouela EN et al. Equivalent therapeutic efficacy and safety of ivermectin and lindane in the treatment of human scabies. Arch Dermatol 1999; 135:651.
117. Glaziou P et al. Comparison of ivermectin and benzyl benzoate for treatment of scabies. Trop Med Parasitol 1993; 44:331.
118. Gulati PV, Singh KP. A family based study on the treatment of scabies with benzyl benzoate and sulphur ointment. Indian J Dermatol Venereol Leprol 1978; 44:269.
119. Orkin M, Maibach HI. Scabies and pediculosis. In: Freedberg IM, Eisen AZ, Wolff K, eds. Fitzpatrick's Dermatology in General Medicine. New York: McGraw-Hill Publishing, 1999:2677.
120. Orion O, Matz H, Wolf R. Ectoparasitic sexually transmitted diseases: scabies and pediculosis. Clin Dermatol 2004; 22:513.
121. McLeod WA. Acute lindane poisoning (letter). Can Med Assoc J 1978; 118:123.
122. Elgart ML. A risk-benefit assessment of agents used in the treatment of scabies. Drug Safety 196; 14:386.
123. Rauch AE et al. Gamma benzene hexachloride (Kwell) induced aplastic anemia. Arch Intern Med 1990; 150:2393.
124. Ramussen JE. The problem of lindane. J Am Acad Dermatol 1981; 5:507.
125. U.S. Food and Drug Administration, FDA Talk Paper, FDA issues health advisory regarding labeling changes for lindane products. Available at: http:www.fda.gov/bbs/topics/ANSWERS/2003/ANS01205.html. Accessed Sept 21, 2005.
126. Chosidow O. Scabies and pediculosis. Lancet 2000; 355:819.

127. Karthikeyan K. Treatment of scabies: newer perspectives. Postgrad Med J 2005; 81:7.
128. Roth WI. Scabies resistant to lindane 1% lotion and crotamiton 10% cream. J Am Acad Dermatol 1991; 24:502.
129. Meinking T et al. The treatment of scabies with ivermectin. N Engl J Med 1995; 333:26.
130. Vaidhyanathan U. Review of ivermectin in scabies. J Cutan Med Surg 2001; 5:496.
131. Macotela-Ruiz E, Islas CCM, Ramos N. Tratamiento de escabiasis con Ivermectina por via oral en una comunidad rural cerrada. Implicaciones epidemiologicas. Dermatologica Rev Mex 1996; 40:179.
132. Dunne CL, Malone CJ, Whiworth JAG. A field study of the effects of ivermectin on ectoparasites of man. Trans R Soc Trop Med Hyg 1991; 85:550.
133. Barkwell R, Shields S. Deaths associated with ivermectin treatment of scabies. Lancet 1997; 349:1144.
134. Paasch U, Haustein U. Management of endemic outbreaks of scabies with allethrin, permethrin, and ivermectin. Int J Dermatol 2000; 39:463.
135. Gulati PV, Singh KP. A family based study on the treatment of scabies with benzyl benzoate and sulphur ointment. Indian J Dermatol Venereol Leprolo 1978; 44:269.
136. Ko CJ, Elston DM. Pediculosis. J Am Acad Dermatol 2004; 50:1.
137. Joura EA. Epidemiology, diagnosis and treatment of vulvar intraepithelial neoplasia. Curr Opin Obstet Gynecol 2002; 14:39.
138. Ferenczy A, Wright TC Jr, Richart RM, Comparison of CO_2 laser surgery and loop electrosurgical excision/fulguration procedure (LEEP) for the treatment of vulvar intraepithelial neoplasia (VIN). Int J Gynecol Cancer 1994; 4:22.
139. Tyring S. Vulvar squamous cell carcinoma: guidelines for early diagnosis and treatment. Am J Obstet Gynecol 2003; 189:S17.
140. Kelley J et al. Minimally invasive vulvar carcinoma: an indication for conservative surgical therapy. Gynecol Oncol 1992; 44:240.
141. Stehman F et al. Early stage I carcinoma of the vulva treated with ipsilateral superficial inguinal lymphadenectomy and modified radical hemivulvectomy: a prospective study of the Gynecologic Oncology Group. Obstet Gynecol 1992; 79:490.
142. Keys H. Gynecologic Oncology Group randomized trials of combined technique therapy for vulvar cancer. Cancer 1993; 71:1691.
143. Spirtos NM, Smith LH, Teng NN. Prospective randomized trial of topical alpha-interferon (alpha-interferon gels) for the treatment of vulvar intraepithelial neoplasia III. Gynecol Oncol 1990; 37:34.
144. Fehr MK et al. Photodynamic therapy of vulvar intraepithelial neoplasia III using topically applied 5-aminolevulinic acid. Gynecol Oncol 2001; 80:62.
145. Berek JM et al. Concurrent cisplatin and 5-fluorouracil chemotherapy and radiation therapy for advanced-stage squamous carcinoma of the vulva. Gynecol Oncol 1991; 42:197.
146. Moore D et al. Preoperative chemoradiation for advanced vulvar cancer: a phase II study of the Gynecologic Oncology Group. Int J Radiat Oncol Biol Phys 1998; 42:79.
147. National Cancer Institute. Vulvar cancer (PDQ) treatment. Available at: http://www.cancer.gov/cancertopics/pdq/treatment/vulvar/healthprofessional. Accessed Sept 21, 2005.

148. Jayne CJ, Kaufman RH. Treatment of vulvar intraepithelial neoplasia 2/3 with imiquimod. J Reprod Med 2002; 47:395.
149. Thuis YN et al. Contemporary experience with the management of vulvar intraepithelial neoplasia. Int J Gynecol Cancer 2000; 10:223.
150. Herod J et al. Vulvar intraepithelial neoplasia: long term follow up treated and untreated. Br J Obstet Gynaecol 1996; 103:446.
151. Sideri M et al. Evaluation of CO_2 laser excision or vaporization for the treatment of vulvar intraepithelial neoplasia. Gynecol Oncol 1999; 75:277.
152. Vlastos A et al. Loop electrosurgical excision procedure in vulvar intraepithelial neoplasia treatment. J Lower Gen Tract Dis 2002; 6:232.
153. Marren OM et al. Failure of cryosurgery to eradicate vulval intraepithelial neoplasia: a pilot study. J Eur Acad Dermatol Venereol 1993; 2:247.
154. Grendys EC Jr, Fiorica JV. Innovations in the management of vulvar carcinoma. Curr Opin Obstet Gynecol 2000; 12:15.
155. Farias-Eisner FD et al. Conservative and individualized surgery for early squamous carcinoma of the vulva: the treatment of choice for stage I and II (T1-2N0-1M0) disease. Gynecol Oncol 1994; 53:55.
156. Ansink A, van der Velden J. Surgical interventions for early squamous cell carcinoma of the vulva. Cochrane Database Syst Rev 2000; CD002036.
157. Burke TW et al. Surgical therapy of T1 and T2 vulvar carcinoma: further experience with radical wide excision and selective inguinal lymphadenectomy. Gynecol Oncol 1995; 57:215.
158. DiSaia PJ, Creasman WT, Rich WM. An alternate approach to early cancer of the vulva. Am J Obstet Gynecol 1979; 133:825.
159. Hacker NF, van der Velden J. Conservative management of early vulvar cancer. Cancer 1993; 71:1673.
160. Andreasson B et al. Verrucous carcinoma of the vulval region. Acta Obstet Gynecol Scand 1983; 62:183.
161. Shepherd V, Davidson E, Davies-Humphreys J. Extramammary Paget's disease. BJOG 2005; 112:273.

10

The Menstrual Cycle, the Composition of Menses, and the Effect of Menses on the Skin

Miranda A. Farage
Feminine Care Clinical Sciences, The Procter & Gamble Company, Cincinnati, Ohio, U.S.A.

William H. Hood
Feminine Care Analytical Sciences, The Procter & Gamble Company, Cincinnati, Ohio, U.S.A.

Paula J. Adams Hillard
Department of Pediatrics, Obstetrics, and Gynecology, University of Cincinnati College of Medicine, Cincinnati, Ohio, U.S.A.

INTRODUCTION

A discussion of vulvar physiology in the reproductive years is incomplete without reference to the menstrual cycle. This chapter describes hormonal and endometrial cycling leading to menstruation, the physical properties and composition of menses fluid, and investigations of the effects of menses and blood on vulvar skin.

A portion of this review appeared in Farage M, Warren R, Wang-Weigand S. The vulva is relatively insensitive to menses-induced irritation. Cutaneous Ocular Toxicol 2005; 24(4):243–246. Reprinted with permission from Taylor & Francis Group.

THE MENSTRUAL CYCLE

The hypothalamic-pituitary-ovarian axis is central to female reproductive function. It regulates the cyclic secretion and feedback mechanisms of a hierarchy of hormones from the pituitary gland and the ovary that (*i*) result in the cyclic production of the steroid hormones, estrogen and progesterone, and (*ii*) promote endometrial growth in preparation for conception, with resulting menstrual cyclicity and endometrial shedding in the absence of conception. The cyclic production of these hormones ensures that a mature ovum is released from the ovaries approximately once a month and that the endometrium is concurrently receptive to the implantation of a fertilized ovum (embryo) should fertilization occur. If fertilization does not occur, the endometrium is shed in an orderly fashion, menstruation ensues, and the cycle proceeds anew. In adult women, the average cycle lasts 28 days, but ranges from 21 to 35 days; cycles shorter or longer are statistically uncommon (1,2).

The hierarchy of hormones that governs the menstrual cycle is produced by the hypothalamus, the pituitary gland, and the ovary, as follows:

1. Gonadotrophin-releasing hormone (GnRH), secreted by the hypothalamus, stimulates production of the gonadotrophic hormones, follicle-stimulating hormone (FSH), and luteinizing hormone (LH), by the anterior pituitary gland.
2. FSH and LH modulate ovarian function to promote follicular growth, follicular maturation, and release of the ovum (*ovulation*).
3. Estrogen (secreted by the ovaries in response to the gonadotrophic hormones) and progesterone (produced by the corpus luteum that develops at the site of a ruptured ovarian follicle) stimulate the proliferation and secretory development of the endometrium. Along with non-steroidal factors such as inhibin, estrogen and progesterone also modulate pituitary production of the gonadotrophic hormones through feedback inhibition.

Concentrations of these gonadotrophic and ovarian hormones vary cyclically in a characteristic pattern over the course of the menstrual cycle (Fig. 1, top and center panels). Convention dictates that the first day of menstruation is considered day 1. Modulation of ovarian function by FSH and LH, leading to follicular maturation and ovulation, is known as the ovarian cycle. Concurrent phases of endometrial development to sustain an embryo, induced by estrogen and progesterone, are known as the endometrial cycle (Fig. 1, bottom panel).

The Ovarian Cycle

The ovarian cycle describes hormonally induced changes in ovarian function that follow the onset of menstrual flow. The first half of the cycle, referred to as the follicular phase, is marked by a rise in FSH and LH concentrations stimulated by the pulsatile release of GnRH. During the follicular phase, a pattern of low

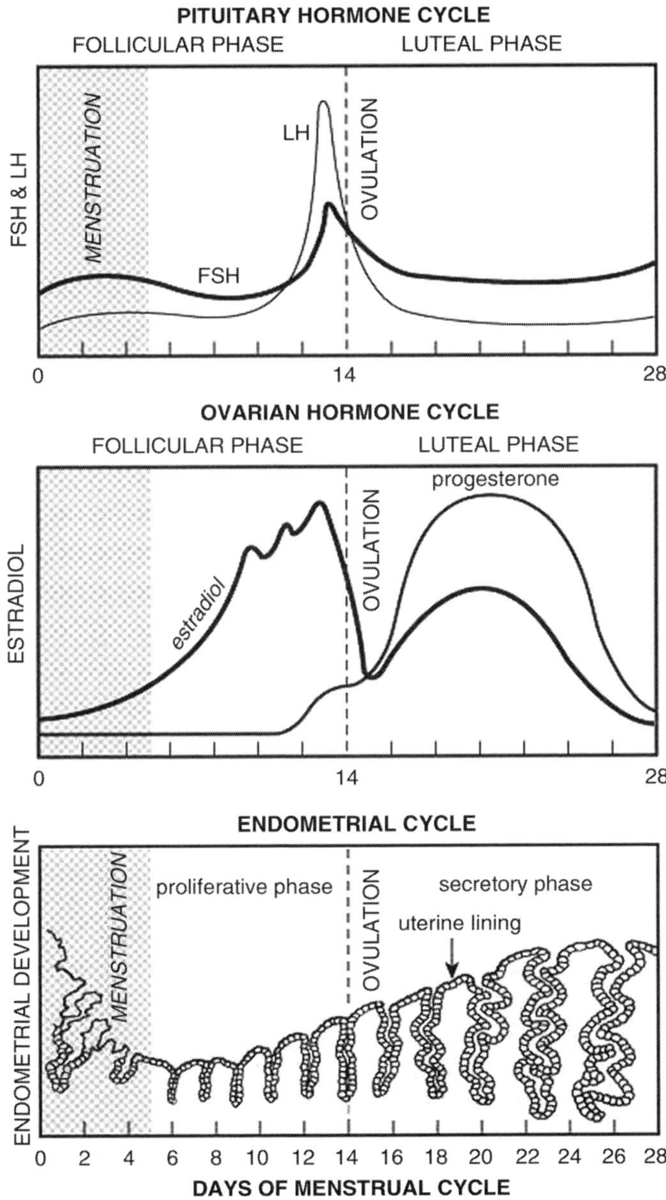

Figure 1 An idealized menstrual cycle of 28 days. *Top panel*—the pituitary hormone cycle: cycling of gonadotrophins (FSH, LH). *Center panel*—the ovarian hormone cycle: cycling of ovarian hormones (estradiol, progesterone). *Bottom panel*—The endometrial cycle: corresponding cyclical development of the endometrium. *Abbreviations*: FSH, follicle-stimulating hormone; LH, luteinizing hormone.

amplitude, high-frequency GnRH pulses is thought to preferentially stimulate the secretion of FSH relative to LH. The rise of FSH and LH causes the follicles within the ovaries to grow. After a week or more of follicular growth—but before ovulation occurs—usually, a single follicle outgrows the others, begins to secrete high concentrations of estrogens (notably estradiol), and then matures. Heightened estrogen production by this dominant follicle creates feedback inhibition of the pituitary secretion of FSH and LH, which in turn causes the remaining ovarian follicles to involute (a process known as atresia).

In an idealized 28-day cycle, ovulation occurs at midcycle, 14 days after the onset of menstruation. An elevated concentration of LH is necessary for final follicular growth and ovulation. High amplitude, low-frequency GnRH pulses mediate the preferential stimulation of LH. In response, approximately two days before ovulation, the rate of secretion of LH increases markedly (6 to 10 fold), peaking about 18 hours prior to ovulation (the LH surge) (Fig. 1, top panel). Concurrently, FSH increases about 2-fold. FSH and LH act synergistically to induce ovulation, that is, the rupture of the mature follicle and release of the mature ovum.

The LH surge is a marker of ovulation. Mild unilateral abdominal pain experienced around the time of ovulation by some women, known as *Mittleschmerz* (German for "midpain"), may be related to the leakage of blood and fluid from the ruptured follicle.

The second half of the ovarian cycle is known as the luteal phase. Most of the variation in menstrual cycle length (21–35 days) is due to variation in the follicular phase; the luteal phase is relatively constant at 14 days from ovulation to menses (3). Under the influence of LH during the last few days prior to ovulation, and continuing for a day or so after ovulation, the granulosa cells of the follicle undergo a physical and biochemical change called luteinization. The mass of cells remaining at the site of the ruptured follicle becomes the corpus luteum and begins secreting large quantities of the hormones progesterone and estrogen (Fig. 1, center panel). A small increase in body temperature occurs because of heightened progesterone secretion. Feedback inhibition by these hormones, and by other nonsteroidal factors such as inhibin, reduce the secretion of FSH and LH, thereby, preventing the growth of the new ovarian follicles.

At about day 26 of the idealized cycle, the corpus luteum degenerates. The resulting drop in progesterone and estrogen is followed by menstruation. The loss of progesterone acts as a trigger for endometrial desquamation and the onset of menstrual flow. Concurrently, feedback suppression of the gonadotrophic hormones is lost. As a result, the anterior pituitary once again secretes high levels of FSH and moderate levels of LH in response to GnRH stimulus, re-initiating the ovarian cycle.

The Endometrial Cycle

The cyclic production of estrogen and progesterone during the ovarian cycle induces a corresponding cycle of endometrial proliferation and development

(Fig. 1, bottom panel). This endometrial cycle includes a proliferative phase lasting about 11 days, a secretory phase lasting about 12 days, and a desquamative or menstrual phase of about five days during which menstruation ensues.

During the follicular phase of the ovarian cycle, the endometrium proliferates and increases in thickness under the influence of estradiol. This marks the proliferative phase of the endometrial cycle. During the luteal phase of the ovarian cycle, progesterone stimulates further endometrial cell proliferation, differentiation, and secretory development to support implantation and to nourish the developing conceptus. This is the secretory phase of the endometrial cycle. Progesterone also promotes secretory changes in the lining of the fallopian tubes that will support the fertilized egg as it travels down the fallopian tube prior to implantation.

If fertilization occurs, human chorionic gonadotrophin produced by the developing placenta maintains the corpus luteum, thereby sustaining progesterone secretion. If fertilization does not occur, the corpus luteum is lost, causing a sudden drop in progesterone. This triggers endometrial desquamation, in an ordely fashion, resulting in menstruation.

Total menstrual blood loss varies from cycle to cycle, among individual women, and at different stages of reproductive life. Average menstrual blood loss is about 50 to 60 mL, but may vary from 10 mL to over 100 mL (4,5). Chronic menstrual blood loss greater than 80 mL results in anemia. A loss of 60 to 80 mL has served to define "heavy flow" (4,5), although the clinical utility of this definition is negligible because most women cannot accurately assess their flow level (4).

COMPOSITION AND PROPERTIES OF MENSES

Menses principally consists of blood, desquamated endometrial tissue, sloughed vaginal epithelial cells, cervico-vaginal secretions, and endogenous vaginal microbes. Consequently, menses differs from venous blood both in its composition (Table 1) and in its physical properties. The composition and physical properties of menses vary among individuals and over the course of menstrual flow. Hence, mean values for menses reported in the accompanying table represent values obtained from sample populations and may not broadly reflect population norms.

Menses may be considered a suspension of blood- and tissue-derived solids within a mixture of serum and cervico-vaginal fluid. Agglomerates of tissue debris, red blood cells, and mucins are scattered throughout a serum-like phase. Figure 2 shows microscopic images obtained from two locations within the same sample of menses. The images show intact and ruptured red blood cells, finer particulate matter, as well as predominantly fluid regions, demonstrating the nonhomogenous nature of menses (6).

The blood content of menses depends on the extent of endometrial breakdown and dilution of blood- and tissue-derived constituents with cervico-vaginal fluid. Vaginal fluid in menses contributes principally water, common electrolytes,

Table 1 Composition of Venous Blood and Menses[a]

Component	Venous blood		Menses		Reference[b]
	Mean	Range[c]	Mean	Range	
Hematological components					
Red blood cells (cells per mm^3)	N/A	$4.8 \pm 2.0 \times 10^6$	N/A	$2.4–3.9 \times 10^6$	(31,32)
White blood cells (cells per mm^3)	N/A	$2.4–2.8 \times 10^6$	N/A	$2.1–3.6 \times 10^4$	(31,32)
Platelets (cells per mm^3)	N/A	$1.4–3.5 \times 10^5$	3.0×10^4	$3.1–3.3 \times 10^4$	(15,32)
Hemoglobin (g/dL)	14	12–18	10	2–20	(10)
Albumin (g/L)	44 ± 8.8	N/A	43.6 ± 11.8	N/A	(11)
Hematological components (coagulation factors)					
Prothrombin	Present in 24/24 subjects studied	N/A	Not detected	Not detected	(12)
Plasminogen activator (CTA units/mL)	0.15	0–0.2[d]	1.04	0–3.5	(11)
Plasmin(ogen) protein (g/L)	0.15 ± 0.03	N/A	0.17 ± 0.05	N/A	(11)
Plasmin activity (μmol/L)	0	0	0.83 ± 0.97	N/A	(11)
α_2-antiplasmin activity	Present in 24/24 subjects studied	N/A	Not detected	N/A	(11)
Fibrinogen (mg/100 mL)	N/A	200–400	Not detected	Not detected	(14)

Fibrinogen degradation products (μg/mL)	10.5 ± 0.8	N/A	>1280	N/A	(14)
Inorganic materials					
Sodium (ppm)	3300	N/A	2600	2300–3100	(33)
Calcium (ppm)	105	85–105	100	90–110	(33)
Iron (ppm)[e]	455	390–585[f]	320	60-650	(10)
Phosphate (ppm)	270	N/A	360	320–450	(33)
Chloride (ppm)	3600	N/A	3500	3200–3900	(33)
Organic materials					
Serum protein (g/100 mL)	7	6.0–8.0	6.5	5.9–7.5	(33)
Amino acids (ppm)	100	N/A	250	160–350	(33)
Nitrogen (ppm)	350	N/A	800	600–1000	(33)
Urea (ppm)	400	N/A	150	100–200	(33)
Bilirubin (ppm)	7	2–9	4	3–7	(33)
Fatty acids (ppm)	3500	N/A	3000	2200–3300	(33)
Total cholesterol (ppm)	1750	1400–3100[g]	1500	1350–1700	(33)
Blood sugar (ppm)	900	700–1100[h]	500	300–500	(33)
Glycogen (ppm)	350	N/A	500	400–600	(33)
Lactic acid (ppm)	110	60–160	300	240–370	(33)

[a]Cited values for menses are based on sample populations and do not necessarily represent population norms. N/A: not available.
[b]References for menses values only.
[c]Normal clinical ranges according to (34), unless otherwise referenced.
[d]From Ref. 11.
[e]Calculated from hemoglobin content.
[f]From Ref. 9.
[g]For ages 30 to 49, as observed clinically (34). Values skew higher with age.
[h]Fasting glucose.
Abbreviation: ppm, parts per million (or μg/mL).

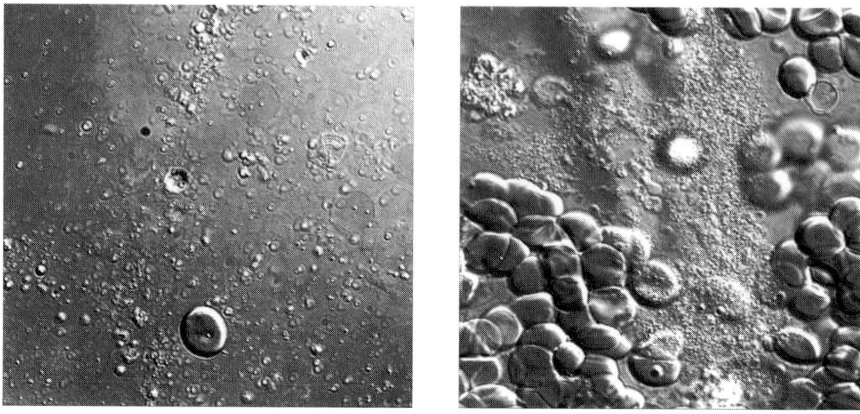

Figure 2 Images of menses obtained by differential interference contrast microscopy (approximately 1000× magnification), demonstrating cellular agglomerates and a predominantly fluid phase within the same menses sample.

organic moieties, and at least 14 proteins (7), including glycoproteins with molecular weights up to 82 kDa (8).

Consequently, the concentrations of many elements in menses are lower than in venous blood. For example, solid matter in venous blood after evaporation of water is typically 20% of the mass, but the solid matter in menses ranges from 7% to 23% of the total mass; hence, menstrual fluid often has a higher water content than venous blood (9). Likewise, the hemoglobin and iron content of menses depend on the extent of endometrial breakdown and display a far broader range than that of venous blood (Table 1). The blood content of menses averaged over all days of menstrual flow is close to 50% (5). The average hemoglobin content of venous blood is about 14 g/dL, but the hemoglobin content of menses samples obtained at the time of peak flow was closer to 10 g/L, with a range of 1.5 g/dL to 19.9 g/dL (10). White blood cell and platelet counts in menses are as much as 100-fold lower than those of venous blood (Table 1).

The pH of menses is similar to that of venous blood, reflecting the serum content of its fluid phase. The median pH measured in a range of menses samples was 7.2 with a skewed distribution tailing into the range of pH 5 to 6 (measured at 25°C using a small diameter glass electrode) (9).

The concentrations of certain serum-derived constituents, such as serum proteins, total cholesterol, and bilirubin, fall within the range found in venous blood (Table 1). The absence of clotting is the most notable biochemical difference between menses and venous blood. What appear to be menstrual blood clots actually represent large samples of the aforementioned blood-tissue agglomerates.

In venous blood, clotting involves three broadly defined steps:

1. Prothrombin activator complex is formed in response to vessel or blood damage.

2. Prothrombin activator complex catalyzes the activation of prothrombin into the proteolytic enzyme, thrombin.
3. Thrombin cleaves fibrinogen into peptides, which polymerize into fibrin threads that enmesh platelets, blood cells, and plasma to form the clot itself.

Other coagulation factors participate in the process. Clot lysis requires the activation of plasminogen to plasmin, a proteolytic enzyme that digests fibrin threads in the blood clot. Unlike venous blood, menses is depleted of key clotting factors, has lower platelet counts and reduced platelet activity, but is high in fibrinolytic activity (Table 1). Prothrombin, free thrombin, fibrinogen, and fibrin are absent from menstrual blood (11–13). Instead, high levels of tissue plasminogen activator and fibrin degradation products are found (11,13,14). The plasmin present in menses, though comparable in concentration to that of venous blood, is no longer fibrinolytically active. Moreover, platelets in menses differ from platelets in venous blood in that they fail to aggregate in response to stimuli or to produce chemical messengers involved in the clotting response (15). These data suggest that clots initially formed in endometrial blood are degraded during menstruation.

Besides these differences in coagulation components, menses but not venous blood contains matrix metalloproteinases (MMPs), enzymes that catalyze endometrial breakdown through proteolysis of the stromal extracellular matrix (16–19). Examples include MMP-1 (interstitial collagenase), MMP-2 (gelatinase-A), MMP-3 (stromelysin 1), MMP-9 (gelatinase-B), and MMP-10 (stromelysin-2). MMPs are secreted as inactive proenzymes. In the endometrium, they are expressed and activated during the late secretory and menstrual phases of the cycle in response to progesterone withdrawal, the hormonal trigger for menstruation (20,21).

The physical properties of menses are highly dependent on its composition. Because the proportions of proteins, lipids, mucins, blood, and tissue-derived constituents vary temporally over the course of menstrual flow, it is not meaningful to cite average values for physical properties such as viscosity and elasticity. Rather, the following discussion highlights the tremendous range in these properties.

For example, menses viscosity (measured at a given shear rate) varies dramatically, as much as an order of magnitude in a single set of samples (data not shown). The thinnest samples, collected when menstrual flow was greatest, had a viscosity similar to that of venous blood; samples collected during times of low menstrual flow were more viscous; indeed, some could be described as more gelatinous than liquid in nature. It is fair to say that a large proportion of menses samples are considerably more viscous than blood or water—about four times as viscous as venous blood and 35 times as viscous as water (22).

The elasticity of menses also varies considerably. *Spinnbarkeit*, a clinical term applied to the elasticity of cervical mucous, can be used describe the elasticity of menses. As background, cervical mucous responds to estrogen with a

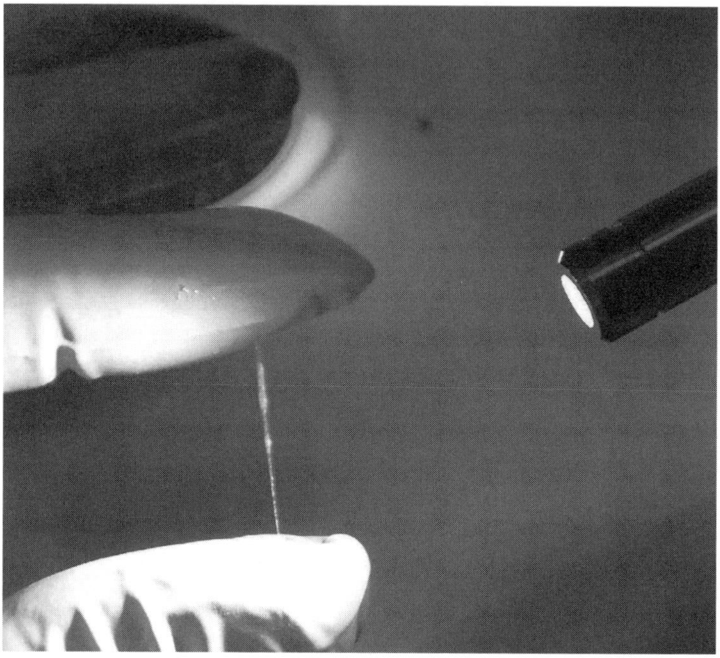

Figure 3 Spinnbarkeit test for menses elasticity. (*See color insert p. 7.*)

decrease in viscosity, which results in a clinically important observation that the elasticity of cervical mucous, i.e., the length of a strand formed when cervical mucous is extended, is greatest at the time of ovulation. (This observation that can be helpful in either avoiding or planning conception.) Spinnbarkeit, or the ability to form a strand, can also be used to measure the elasticity of menses (Fig. 3). The length of a "strand" formed when menses fluid is rapidly extended often reaches 30 mm before it breaks; however, strand length can range from 0 mm (no elasticity) to 70 mm (more elastic than maple syrup) (23).

In conclusion, menses differs in important respects from venous blood because its constituents are derived from endometrial breakdown and passage through the vaginal tract. Besides red blood cells and serum constituents, menses contains tissue agglomerates, endometrial proteases, and cervico-vaginal secretions not found in venous blood. Menses is also depleted of certain clotting factors. Consequently, menses exhibits a broader range in physical characteristics and chemical composition than does venous blood.

EFFECTS OF MENSES AND VENOUS BLOOD ON THE SKIN

Some women report vulvar irritation during the menstrual period. To assess whether menses contributes to vulvar irritation, we performed a four-day skin patch test of menses and venous blood on the labia majora and on the upper arm in 20 women volunteers (24). Compositional differences between blood and menses (e.g., proteinase content) (25) and anatomical differences in irritant susceptibility (26,27) could affect the erythema response.

In brief, physiologic saline (non-irritant control), aqueous sodium lauryl sulphate (SLS, 0.6% weight/volume, irritant control), and each volunteer's own venous blood and menses (collected overnight with an intravaginal cup) (0.3 mL each) were applied for two, consecutive 24-hour periods to the lateral labia majora (randomized across two clipped sites on each labium) and to the upper arm (randomized across five sites per arm). Occlusive patches were applied to the labia and to one upper arm; semi-occlusive patches were applied to the alternate arm. The fifth site on each arm was pretreated with a proprietary, petrolatum-based emollient prior to menses application. A standard five-point erythema scale was used to score skin irritation (28,29).

Effect of Anatomical Site

The labia majora were less responsive than the upper arm to all applied materials (Figs. 4A and B). On the labia majora, menses and venous blood elicited no significant erythema at either time point; SLS, the irritant control, elicited significant, mild erythema (0.6 ± 0.08 and 1.2 ± 0.15 at 24 and 48 hours, respectively).

On the upper arm, menses and venous blood elicited mild erythema at the 48-hour time point only (Fig. 4B: 0.7 ± 0.14 and 1.1 ± 0.14, respectively). SLS elicited moderate to severe erythema at both the 24- and 48-hour time points (Figs. 4A and B: 2.3 ± 0.09 and 3.4 ± 0.14, respectively). Mean scores to SLS on the arm were three- to four-fold higher than those observed on the labia; this is consistent with prior reports that the arm is more susceptible to SLS-induced skin irritation than the labia (27,30).

Effect of Occlusion

Semi-occlusive conditions attenuated the erythematous response to all materials (Fig. 5, upper arm, 48 hours). Notably, SLS-induced erythema was reduced almost six-fold (mean scores of 0.6 ± 0.1 vs. 3.4 ± 0.14, semi- and full-occlusion, respectively). Pretreatment of the upper arm with emollient prevented menses-induced skin irritation, regardless of the degree of occlusion.

Taken together, these observations suggest that the vulva (labia majora) is adapted to be less sensitive to menses-induced skin irritation and that pretreatment with a petrolatum-based emollient attenuates potential skin irritation from menses.

These findings suggest that vulvar skin may have unique properties relative to skin at other sites. This investigative approach may have clinical utility in addressing women's complaints about vulvar irritation. For example, similar methods may be used to assess the responsiveness of prepubertal and

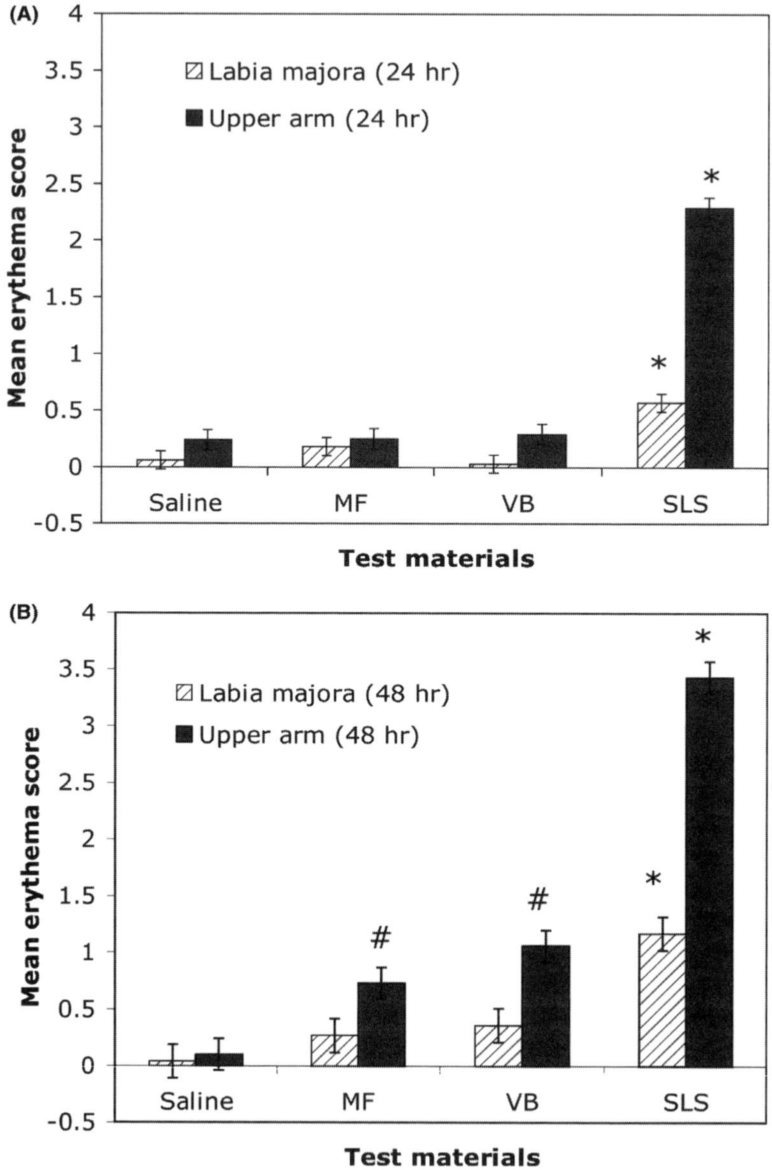

Figure 4 Skin erythema of the labia majora and upper arm, following the application of test materials under occlusive patch for 24 and 48 hours. (**A**) 24-hour exposure. (**B**) 48-hour exposure. *Note*: *, significantly different from other test materials applied to that anatomical site. #, significantly different from the nonirritant control (saline) applied to that anatomical site. Test materials, Saline (nonirritant control); *Abbreviations*: MF, menses fluid; VB, venous blood; SLS, 0.6% aqueous sodium lauryl sulfate (irritant control). *Source*: Adapted from Ref. 24.

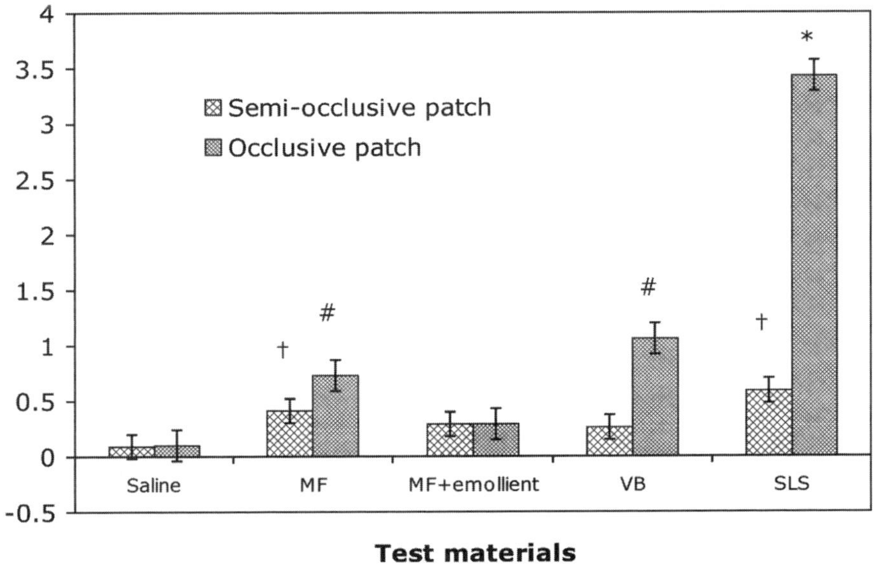

Figure 5 Skin erythema of the upper arm induced by test materials applied for 48 cumulative hours under semi-occlusive or occlusive patch. *Note*: †, significantly different from the non-irritant control (saline) under semi-occlusive conditions. #, significantly different from the non-irritant control (saline) under occlusive conditions. *, significantly different from other test materials under occlusive conditions. Test materials, Saline (non-irritant control); *Abbreviations*: MF, menses fluid; MF + emollient, menses fluid applied to emollient-treated skin, VB, venous blood; SLS = 0.6% aqueous sodium lauryl sulfate (irritant control). *Source*: Adapted from Ref. 24.

postmenopausal skin to vaginal bleeding, or to investigate the response of vulvar skin to menses in the presence or absence of pathological conditions such as candidal vulvitis, lichen sclerosus, or vulvar ulcers associated with herpes simplex infection. The pursuit of such questions will add to our knowledge of vulvar reactions in health and disease.

CONCLUSION

The menstrual cycle is central to female reproductive function. In an idealized cycle, cyclical variations in the production and concentrations of hypothalamic, pituitary, and ovarian hormones over a 28-day period lead to the release of a mature ovum at approximately midcycle and to the concurrent development of the endometrium in anticipation of fertilization. When fertilization does not occur, the endometrium is shed, menstruation ensues, and the cycle begins anew.

Menses is composed of blood that is depleted of clotting factors as well as desquamated endometrial tissue, sloughed vaginal cells, and cervico-vaginal secretions. The composition and physical properties of menses vary both temporally and among individuals because the concentration of menses constituents changes as flow progresses. Menses and blood might be expected to differ in their potential effects on vulvar skin because menses is more complex and contains endometrial metalloproteinases not present in blood. However, vulvar patch testing of blood and menses revealed minimal vulvar irritation in response to these substances when compared to patch testing on the upper arm. These findings suggest that vulvar skin may be uniquely adapted to be less sensitive to the cyclical exposure to menses that occurs during women's reproductive years.

REFERENCES

1. Arey LB. The degree of normal menstrual irregularity. Am J Obstet Gynecol 1939; 37(12):12–29.
2. Treloar AE, Boynton RE, Behn BG, Brown BW. Variation of the human menstrual cycle through reproductive life. Int J Fertil 1967; 12(1 Pt 2):77–126.
3. Nussey SS, Whitehead SA. Endocrinology: An Integrated Approach. 1st ed. Oxford, U.K.: Bios Scientific Publishers Limited, Taylor & Francis Group, 2001.
4. Chimbira TH, Anderson ABM. Relation between measured menstrual blood loss and patient's subjective assessment of loss, duration of bleeding, number of sanitary towels used, uterine weight and endometrial surgace area. Br J Obstet Gynaecol 1980; 87:603–609.
5. Fraser IS, Warner P, Marantos PA. Estimating menstrual blood loss in women with normal and excessive menstrual fluid volume. Obstet Gynecol 2001; 98(5 Pt 1): 806–814.
6. Flood JA. The Procter & Gamble Company. 2003; Unpublished data.
7. Moghissi KS. Vaginal fluid constituents. In: Beller FK, Schumacher GFB, eds. The Biology of The Fluids of the Female Genital Tract. New York, NY: Elsevier/North Holland, 1979:13–22.
8. Rajan N, Cao Q, Anderson BE, et al. Roles of glycoproteins and oligosaccharides found in human vaginal fluid in bacterial adherence. Infect Immun 1999; 67(10):5027–5032.
9. Hood WH. The Procter & Gamble Company. 2004; Unpublished data.
10. Ventura AM. The Procter & Gamble Company. 2003; Unpublished data.
11. Cederholm-Williams SA, Rees MC, Turnbull AC. Consumption of fibrinolytic proteins in menstrual fluid from women with normal menstrual blood loss. J Clin Pathol 1984; 37(8):879–881.
12. Cederholm-Williams SA, Rees MC, Turnbull AC. Examination of certain coagulation factors in menstrual fluid from women with normal blood loss. Thromb Haemost 1984; 52(3):224–225.
13. Rees MC, Cederholm-Williams SA, Turnbull AC. Coagulation factors and fibrinolytic proteins in menstrual fluid collected from normal and menorrhagic women. Br J Obstet Gynaecol 1985; 92(11):1164–1168.
14. Dockeray CJ, Sheppard BL, Daly L, Bonnar J. The fibrinolytic enzyme system in normal menstruation and excessive uterine bleeding and the effect of tranexamic acid. Eur J Obstet Gynecol Reprod Biol 1987; 24(4):309–318.

15. Rees MC, Demers LM, Anderson AB, Turnbull AC. A functional study of platelets in menstrual fluid. Br J Obstet Gynaecol 1984; 91(7):667–672.
16. Marbaix E, Vekemans M, Galant C, et al. Circulating sex hormones and endometrial stromelysin-1 (matrix metalloproteinase-3) at the start of bleeding episodes in levonorgestrel-implant users. Hum Reprod 2000; 15(suppl 3):120–134.
17. Marbaix E, Kokorine I, Moulin P, Donnez J, Eeckhout Y, Courtoy PJ. Menstrual breakdown of human endometrium can be mimicked in vitro and is selectively and reversibly blocked by inhibitors of matrix metalloproteinases. Proc Natl Acad Sci USA 1996; 93(17):9120–9125.
18. Marbaix E, Kokorine I, Henriet P, Donnez J, Courtoy PJ, Eeckhout Y. The expression of interstitial collagenase in human endometrium is controlled by progesterone and by oestradiol and is related to menstruation. Biochem J 1995; 305(Pt 3):1027–1030.
19. Kokorine I, Marbaix E, Henriet P, et al. Focal cellular origin and regulation of interstitial collagenase (matrix metalloproteinase-1) are related to menstrual breakdown in the human endometrium. J Cell Sci 1996; 109(Pt 8):2151–2160.
20. Marbaix E, Kokorine I, Donnez J, Eeckhout Y, Courtoy PJ. Regulation and restricted expression of interstitial collagenase suggest a pivotal role in the initiation of menstruation. Hum Reprod 1996; 11(suppl 2):134–143.
21. Rigot V, Marbaix E, Lemoine P, Courtoy PJ, Eeckhout Y. In vivo perimenstrual activation of progelatinase B (proMMP-9) in the human endometrium and its dependence on stromelysin 1 (MMP-3) ex vivo. Biochem J 2001; 358(Pt 1):275–280.
22. Hartt WH. The Procter & Gamble Company. 2004; Unpublished data.
23. Minoguchi R. The Procter & Gamble Company. 2003; Unpublished data.
24. Farage M, Warren R, Wang-Weigand S. The vulva is relatively insensitive to menses-induced irritation. Cutaneous Ocular Toxicol 2005; 24(4):243–246.
25. Beller FK, Schweppe KW. Review of the biology of menstrual blood. In: Beller RK, Schumacher GFB, eds. The Biology of the Fluids of the Female Genital Tract. New York, NY: Elsevier/North Holland, 1979:231–235.
26. Britz MB, Maibach, HI. Human cutaneous vulvar reactivity to irritants. Contact Dermatitis 1979; 5(6):375–377.
27. Elsner P, Wilhelm D, Maibach HI. Effect of low-concentration sodium lauryl sulfate on human vulvar and forearm skin. Age-related differences. J Reprod Med 1991; 36(1):77–81.
28. Patrick E, Maibach HI. Dermatotoxicology. In: Hayes A, ed. Principles and Methods of Toxicology. 2nd ed. New York: W. Raven Press, 1989:383–405.
29. Phillips L, 2nd, Steinberg M, Maibach HI, Akers WA. A comparison of rabbit and human skin response to certain irritants. Toxicol Appl Pharmacol 1972; 21(3):369–382.
30. Elsner P, Wilhelm D, Maibach HI. Irritant effect of a model surfactant on the human vulva and forearm. Age-related differences. J Reprod Med 1990; 35(11):1035–1039.
31. Stickle M, Zondok B. Dus Menstruationsblut. Z Geburtsh u Gynåkol 1920; 83:1–26.
32. DeMerre LJ, Moss JD, Pattison DS. The hemalogical study of menstrual discharge. Obstet Gynecol 1967; 30:830.
33. Büssing HJ. Zur Biochemie des menstrualblutes. Zbl Gynaec 1957; 79:456.
34. Wallach J. Interpretation of Diagnostic Tests. A Handbook Synopsis of Laboratory Medicine. 3rd ed. Boston: Little, Brown and Company, 1978.

11

The Menstrual Cycle and the Skin

Birgit Drexler, Michael Landthaler, and Silvia Hohenleutner
Clinic and Outpatient Clinic of Dermatology, Clinical Center of the University of Regensburg, Regensburg, Germany

INTRODUCTION

The menstruation of a sexually mature woman is a sign of a cyclic hormonal stimulation of the endometrium. It is well documented that the menstrual cycle influences many systemic disorders, such as asthma, porphyria, epilepsy, migraine, myasthenia gravis, and allergic rhinitis (1). Estrogen and progesterone, the two female sex hormones, can also lead to cycle-dependent variations in the activity of many skin disorders. Although detailed data on the cycle-associated hormonally mediated changes in the target organs, such as the uterus, vagina, cervix, and mammary glands, are available, little is known about the effects of the menstrual cycle on the skin (2). It is the goal of this chapter to provide an overview of the most important skin disorders with cycle-dependent variations.

HORMONAL CHANGES IN THE COURSE OF THE MENSTRUAL CYCLE

The menstrual cycle is controlled by two ovarian hormones. Under the stimulating and determinant influence of the gonadotrophins follicle-stimulating hormone (FSH) and luteinizing hormone (LH), cyclic morphological changes take place in the ovaries of the sexually mature woman. At the beginning of the cycle, after completion of menstruation, the buildup of the endometrium and the synthesis of the endometrial progesterone and estrogen receptors are triggered as a result of an increasing secretion of estradiol. The ovarian estrogen synthesis takes place via the intermediate products androstenedione and testosterone, which are aromatized to estrone and estradiol subsequently.

The processes are stimulated by LH in synergy with FSH, which is presumably responsible for the development of a large number of primary follicles in the early follicular phase. Via negative feedback, estrogen production—which increases in the preovulatory phase and reaches the first peak at the time of ovulation—causes FSH to decrease, which leads to a regression of most of the stimulated follicles. Only a dominant follicle becomes independent of the stimulation by pituitary FSH and reaches ovulation maturity. The ovulation in the middle of the cycle is associated with a peak in the LH production and a peak in the FSH production, although the latter is less pronounced. The LH peak lasts approximately 36 hours and is controlled by the pulsatile release of gonadotrophin-releasing hormone (GnRH) from the hypothalamus. After ovulation, the corpus luteum develops, accompanied by an increasing secretion of gestagen, which is responsible for the increase in the thickness of the endometrium and which, via negative feedback, inhibits the release of FSH from the pituitary gland and, thus, the further maturation of the follicles in the corpus luteum phase. As the luteal phase progresses, estradiol reaches the second peak. The new premenstrual increase in FSH, which is the result of a decrease of the progesterone formation in the corpus luteum, causes the stimulation of a new generation of follicles in the ovaries. The secretory phase is controlled jointly by estradiol and progesterone. The endometrial breakdown that causes menstrual bleeding is caused by decreases in the levels of these two sex hormones. Cyclic hormonal changes, however, have an influence not only on the endometrium but also on the vaginal epithelium and the skin (2). Figure 1 shows the pattern of the pituitary hormones LH/FSH and the two sex hormones estradiol/progesterone during a normal menstrual cycle.

INFLUENCE OF THE SEX HORMONES ON THE SKIN

The skin contains receptors for estrogen and progesterone and is as highly sensitive to the effect of these two steroid sex hormones as it is to androgens (3).

Estrogens

At a high concentration, estrogens suppress sebum production but have only an insignificant or no influence on the apocrine glands (4). The sebum content of the skin is related to the menstrual cycle, with the lowest sebum level following the peak of the estrogen level (5). Estrogens improve the water-binding capacity of the stratum corneum and, through an increase in acid mucopolysaccharides and hyaluronic acid, that of the dermis as well (6). There is a significant increase in the thickness of the skin with the increase in the estradiol level in the middle

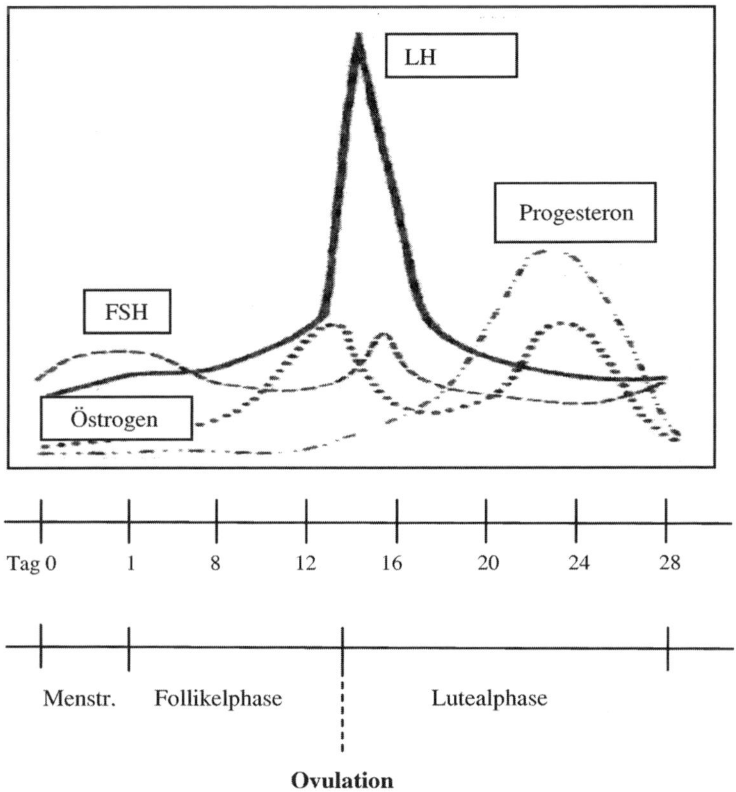

Figure 1 Serum levels of pituitary and sexual steroid hormones during a normal menstrual cycle. *Abbreviations*: FSH, follicle-stimulating hormone; LH, luteinizing hormone. *Source*: Modified from Ref. 4.

and at the end of the menstrual cycle, which can be explained by an increased fluid retention under the influence of estradiol (7).

By increasing the transformation of soluble collagen into the cross-linked insoluble form, estrogens slow the breakdown of dermal collagen. Eighty percent of the collagen of the skin is made up of type I collagen and 15% of type III collagen, with type I collagen being principally responsible for the skin's thickness and type III collagen for its elasticity. A deficiency of estrogen leads to a decrease of types I and III collagen, which leads to a shift of the type I : type III ratio in the direction of type III collagen, and to a corresponding decrease of the skin thickness (6).

Estrogens stimulate epidermal melanogenesis, which can lead to a transient hyperpigmentation that generally appears in the premenstrual phase, especially around the eyes and nipples (3,4,8). The anti-inflammatory effect of estrogens alone seems to be more pronounced than when combined with the effect of progesterone, which is the case in the premenstrual phase and which is attributable to the antiestrogenic effect of progesterone (2,4). Estrogens suppress the cellular immune response, which may be due to an influence on the regulatory T cells. Furthermore, estrogens inhibit the activity of natural killer cells and neutrophilic granulocytes and have a regulatory influence on the interferon-gamma promoter. Together with the previously mentioned effects on the skin barrier, this immunological effect of estrogen gives rise to cyclic changes in the activity of the skin (9,10). The general effects of estrogen on the skin are:

1. Decreased sebum
2. Increased water-binding capacity (stratum corneum, dermis)
3. Increased skin thickness
4. Increased fluid retention
5. Decreased collagen breakdown
6. Increased epidermal hyperpigmentation
7. Decreased cellular immune response
8. Increased vasodilation (in combination with gestagen)

Progesterone

The influence of progesterone on the skin is less understood. Research has demonstrated an immunosuppressive effect of progesterone that is potentially caused by the inhibition of monocytic functions (10). As progesterone is the dominating circulating hormone in the premenstrual phase, it is hypothesized that the premenstrual exacerbation of many skin disorders is caused by the influence of this hormone.

The blood supply to the skin increases in the second phase of the menstrual cycle. Harvell, et al. (11), demonstrated that the basal blood flow at the time of maximum progesterone secretion was significantly higher than on the day of maximum estrogen secretion. In another study, researchers observed a gradual dilation of the venous lumen, which reached its maximum diameter approximately one week prior to the onset of menstrual bleeding. This phenomenon also may be responsible for the subjective symptoms of chronic venous insufficiency in patients with varicose veins, in whom symptoms often increase in the second half of the cycle (12). In the premenstrual phase, not only does progesterone reach its highest level, but a high estrogen concentration is present as well; the combined effect of both hormones may be causally responsible for dilation of the vessels (12).

More recent studies demonstrate that the combination of high estrogen and gestagen levels, such as seen in the middle of the luteal phase, influences the vasodilatory system of the skin. Independently of the sympathetic innervation, local warming of the skin leads to vasodilation, which is mediated presumably by the formation of nitric oxide. This vasodilatory response to local thermal stimuli is intensified by high estrogen and gestagen levels. An effect on the active, adrenergically controlled vasoconstriction following cold application does not appear to be present (13).

PREMENSTRUAL SYNDROME

Premenstrual syndrome (PMS) is accompanied by cutaneous manifestations that emerge in the premenstrual phase of the menstrual cycle. Accordingly, approximately 70% of women report that prior to the onset of menstrual bleeding, they suffer from mild acne eruptions, often in association with an increased greasiness of the skin and hair; a premenstrual exacerbation of perioral dermatitis is reported frequently, especially by young women (4). Additional clinical symptoms of PMS include:

1. Migraine and other forms of headache
2. Tiredness, lethargy
3. Depression
4. Irritability and nervousness
5. Feeling of tenseness in and swelling of the breasts
6. Abdominal pain, feeling of fullness
7. Increased thirst, appetite, and weight gain
8. Constipation and flatulence
9. Hot flush symptoms
10. Acneiform cutaneous efflorescences, perioral dermatitis
11. Oily skin and hair
12. Hyperpigmentation of the skin

To date, the definite endocrinologic mechanism responsible for PMS has not been found. Given the temporal association of the symptoms with the luteal phase of the menstrual cycle, it is possible that progesterone plays an important role. Various hypotheses have been offered to explain the pathogenesis, such as an individual progesterone deficiency, an imbalance between the estrogen and progesterone levels, and even an allergy to progesterone (4,14). One confirmed fact is that the β-endorphin level in the premenstrual phase is decreased in patients with PMS (2). Research has confirmed the thesis of an immunological mechanism of PMS by the finding of a positive intracutaneous test reaction to female sex hormones in women with PMS and associated cutaneous manifestations (15). A hypersensitization treatment led to a significant reduction of the PMS symptoms, as well as to an improvement of the cutaneous manifestations. A connection with autoimmune progesterone and autoimmune estrogen dermatitis seems possible.

MENSTRUAL CYCLE AND ASSOCIATED SKIN DISORDERS

Chloasma and Hyperpigmentation

The stimulation of epidermal melanogenesis by means of hormones has long been known. During pregnancy, for example, hormonal influences can cause an increased pigmentation in the face (chloasma), the areolae, the linea alba, and the perineal skin. After administration of estrogen-containing oral contraceptives, facial hyperpigmentation was observed in 8% to 29% of women. The application of estrogen-containing ointments to children can also lead to hyperpigmentations in the genital area and in the area of the nipples and the linea alba (3). One study found that of 62% of the women tested, hormonal influences in the premenstrual phase led to increased pigmentation, particularly in the periorbital region (8).

Acne Vulgaris and Rosacea

A high percentage of women with acne vulgaris experience a premenstrual exacerbation. The figures in the literature vary between 27% and 70% (16,17). A study of 400 acne patients found a premenstrual exacerbation in 44% of the cases. Women older than 33 years of age appear to be affected more frequently than younger women between 20 and 33 years of age (18). A comparison of acne lesions in the late follicular phase and the luteal phase found that in the premenstrual phase, 63% of the women studied had an increase of inflammatory acne efflorescences, on average by 25%. In 54% of the women studied, the comedo rate increased by an average of 21% (19).

The definite mechanism of premenstrual exacerbations of acne vulgaris is not known. It is possible that premenstrual skin edema causes a narrowing of the lumen of the ducts of the sebaceous glands, which leads to sebum accumulation and/or to variations in sebum secretion (5,16). Treatment with oral contraceptives with an antiandrogenic component has proved successful, although increased androgen levels in women with acne were found in only some of the relevant studies (18).

Patients with rosacea can also experience premenstrual exacerbation (4). It is possible that the previously mentioned changes in sebum secretion and/or an increased blood supply to the skin in the luteal phase play a pathogenetic role.

Psoriasis

It has long been known that psoriasis can be influenced by hormones. During pregnancy, the cutaneous manifestations frequently improve, but 15% of the cases can experience an exacerbation. After giving birth, more women report an exacerbation rather than an improvement of the cutaneous manifestations (20). In particular, generalized pustular psoriasis can be provoked by pregnancy or by the premenstrual phase (21). Researchers found that it is possible to trigger episodes of general pustular psoriasis through the experimental administration of

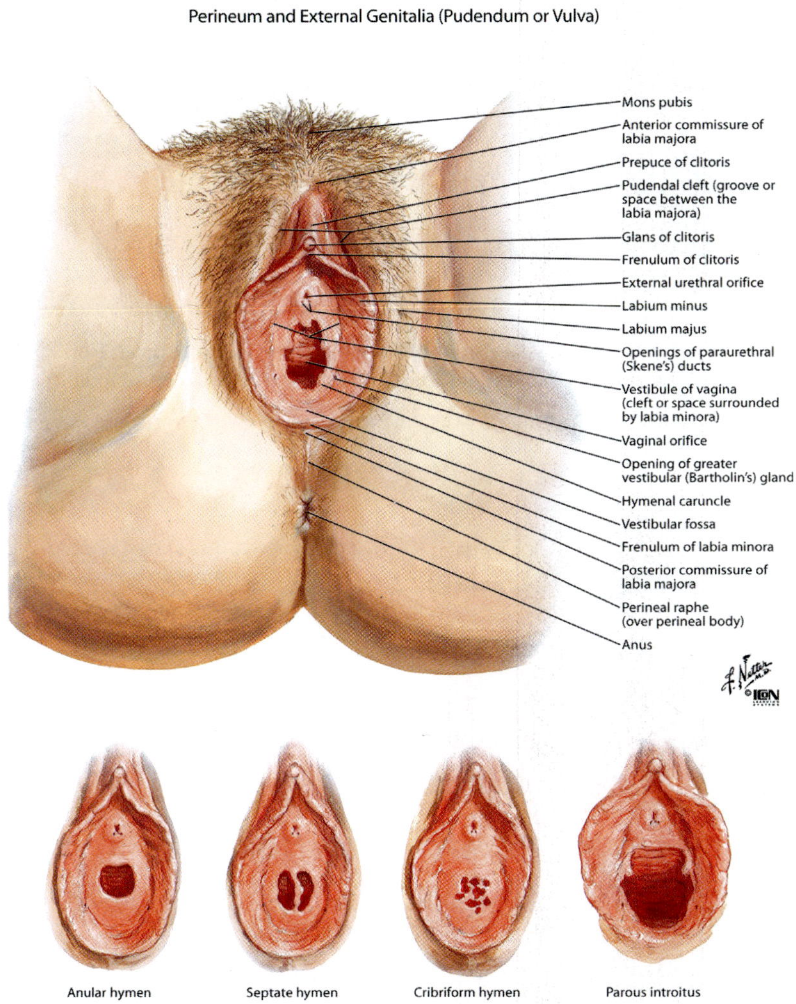

Anatomy of the adult vulva. *Source*: Courtesy of Elsevier.

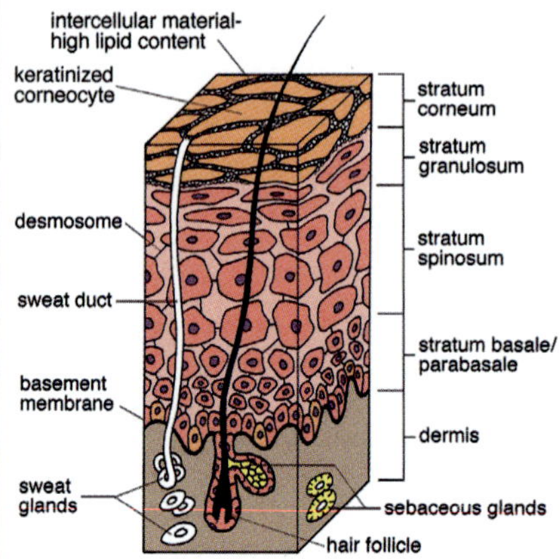

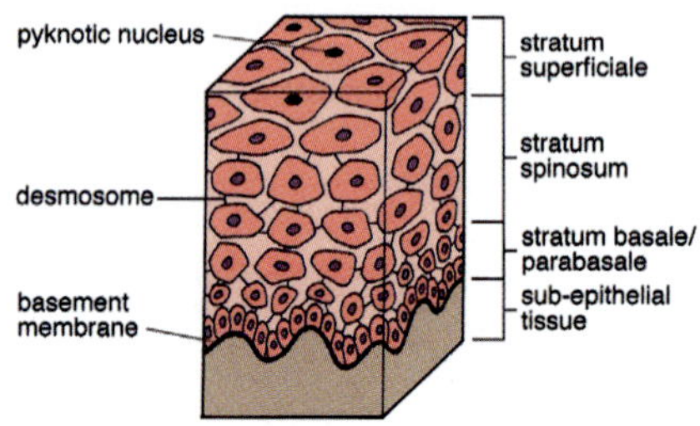

Figure 2.1 (*Left*) Epithelial structure of vulvar skin. *Source*: Adapted from Ref. 85.
Figure 2.2 (*Right*) Epithelial structure of the vulvar vestibule. *Source*: Adapted from Ref. 85.

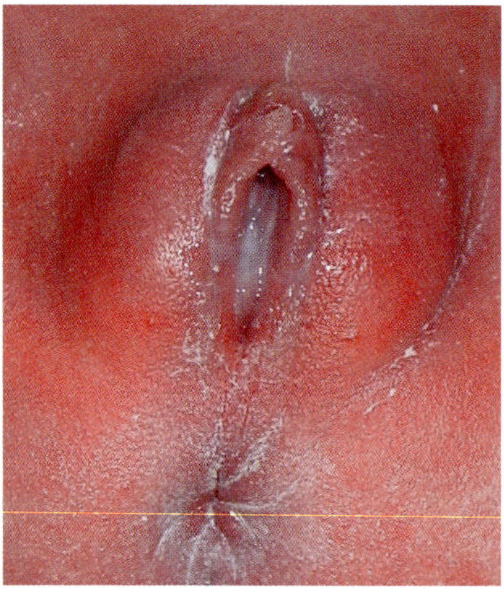

Figure 3.1 Anatomy of the newborn vulva.

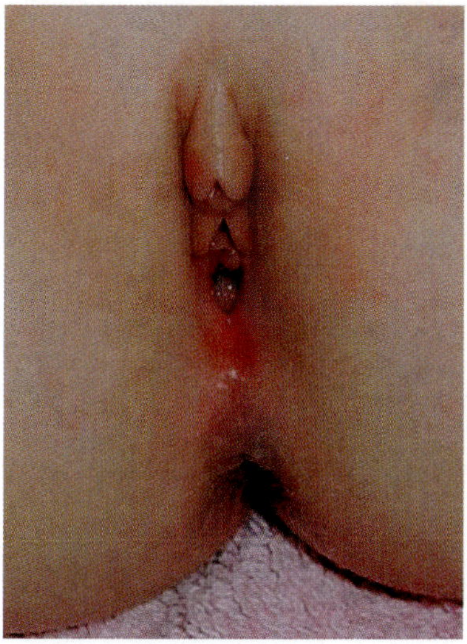

Figure 3.2 Anatomy of the prepubescent vulva.

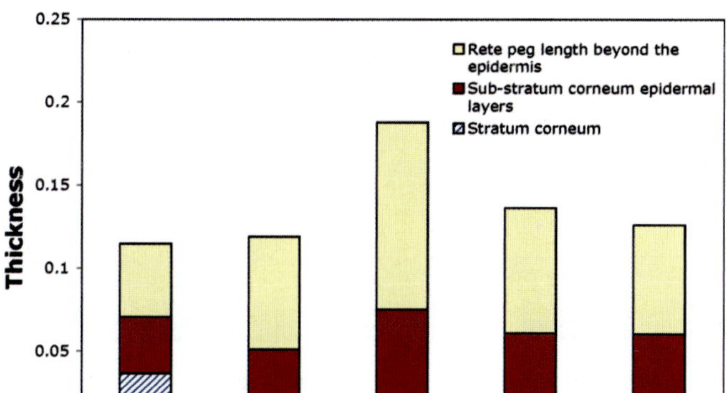

Figure 3.4 Epithelial thickness of labia majora with age. *Source*: Adapted from Ref. 7.

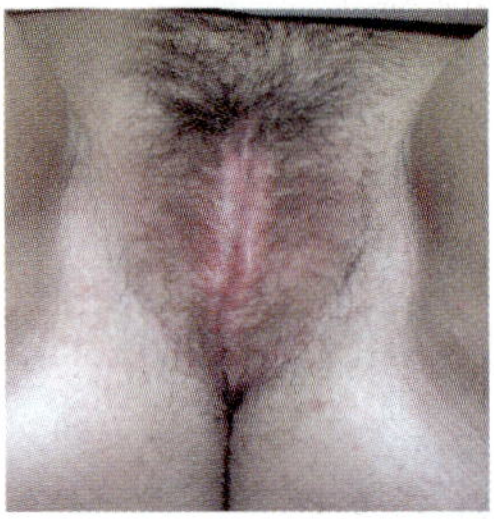

Figure 6.2

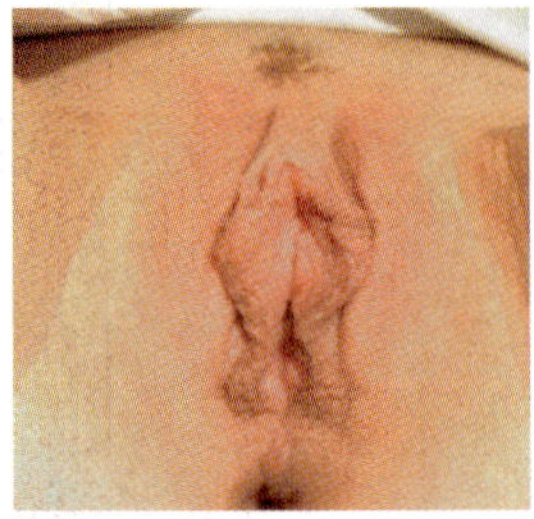

Figure 6.3

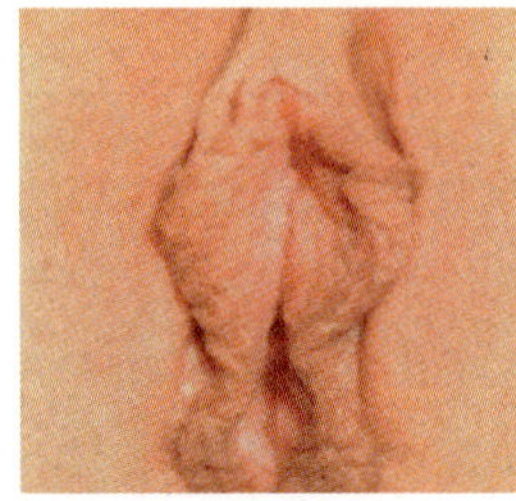

Figure 6.4

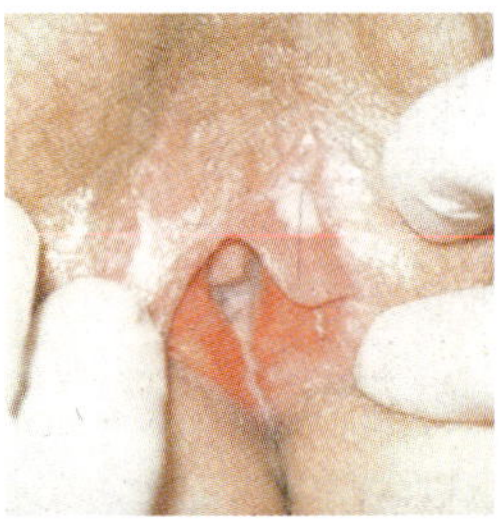

Figure 6.5

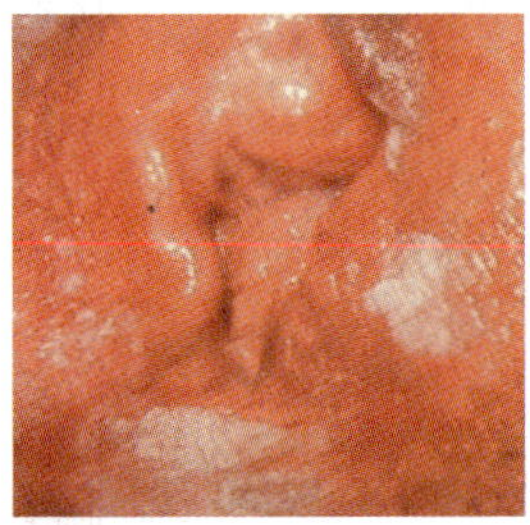

Figure 6.6

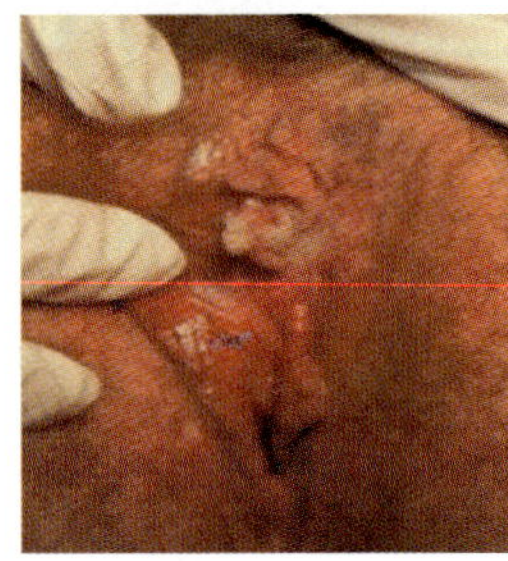

Figure 6.7

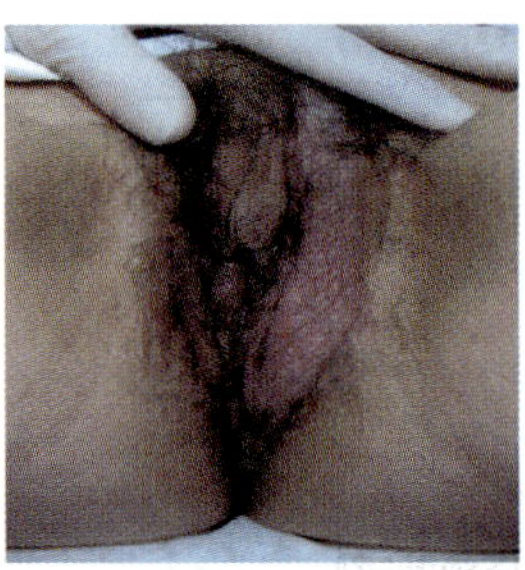

Figure 6.8

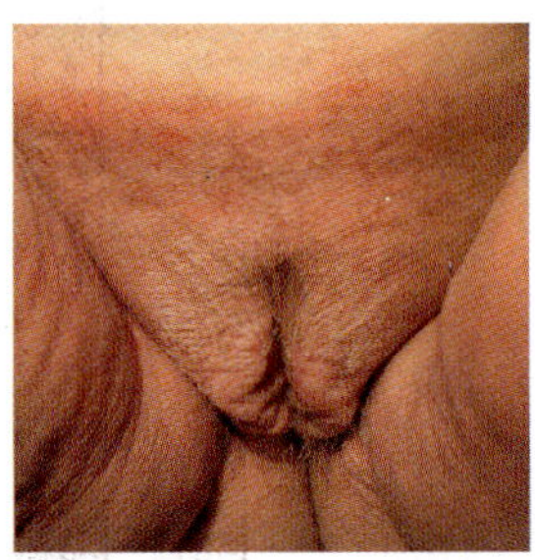

Figure 6.9

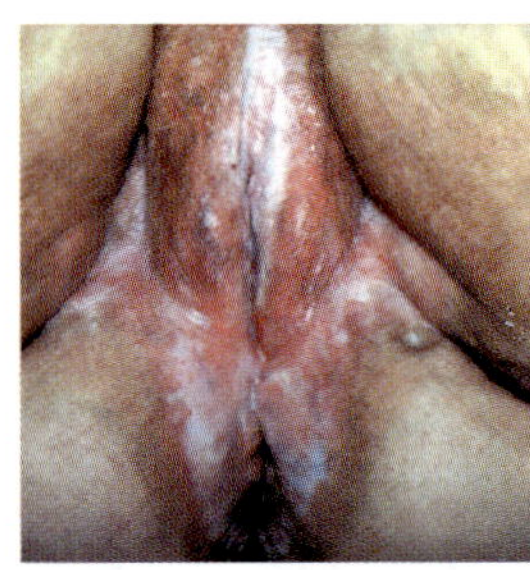

Figure 6.10

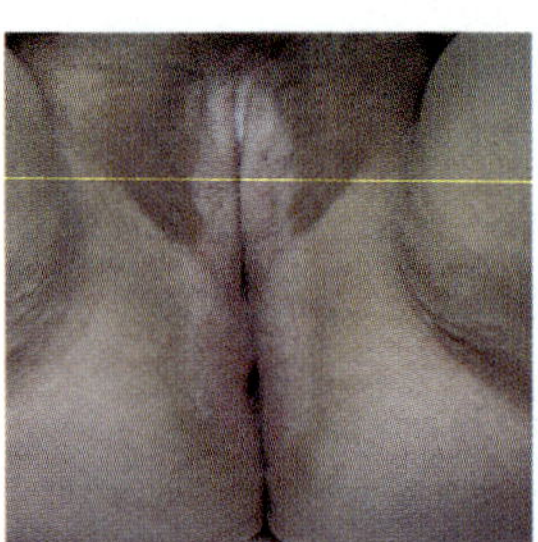

Figure 6.11

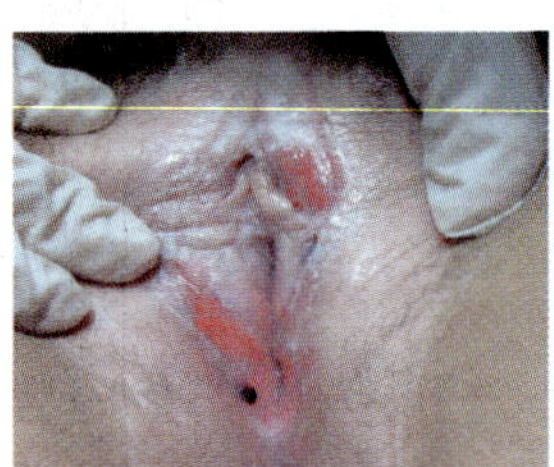

Figure 6.12

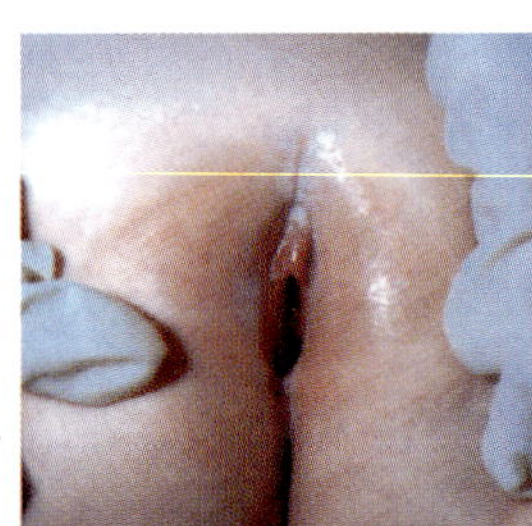

Figure 6.13

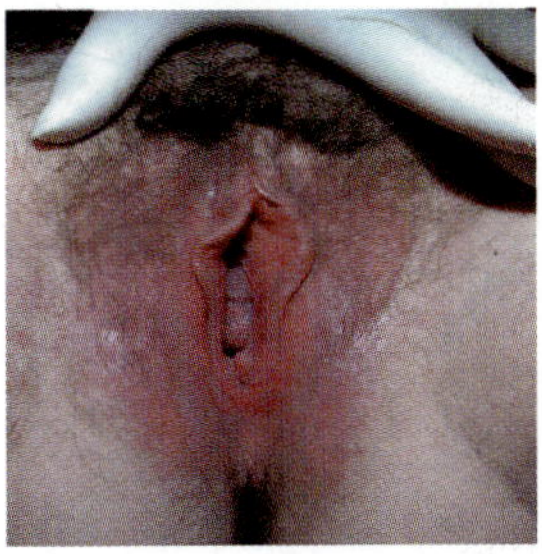

Figure 6.14

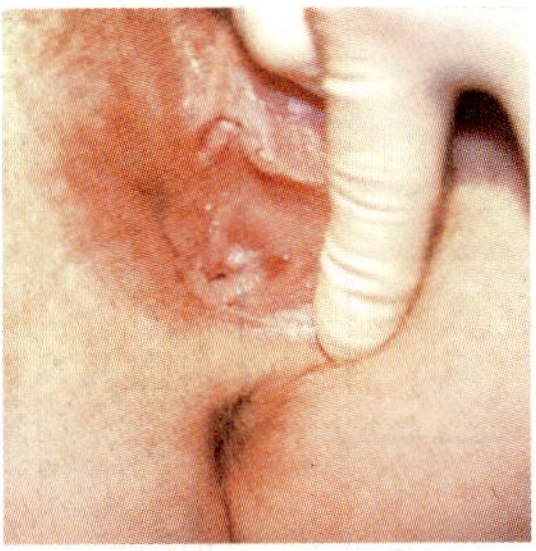

Figure 6.15

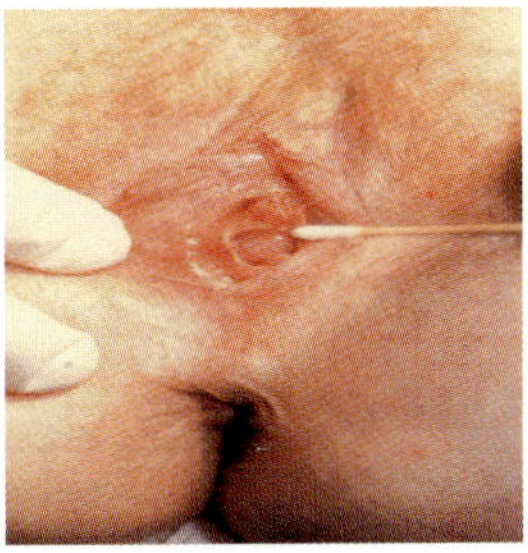

Figure 6.16

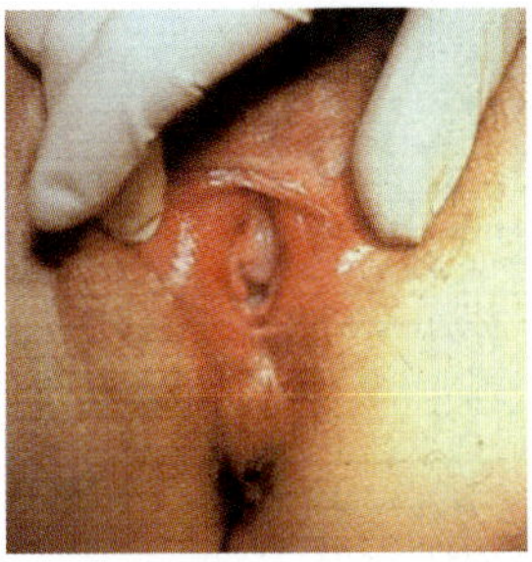

Figure 6.17

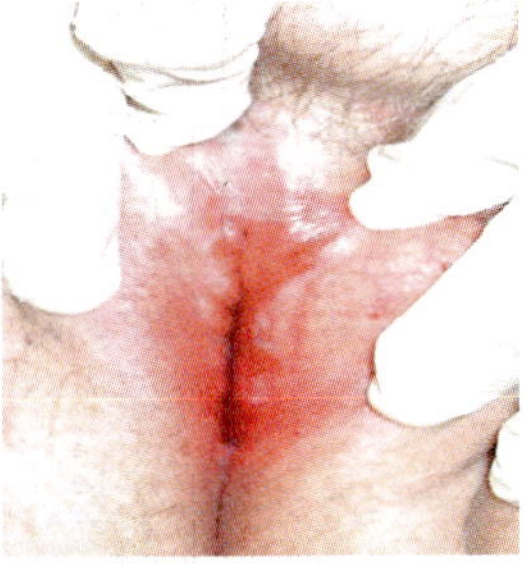

Figure 6.18

Figure 6.2 Contact dermatitis: uniform, well-demarcated erythema of the labia majora and labia minora.
Figure 6.3 Contact dermatitis: uniform erythema and edema of the labia minora and introitus (same patient as in Fig. 2).
Figure 6.4 Contact dermatitis: vulva is shaved, erythema is present in uniform distribution from daily pad wear.
Figure 6.5 Atrophic vaginitis: thin, pale erythematous tissue.
Figure 6.6 VIN I and II: acetowhite changes in the posterior fourchette and the left labia.
Figure 6.7 VIN III: periclitoral dysplastic disease.
Figure 6.8 Lichen simplex: hyperkeratosis and erythema of the left labia majora.
Figure 6.9 Lichen simplex: hyperkeratosis extending from the base of mons pubis to the labia majora bilaterally.
Figure 6.10 Lichen sclerosus: classic changes of lichen sclerosus of the vulva and perianal area in a postmenopausal woman, with areas of thin erythematous skin, white parchment paper-like skin in the perianal area, and thickened white skin.
Figure 6.11 Lichen sclerosus: vulvar and perianal changes of lichen sclerosus in a young woman.
Figure 6.12 Lichen sclerosus: vulvar examination of the same patient as in Figure 10, with thin, erythematous skin and white hyperkeratotic skin.
Figure 6.13 Lichen sclerosus: changes of lichen sclerosus in the periclitoral area and medial aspects of the labia majora in a three-year-old girl.
Figure 6.14 Yeast vulvovaginitis: irregular border of erythema, edema of the labia minora, satellite lesions extending to the right thigh and the perianal area.
Figure 6.15 Vestibulitis: localized erythema in the left vestibule.
Figure 6.16 Vestibulitis: localized erythema in the right vestibule.
Figure 6.17 Vestibulitis: localized erythema in the right periurethral area.
Figure 6.18 Erosive lichen planus: erosive changes of the introitus.

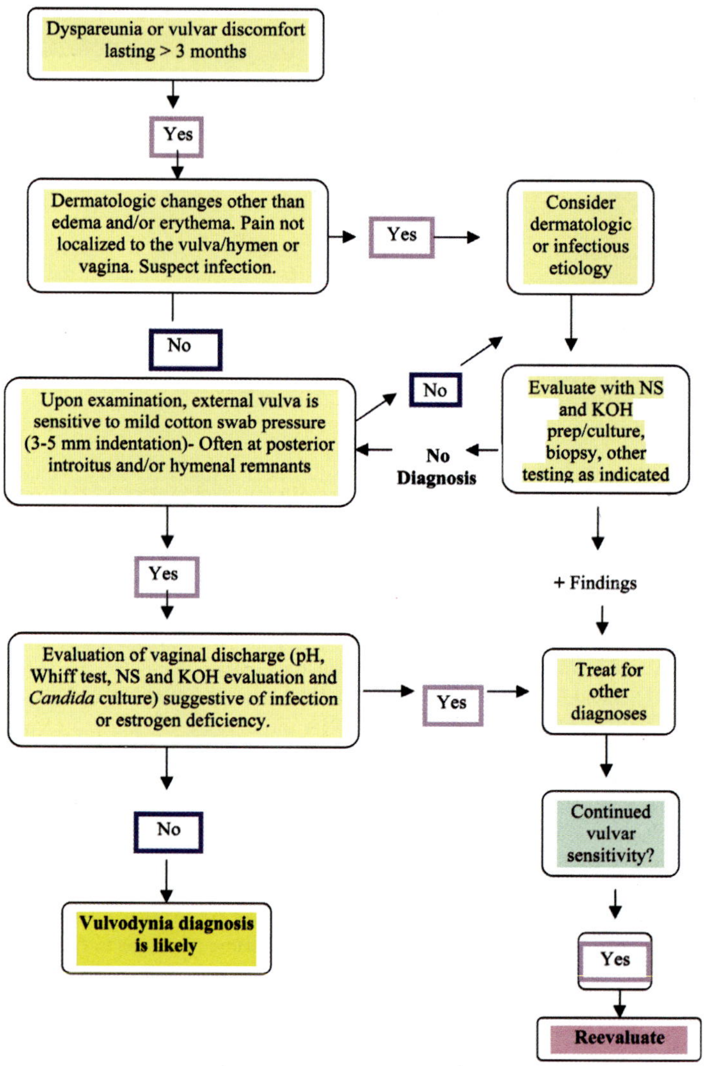

Figure 7.4 Diagnostic algorithm for vulvodynia. *Source*: From Ref. 47.

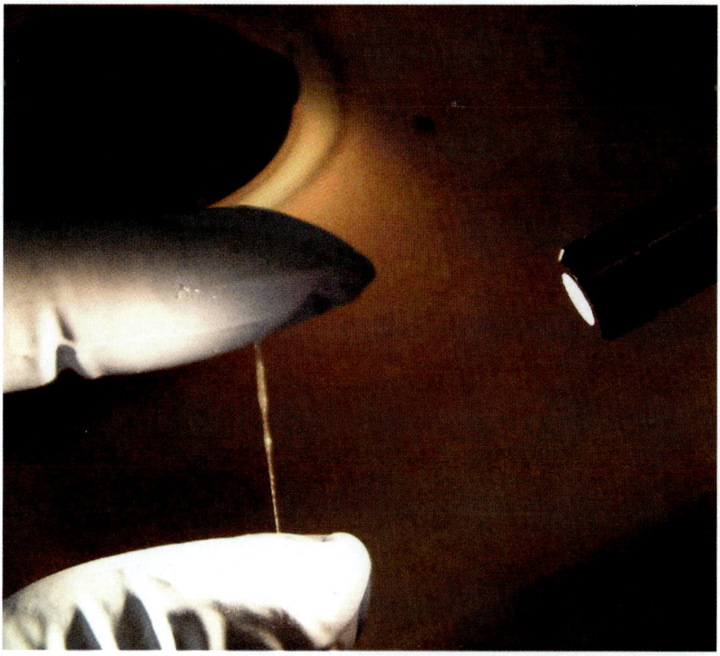

Figure 10.3 Spinnbarkeit test for menses elasticity.

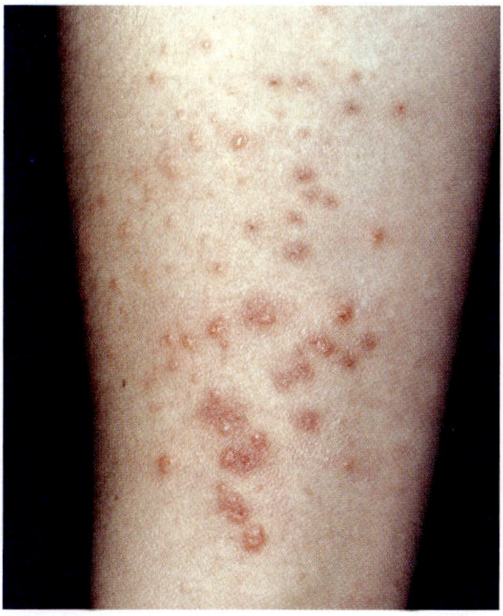

Figure 11.2 Autoimmune progesterone dermatitis, eczema type.

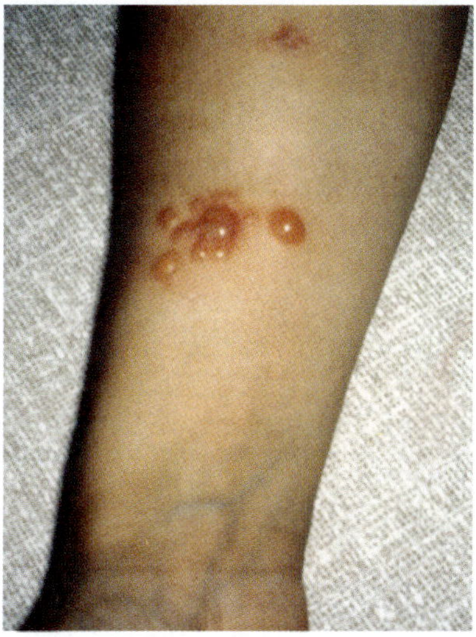

Figure 11.3 Autoimmune progesterone dermatitis, pompholyx type.

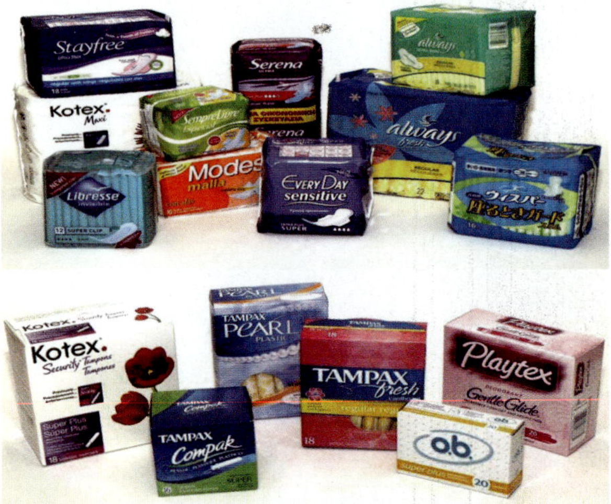

Figure 13.2 Examples of common menstrual protection products.

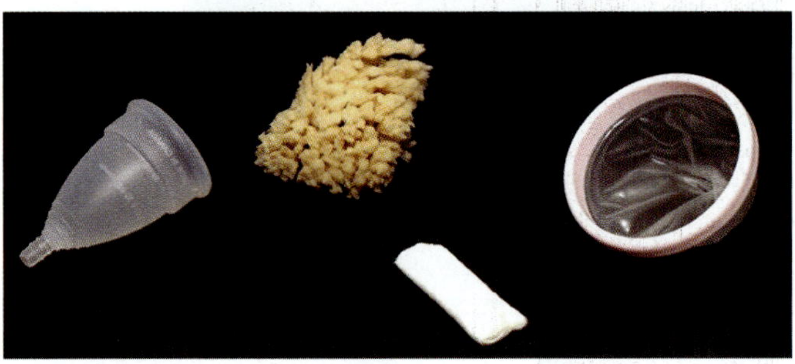

Figure 13.3 Examples of alternative menstrual protection (e.g., Diva Cup, sea sponges, Padette interlabial pad).

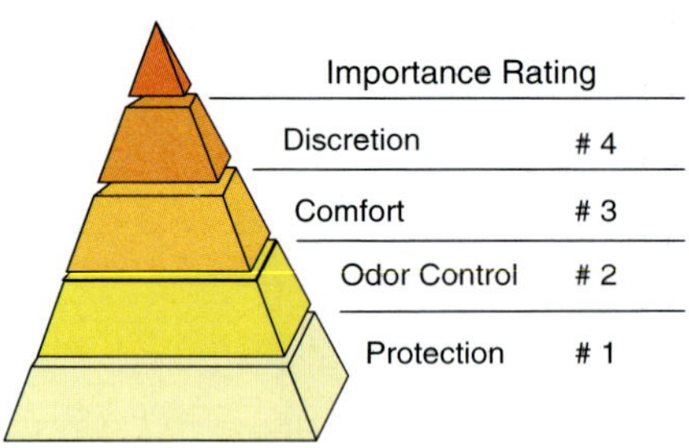

Figure 19.1 Factors of importance sought from a feminine hygiene pad. *Source*: Courtesy of Research International Agency.

progesterone and indirectly by the induction of ovulation by means of clomiphene (21,22). Thus, progesterone appears to play an important role pathogenetically, although the exact pathomechanism remains unknown.

Atopic Dermatitis

An exacerbation of the cutaneous symptoms of atopic dermatitis frequently takes place as a function of the menstrual cycle, although data on the cycle-associated exacerbation of atopic dermatitis vary widely (9–100%) (23,24). Some authors report an exacerbation of the skin condition during menstruation, whereas others report that the skin condition deteriorated approximately one week prior to the onset of menstrual bleeding (23,24). A study involving 286 Japanese women with atopic dermatitis found that 47% reported a monthly exacerbation of the cutaneous symptoms that were observed in 96% of the patients in the premenstrual phase (24). Only 4% reported a deterioration of the skin during menstruation. Interestingly, of all patients affected, a premenstrual deterioration of atopic dermatitis occurred along with other symptoms of PMS (14), such as headaches, a feeling of tenseness in the breasts, abdominal pain, edema of the legs, or psychological symptoms, such as irritability or depression. Another study also reported a significant correlation between a premenstrual exacerbation of atopic dermatitis and PMS and, again, the mechanism was unclear (23). Skin reactivity to antigens and irritating substances increases during the premenstrual phase (25,26); it is possible that the immunological influence of estrogen and progesterone mentioned previously plays a role in the pathogenesis of this disorder.

Aphthous Ulcerations and Herpes Simplex Labialis

In some women, the occurrence of relapsing aphthae of the oral mucous membrane is associated closely with the drop of progesterone in the luteal phase of the menstrual cycle. In these cases, a hormonal treatment with progesterone to suppress ovulation can be successful. The exact hormonal or immunological mechanism, however, again remains unknown (27).

Many women report a monthly eruption of herpes simplex infections, although relapses are not always strictly cycle dependent. Frequently, herpes simplex labialis can erupt both prior to or during menstruation (28), but there are also reports of eruptions in the preovulatory phase (29). Possibly, decreased IL-2 levels as well as an increase in TNF-alpha and IL-6 play a pathogenetic role (30).

Keratosis Follicularis (Darier's Disease)

The intensity of keratosis follicularis can vary in association with hormonal status. One study involving eight women found that the disease presented most often at the beginning of puberty and continued for years without interruptions.

Invariably, the cutaneous manifestations worsened during menstruation. In three patients, treatment with estrogen-containing oral contraceptives led to a marked improvement of the skin condition. Thus, it appears that higher estrogen levels improve the symptoms of keratosis follicularis (31).

Cyclic Vulvovaginitis, *Candida* Vaginitis, Pruritus Vulvae

Cyclic vulvovaginitis is marked by pain during certain cycle phases (luteal phase, perimenstrual phase), although the local findings are in most cases nonpathologic. In the final analysis, the genesis is again unclear, although the hypothesis of a hypersensitive reaction to *Candida albicans* is advanced frequently (32).

There have long been indications that the incidence of *Candida* vaginitis is hormone dependent (2,33). Thus, a *Candida* infection is observed more frequently in pregnant women than in nonpregnant women. The use of ovulation inhibitors, in particular, those with a high estrogen content, also increases the risk of an infection. In postmenopausal women who do not use estrogen replacement therapy, the incidence is low. Relapses of a *Candida* infection with pruritus vulvae occur frequently in the luteal phase prior to the onset of menstruation. Kalo-Klein and Witkin demonstrated an inhibition of the cellular immune response to *C. albicans* during this phase, which they attributed to variations in the progesterone and estradiol levels (33). However, even independent of the menstrual cycle, patients with relapsing *Candida* vaginitis were shown to have a reduced *Candida*-specific T cell reaction. In vitro, both a reduced T cell proliferation and a reduced interferon-gamma secretion were demonstrated after stimulation with *Candida* antigen (10). The immunological effects of progesterone and estrogen discussed previously influence the cycle-dependent occurrence of candida vaginitis. In addition, the presence of an estrogen-binding protein on *C. albicans* was demonstrated. It is via this estrogen-binding protein that the transformation of *C. albicans* into the invasive hyphal form is directly stimulated (10).

Lupus Erythematosus

A premenstrual exacerbation of the cutaneous manifestations of lupus erythematosus (LE) was described in 25% of patients with systemic LE (34) and in 13% to 16% of patients with discoid LE (34,35). There are several indications that estrogen is an important cofactor for the development or exacerbation of LE. This is corroborated by the facts that the disorder affects females predominantly, that it is well known that estrogen-containing oral contraceptives may cause an exacerbation, as well as by the described association of LE with Klinefelter syndrome. In an in vitro study, the administration of estrogen was shown to lead to an upregulation of the binding capacity of antiRo/SSA antibodies to keratinocytes (34).

It is hypothesized that in patients with LE, a changed estrogen metabolism with increased estrogen and decreased androgen levels acts as an etiopathogenetic cofactor. In conjunction with these suggestions, the physiologically increased premenstrual estrogen levels would lead to a perimenstrual exacerbation of LE (34).

Porphyria Cutanea Tarda

Porphyria cutanea tarda (PCT) is a defect of uroporphyrinogen decarboxylase that can be acquired or inherited through autosomal dominant transmission. This disorder becomes active only after additional liver-specific precipitating factors, such as alcohol, drugs, or viral infections (hepatitis, HIV) are present. Among the precipitating factors of hepatic porphyria, estrogens also play an important role; estrogen-containing contraceptives have been implicated in the manifestation of PCT in young women. It is known that all of these factors either inhibit uroporphyrinogen decarboxylase or lead to liver damage as a result of direct or indirect deposition of iron in the liver. Perimenstrual improvement of PCT has been explained by menstrual bleeding, which, similar to therapeutic bloodletting, leads to a reduction of iron (36).

Herpes Gestationis

Herpes gestationis (HG) is a rare pruriginous, blister-forming disorder that occurs, in most cases, in the second or third trimester of pregnancy (37). It can also occur in association with a cystic mole or a chorionic carcinoma (37). Both in pregnancy and in the presence of trophoblastic tumors, the immune system is confronted with foreign antigens of the sex partner, which may potentially play an important role in the pathogenesis of HG. In addition to a certain constellation of human leucocyte antigen (HLA) antigens in the mother and father, hormonal effects also have an important pathogenetic influence. For example, administering oral contraceptives with a high estrogen level to treat trophoblastic tumors cam exacerbate HG. Furthermore, the ovulation phase of the cycle may cause an exacerbation of HG, possibly because of estrogen's immunostimulating effects at certain concentrations (37). In most patients, however, an exacerbation of HG occurs more frequently in the premenstrual phase, possibly because of the steep decline of the high progesterone level prior to the onset of menstrual bleeding. The clinical activity of HG during pregnancy is also dependent on hormonal changes. In the last weeks of pregnancy, for example, when the progesterone level is high, there is a relative remission of the cutaneous manifestations, which are exacerbated immediately after delivery, when the progesterone level decreases markedly (37).

Dermatitis Herpetiformis

Although a report describing a premenstrual exacerbation of dermatitis herpetiformis was published in 1906 (38), the medical literature contains few reports that refer to the influence of the menstrual cycle on the activity of this disease.

Clinically, it is difficult to distinguish the perimenstrual exacerbation of dermatitis herpetiformis from an autoimmune progesterone dermatitis. The diagnosis must be based on histopathology, direct immunofluorescence, and the lack of evidence for an autosensitization to progesterone (39).

Autoimmune Progesterone Dermatitis

Autoimmune progesterone dermatitis (APD) is a rare skin disorder that is marked by relapsing cyclic eruptions during the luteal phase of the menstrual cycle when the serum progesterone level increases (40). Pathogenetically, an autoallergic reaction to endogenous progesterone is involved in APD, which can be demonstrated by a positive intracutaneous test reaction to progesterone. An allergic genesis of the skin disorder is also corroborated by a positive basophilic degranulation test following provocation with progesterone (41). Cutaneous manifestations can also be provoked by the intramuscular or oral administration of progesterone. Indirect immunofluorescence can detect progesterone antibodies in the serum of some women affected with APD. Ovulation-inhibiting drugs can suppress the clinical symptoms of APD (40).

There are several hypotheses concerning the mechanism of autosensitization. One is based on the assumption that the previous use of exogenous progesterone leads to the formation of antibodies, which, as a result of cross-reactivity with endogenous progesterone, subsequently leads to premenstrual cutaneous manifestations (4,42). However, not all women with APD have taken synthetic progesterone preparations previously. Alternatively, a cross-reactivity to steroids has been proposed as the mechanism of sensitization (4). The clinical morphological picture of APD is extremely variable (Figs. 2 and 3).

The cutaneous manifestations of APD include:

1. Eczema (42)
2. Erythema multiforme (42,43)
3. Urticaria (42,44)
4. Angioedema, anaphylaxis (1)
5. Pompholyx (42)
6. Stomatitis (45)
7. Dermatitis herpetiformis (39)
8. Erythema annulare centrifugum (46)
9. Prurigo simplex subacuta (41)
10. Nonspecific maculopapulous exanthemas (40)

However, the cutaneous manifestations differ neither morphologically nor histologically from the cycle-independent variants. One characteristic feature, however, is that they occur in the premenstrual phase. As a rule, the different manifestations of APD do not respond to conventional therapeutic regimens of the individual disorders. Treatment options include the use of conjugated estrogen-containing preparations, the ovulation-inhibiting antiestrogen

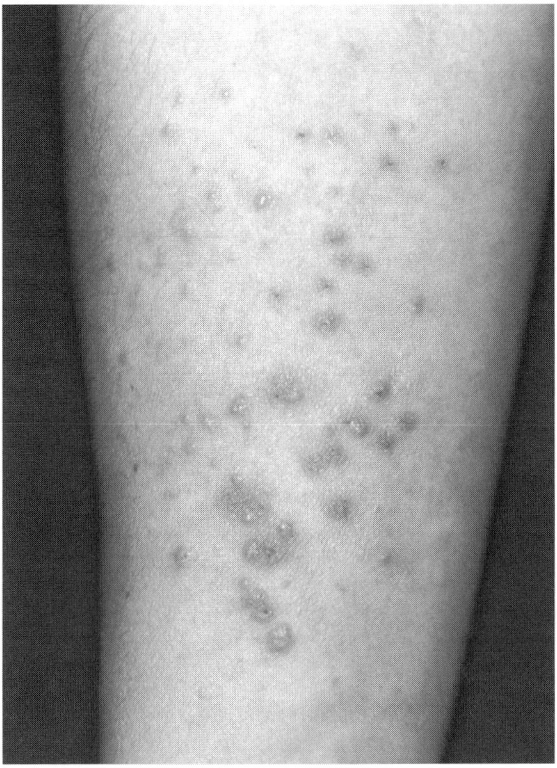

Figure 2 Autoimmune progesterone dermatitis, eczema type. (*See color insert p. 7.*)

tamoxifen, the androgen danazole (4,40), or—in severe cases—an elimination of the ovaries by bilateral oophorectomy or by administering buserelin, an analog of the GnRH (4,47).

Autoimmune Estrogen Dermatitis

Estrogen sensitivity also can imitate the clinical picture of APD. Clinical manifestations include papulovesicular exanthemas, eczemas, urticaria, and localized or generalized pruritus. The face, upper arms, and trunk are the regions affected principally, which may be attributable to an increased density of estrogen receptors in these regions. This disorder is considerably more rare than APD but, like APD, it is marked by the cyclic occurrence prior to menstruation (48). Murano and Koyano (49) described a patient in whom an exacerbation of the cutaneous manifestations occurred twice within the course of each menstrual cycle, i.e., premenstrually and at the time of ovulation. This can be explained by the two-peak course in the estrogen curve within the menstrual cycle. The diagnosis of autoimmune estrogen dermatitis can be corroborated by a positive

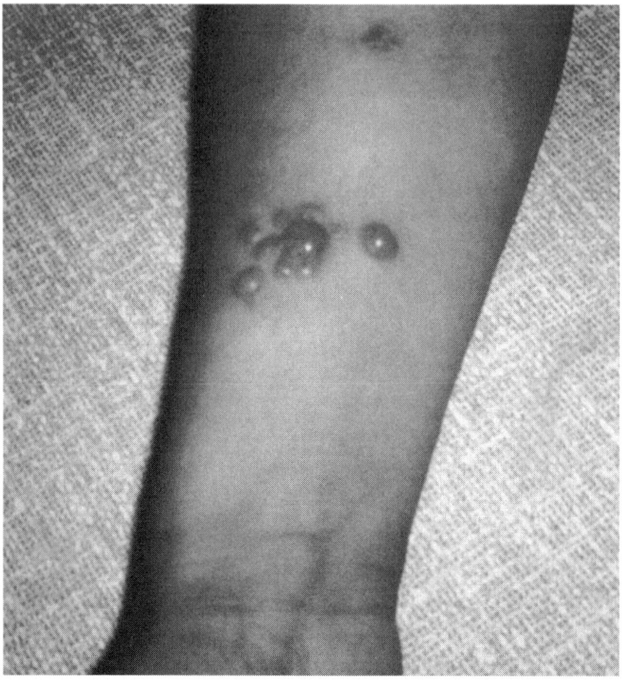

Figure 3 Autoimmune progesterone dermatitis, pompholyx type. (*See color insert p. 7.*)

intracutaneous test to estrogen; progesterone provocation will be negative. Treatment options include antihistamines, corticosteroids, tamoxifen, progesterone, and a surgical- or drug-induced elimination of ovarian function (48).

Hereditary Angioedema and Urticaria

Hereditary angioedema results from an inherited autosomal dominant deficiency or a functional defect of the C1 esterase inhibitor. A study to examine the influence of the steroid sex hormones found a positive correlation between the frequency of angioneurotic edema episodes and the serum progesterone level, with an increase in the incidence during the luteal phase of the menstrual cycle.

The mechanism by which progesterone influences angioedema is largely unknown. It has been hypothesized that progesterone influences the equilibrium between the coagulation and the complement cascade and, thus, enables the cleavage of the C1 esterase inhibitor by proteases. An inhibition of the synthesis of the C1 esterase inhibitor in the liver has also been discussed (50).

Wilkinson, et al. described a patient with relapsing urticaria in the premenstrual phase. In spite of the possibility of provoking such cutaneous manifestations by systemic progesterone or estrogen administration, it was not possible to demonstrate an immunological reaction to progesterone or estrogen either in the epicutaneous test or in the intracutaneous test. Therefore, it appears more likely that metabolic rather than direct autoimmunological mechanisms are responsible for triggering urticaria in the premenstrual phase. In predisposed women, independent of an autoimmunological reaction, progesterone-induced urticaria can be provoked by hormonally triggered changes in the immune system. There are indications that, as a result of a metabolic effect, increased progesterone levels in the premenstrual phase of the menstrual cycle can lead to an intensification of Type I and IV hypersensitivity reactions (51).

Contact Dermatitis and Skin Reactivity

Contact dermatitis can be exacerbated in the premenstrual phase. Alexander described a patient whose patch test of fragrance mixture led to positive results only in the premenstrual phase but was negative one week after menstrual bleeding (26). This can be explained by the suppression of the cellular immune response by estrogens mentioned previously (9). Considering the increased skin reactivity to contact allergens during the premenstrual phase, in special cases of premenstrual aggravated contact dermatitis, clinicians are advised to consider the phase of the menstrual cycle when interpreting the results of epicutaneous tests (25,26,51). In case of negative skin testing, the repetition of epicutaneous tests during the premenstrual phase might yield positive results.

CONCLUSION

Many skin disorders are associated with various phases of the menstrual cycle. Although there are many indications that female sex hormones influence the disease activity via both direct immunological and metabolic mechanisms, an examination of the relevant literature shows that in the final analysis, the pathogenesis of these cycle-associated changes can be explained only in very rare instances. With regard to potential therapeutic approaches, this topic should be the focus of further dermatological research.

REFERENCES

1. Snyder JL, Krishnaswamy G. Autoimmune progesterone dermatitis and its manifestation as anaphylaxis: a case report and literature review. Ann Allergy Asthma Immunol 2003; 90:469.
2. Schmidt-Matthiesen H, Hepp H. Gynäkologie und Geburtshilfe [Gynecology and Obstetrics]. 9th ed. Stuttgart, New York: Schattauer Verlag, 1998.
3. Thornton MJ. The biological actions of estrogens on the skin. Exp Dermatol 2002; 11:487.
4. Stephens CJM. Perimenstrual eruptions. Clin Dermatol 1997; 15:31.

5. Burton JL, Cartlidge M, Shuster S. Variations in sebum excretion during the menstrual cycle. Acta Dermatol Venereol 1973; 53:81.
6. Shah MG, Maibach HI. Estrogen and skin—an overview. Am J Clin Dermatol 2001; 2:143.
7. Eisenbeiss C, Welzel J, Schmeller N. The influence of female sex hormones on skin thickness: evaluation using 20 MHz sonography. Br J Dermatol 1998; 39:462.
8. Snell RS, Turner R. Skin pigmentation in relation to the menstrual cycle. J Invest Dermatol 1996; 47:147.
9. Myers JM, Butler LD, Petersen BH. Estradiol-induced alteration in the immune system. II: suppression of cellular immunity in the rat is not the result of direct estrogen action. Immunopharmacology 1986; 11:47.
10. Carrigan EM et al. Cellular immunity in recurrent vulvovaginal candidiasis. Clin Exp Immunol 1998; 111:574.
11. Harvell J, Hussano-Saeed J, Maibach HI. Changes in transepidermal water loss and cutaneous blood flow during the menstrual cycle. Contact Dermatitis 1992; 27:294.
12. McCausland AM, Holmes F, Trotter AD. Venous distensibility during the menstrual cycle. Am J Obstet Gynecol 1983; 84:640.
13. Charkoudian N et al. Influence of female reproductive hormones on local thermal control of blood skin flow. J Appl Physiol 1999; 87:1719.
14. Reid RL, Yen SSC. Premenstrual syndrome. Am J Obstet Gynecol 1981; 139:85.
15. Itsekson A et al. Premenstrual syndrome and associated skin diseases related to hypersensitivity to female sex hormones. J Reprod Med 2004; 49:195.
16. Williams M, Cunliffe WJ. Explanation for premenstrual acne. Lancet 1972; 10:1055.
17. Shaw JC. Low dose adjunctive spironolactone in the treatment of acne in women: a retrospective analysis of 85 consecutively treated patients. J Am Acad Dermatol 2000; 43:503.
18. Stoll S et al. The effect of the menstrual cycle on acne. J Am Acad Dermatol 2001; 45:957.
19. Lucky AW. Quantitative documentation of premenstrual flare of facial acne in adult women. Arch Dermatol 2004; 140:423.
20. Dunna SF, Findlay AY. Psoriasis: improvement during and worsening after pregnancy. Br J Dermatol 1989; 120:584.
21. Murphy FR, Stolman LP. Generalized pustular psoriasis. Arch Dermatol 1979; 115:1215.
22. Shelley WB. Generalized pustular psoriasis induced by potassium iodide. JAMA 1967; 201:1009.
23. Kemmett D, Tidman MJ. The influence of the menstrual cycle and pregnancy on atopic dermatitis. Br J Dermatol 1991; 125:56.
24. Kiriyama K, Sugiura H, Uehara M. Premenstrual deterioration of skin symptoms in female patients with atopic dermatitis. Dermatology 2003; 206:110.
25. Agner T, Domm P, Skouby SO. Menstrual cycle and skin reactivity. J Am Acad Dermatol 1991; 24:566.
26. Alexander S. Patch testing and menstruation (letter). Lancet 1988; 2:751.
27. Ferguson MM et al. Progesterone therapy for menstrually related aphthae. Int J Oral Surg 1978; 7:463.
28. Spruance SL. The natural history of recurrent oral-facial herpes simplex virus infection. Semin Dermatol 1992; 3:200.

29. Amann W. Mitteilung über präovulatorisches Auftreten von Herpes labialis [Preovulatory appearance of herpes labialis]. Hautarzt 1975; 26:47.
30. Mysliwska J et al. Lower interleukin-2 and higher serum tumor necrosis factor-levels are associated with perimenstrual, recurrent, facial Herpes simplex infection in young women. Eur Cytokine Netw 2000; 11:397.
31. Espy PD, Stone S, Jolly HW. Hormonal dependency in Darier disease. Cutis 1976; 17:315.
32. Paavonen J. Diagnosis and treatment of vulvodynia. Ann Med 1995; 27:175.
33. Kalo-Klein A, Witkin SS. Regulation of immune response to candida albicans by monocytes and progesterone. Am J Obstet Gynecol 1991; 164:1351.
34. Yell JA, Burge SM. The effect of hormonal changes on cutaneous disease in lupus erythematosus. Br J Dermatol 1993; 129:18.
35. Rowell NR, Goodfield MJD. The connective tissue diseases. In: Champion RH, Burton JL, Ebling FJG, eds. Textbook of Dermatology. Oxford: Blackwell Scientific Publications, 1992:2163.
36. Nishioka E et al. Porphyria cutanea tarda with menopausal exacerbation: the possible role of menstruation as natural phlebotomy. J Am Acad Dermatol 2003; 49:547.
37. Holmes RC et al. Clues to aetiology and pathogenesis of herpes gestationis. Br J Dermatol 1983; 109:131.
38. Buckley LD. The Influence of the Menstrual Function on Certain Diseases of the Skin. New York: Rebman, 1906.
39. Leitao EA, Bernhard JD. Perimenstrual nonvesicular dermatitis herpetiformis. J Am Acad Dermatol 1990; 22:331.
40. Herzberg AJ, Strohmeyer CR, Cirillo-Hyland VA. Autoimmune progesterone dermatitis. J Am Acad Dermatol 1995; 32:333.
41. Hoischen W, Steigleder GK. Überempfindlichkeit gegen Progesteron bei Prurigo mit prämenstrueller Exazerbation [Hypersensitivity to progesterone in prurigo with premenstrual exacerbation]. Dtsch Med Wschr 1966; 91:398.
42. Hart R. Autoimmune progesterone dermatitis. Arch Dermatol 1977; 113:426.
43. Wojnarowska F, Greaves MW, Peachey RD. Progesterone induced erythema multiforme. J R Soc Med 1985; 78:407.
44. Farah FS, Shbaklu Z. Autoimmune progesterone urticaria. J Allergy Clin Immunol 1971; 48:357.
45. Moghadam BK, Hersini S, Barker BF. Autoimmune progesterone dermatitis and stomatitis. Oral Surg Oral Med Oral Pathol Oral Radiol Endod 1998; 85:537.
46. Halevy S et al. Autoimmune progesterone dermatitis manifested as erythema annulare centrifugum. Confirmation of progesterone sensitivity by in vitro interferon-γ release. J Am Acad Dermatol 2002; 47:311.
47. Rodenas JM, Herranz MT, Tercedor J. Autoimmune progesterone dermatitis: treatment with oophorectomy. Br J Dermatol 1998; 139:508.
48. Shelley WB et al. Estrogen dermatitis. J Am Acad Dermatol 1995; 32:25.
49. Murano K, Koyano T. Estrogen dermatitis that appeared twice in each menstrual period. J Dermatol 2003; 30:719.
50. Visy B et al. Sex hormones in hereditary angioneurotic oedema. Clin Endocrinol 2004; 60:508.
51. Wilkinson SM, Beck MH, Kingston TP. Progesterone-induced urticaria—need it be autoimmune? Br J Dermatol 1995; 133:792.

12

Genital Hygiene: Culture, Practices, and Health Impact

Miranda A. Farage
Feminine Care Clinical Sciences, The Procter & Gamble Company, Cincinnati, Ohio, U.S.A.

Mario Bramante
Central Product Safety Services, Procter & Gamble Service GmbH, Schwalbach am Taunus, Germany

INTRODUCTION

Hygiene practices are affected by personal preference, cultural norms, and other societal influences. This chapter describes female genital hygiene from infancy to old age, with reference to regional and cultural differences in hygiene practices and to the potential implications for gynecological health.

GENITAL HYGIENE OF INFANTS

Vulvar Anatomy and Vaginal Discharge

The vulva of the newborn exhibits the effects of residual maternal estrogen. Immediately after birth, the labia appear swollen, and a white mucoid discharge is present for the first few weeks of infancy. The discharge is normal and can be cleansed by wiping gently from front to back with a damp washcloth, moistened cotton wool, or wipe. As the influence of the residual maternal hormones declines, slight blood spotting may occur because of endometrial bleeding caused by maternal estrogen withdrawal. These effects cease within three to four weeks of birth once the influence of residual maternal estrogen dissipates fully.

Labial adhesions sometimes occur in late infancy and in the toddler years, most often between the ages of about two months and two years. This condition, related to estrogen deficiency, creates a flat vulvar appearance that may elicit parental anxiety. Labial adhesions are usually asymptomatic and outgrown without the need for treatment. Occasionally, urinary tract or vulvovaginitis symptoms result if there is blockage of the free flow of urine. In this event, topical estrogen is used to promote the separation of the labia.

Diaper Dermatitis

Managing incontinence is the principal urogenital hygiene challenge in infants. Global diapering practices vary: disposable paper diapers are used widely in Western industrialized countries; typically, cloth is used in the developing world.

Prolonged genital skin contact with urine and feces can cause irritant dermatitis on the vulva, the perineum, and the buttocks of the diapered skin (diaper rash). The etiology is multifactorial (Fig. 1) (1–6). In brief, prolonged contact with urine increases skin wetness and skin pH, making the skin vulnerable to damage by friction and local irritants. Wet, occluded skin has a higher coefficient of friction and is more vulnerable to damage from abrasion (6,7). Urinary ammonia, however, is not a primary irritant, as once thought (8,9). Ammonia produced by bacterial action on urea increases the local pH; this, in turn, disturbs the normal acid mantle of the skin, impairs skin barrier function (10), elevates the activity of fecal enzymes that compromise skin integrity (2,5,10), and reduces the acid inhibition of microbial pathogens that cause secondary infections on the compromised skin. Accelerated gastrointestinal transit also raises fecal enzyme activity resulting in more frequent diaper dermatitis after bouts of diarrhea (11).

The etiology of irritant diaper dermatitis provides a scientific basis for recommending the use of barrier preparations and superabsorbent diapers to maintain drier skin and limit the effects of urine and feces (12–15). These recommendations are supported by clinical evidence of efficacy in reducing rash (16–24). Figure 2 illustrates representative results for diapers. However, such products are not always available or affordable in many regions of the world. To limit contact with skin and contact with urine and feces, frequent diaper changes and good perineal hygiene are recommended as a general practice, regardless of the mode of diapering.

GENITAL HYGIENE AMONG PREMENARCHAL GIRLS

General Hygiene

Poor vulvar hygiene may lead to the accumulation of smegma, a pasty agglomeration of epithelial cells and sebum that collects in moist areas of the genitalia such

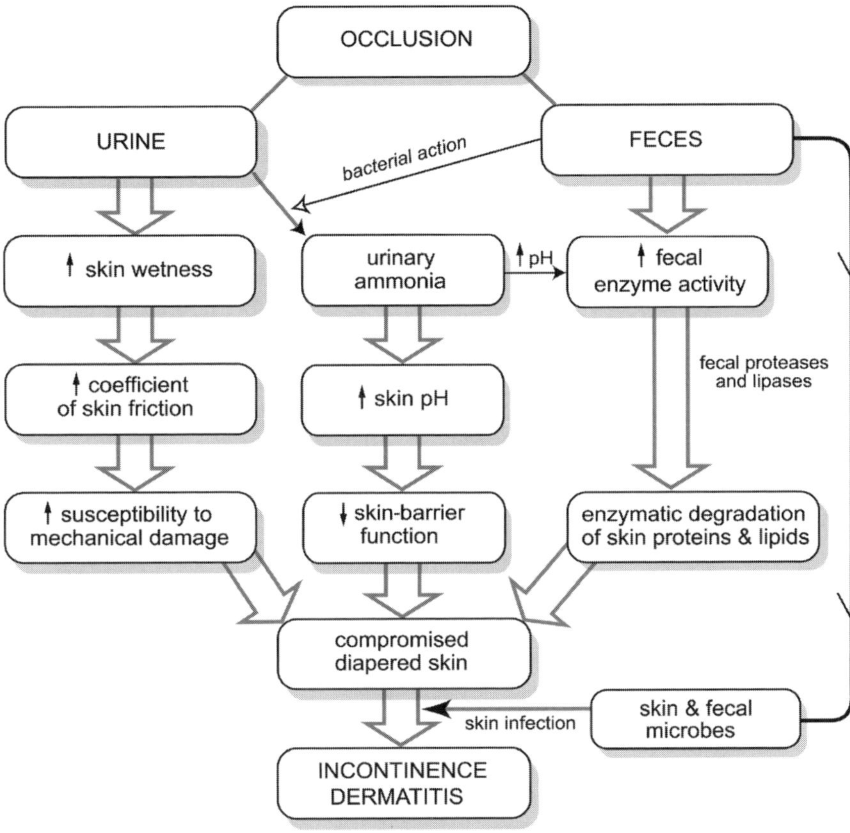

Figure 1 The etiology of diaper dermatitis (diaper rash) in infants. *Source*: Adapted from Refs. 1–6, 10, 189.

as the clitoral folds. Smegma hardens over time, causing itch or pain often exacerbated by scratching. Routine gentle washing of the vulva prevents this condition.

Toilet Habits

Maintaining proper toilet habits and perineal hygiene in young girls can be a challenge when parental supervision is first withdrawn. To avoid vulvar contamination with fecal material, young girls should be taught to consistently wipe from front to back after toileting.

Common sense dictates that establishing good hygiene habits is desirable and healthful, but research on the contribution of hygiene to premenarchal vulvovaginitis has produced mixed results. A case study of 54 patients, drawn from a North American population of low socioeconomic background, concluded that most noninfectious cases of vulvitis in young girls were caused by improper

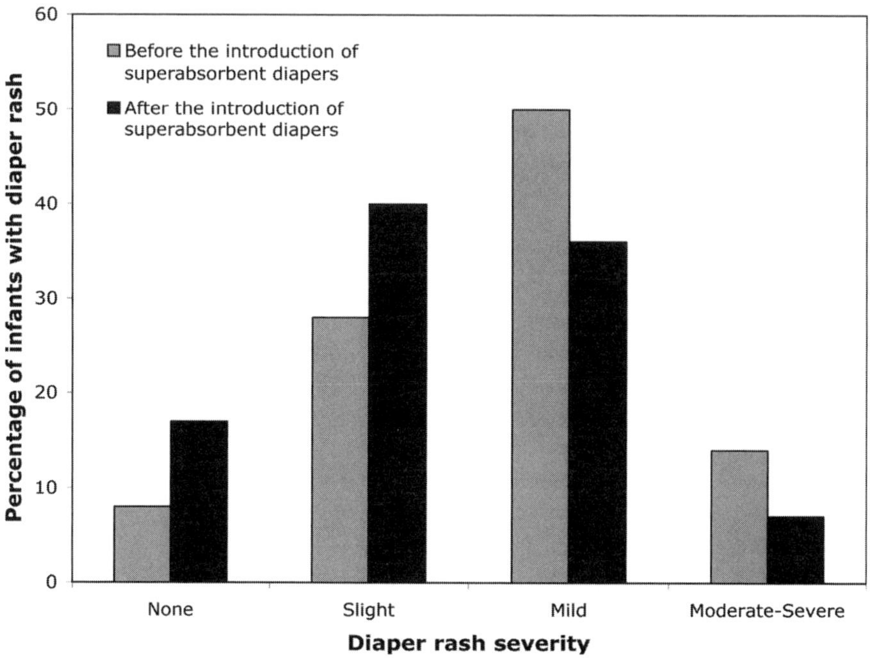

Figure 2 Changes in diaper rash severity before and after the introduction of superabsorbent disposable diapers. *Note*: Data represent the aggregate rash frequency and severity from (*i*) six clinical studies conducted between 1984 and 1988, involving 1850 infants (prior to the introduction of superabsorbents) and (*ii*) six clinical studies conducted between 1988 and 1995, involving 1975 children (after the introduction of superabsorbents). *Source*: Adapted from Ref. 15.

perineal hygiene (25). Only cases with visible inflammation and discharge were confirmed to be of infectious origin. Complaints of vulvitis with no infectious cause were judged to be hygiene-related based either on the clinical observation of stool or smegma or on the resolution of symptoms with improved hygiene and toilet practices.

Conversely, an Australian case-control study of pediatric vulvovaginitis (50 per group) found no difference in personal hygiene habits, consistent with these researchers' empirical experience that most premenarchal girls with vulvovaginitis exhibit good hygiene (26). Because most cases of pediatric vulvitis in this study were neither infectious nor attributable to improper hygiene, the investigators postulated that vulvitis of nonspecific etiology may be common in early childhood.

An alternative hypothesis was proposed by a different group of Australian investigators, who examined 130 young girls with vulvar complaints and determined that the majority had a dermatologic condition of the vulva (irritant or atopic dermatitis, psoriasis, or lichen sclerosus) (27). Poor hygiene was infrequently causative. These researchers proposed that most pediatric vulvar complaints of "nonspecific" etiology may be the result of undiagnosed dermatological conditions (28).

These disparate conclusions probably reflect the demographic differences in the populations from which the study participants were drawn. Inadequate hygiene may contribute to pediatric vulvovaginitis in some groups of patients, whereas when hygiene practices are adequate, other factors may predominate among those with vulvar complaints.

Fecal contamination of the vulva and perineum in young children is not always due to improper hygiene, but can result from fecal overflow around rectal blockage caused by constipation. This often unrecognized cause of fecal soiling is a precipitating or perpetuating factor in recurrent urinary tract infections (UTIs) in young girls. Because the anus and the urethra are closer in premenarchal girls than in mature women, poor hygiene and toilet practices are often emphasized as a primary contributing factor. However, vulvar hygiene does not play a singular role. The most important risk factors for recurrent UTIs unrelated to physical abnormalities are a combination of:

1. Infrequent voiding
2. Inadequate fluid intake
3. Stool retention due to constipation

Inadequate hygiene and toilet habits usually coexist with these variables (29).

Vaginal foreign bodies, a relatively uncommon result of improper toilet practices by the young girls, cause a foul-smelling, occasionally brown or blood-tinged discharge. Bits of cloth or toilet paper, deposited when the child wipes herself after urinating, are the most common culprits. These can be removed with cotton swabs or by vaginal irrigation.

Pinworm Infestation

Inadequate hygiene plays a role in rectal infestation of pinworm (*Enterobius vermicularis*), a common worldwide nuisance in children. The condition causes an intense vulvovaginitis with discharge in up to 20% of afflicted girls (30). Among the risk factors identified in urban and rural regions worldwide are overcrowded schools, day-care settings or dwellings, improper sanitation, lack of handwashing after toileting and before meals, and inadequate water supplies (31–35). Rectal itching that worsens at night (when the female emerges to lay eggs) is the primary symptom. Scratching spreads the eggs to other parts of the child's environment. To eradicate the infection effectively, the entire family must be treated at the same time, with scrupulous attention to cleaning of bedding, clothes, bathrooms, and surfaces in the home. Similar action should also be undertaken at the site of acquisition.

Genital Autoinoculation with Pathogens

Secondary infections of the genitalia resulting in vulvovaginitis can occur when a child inoculates herself with organisms from an upper respiratory tract, pharyngeal, or skin infection. The most common organism is the Group A β-hemolytic streptococcus (28,30,36). Vaginal discharge should be cultured to determine whether a specific organism is involved. The discovery of sexually transmitted organisms points to sexual abuse.

Aberrant Hygiene Practices

Rare cases of aberrant genital hygiene practices in young girls have been reported in the North American medical literature (37,38). They involve three classes of behavior. The first is a ritualistic focus by the parent on invasive and sometimes painful inspection and washing of the child's genitalia. This may be related to parental suspicion of sexual abuse. The second is a form of Munchausen syndrome by proxy, whereby the parent repeatedly solicits medical intervention for perceived or fabricated genital problems in the child. The third is an overt form of abuse, usually by a male, involving the application of creams or ointments to the child's genitalia for the purpose of the perpetrator's sexual gratification. All three classes are forms of abuse requiring intervention, which may include referral of the child and the caregiver for treatment and, when appropriate, reporting to child protective services.

GENITAL HYGIENE AMONG WOMEN OF REPRODUCTIVE AGE

Menstrual Hygiene

In many cultures, menstruation is a taboo subject considered the private province of women (39,40). Theories abound about the historical and cultural underpinnings of this pervasive attitude. Perhaps, the link to reproduction and birth imbues the menstrual cycle with a certain mystique. Bleeding is usually a sign of injury: our ancestors may have viewed cyclical bleeding—without dying—as a supernatural event. The notion that blood flow carries a basic life principle, with both beneficial and harmful consequences, is powerful in some parts of the world (41,42). From the first century Rome to the 19th century England, menstruation was thought to render women periodically dangerous (43). In the 1920s, scientists reported isolating a lethal toxin from menses (44), a finding discredited in the 1950s as an artifact of bacterial contamination (45). As recently as 1985, a quarter of young Australian women believed that menstrual flow rids the body of wastes (46). This view is held by many cultures worldwide. Some orthodox religious traditions consider the menstruating woman to be spiritually unclean (46). Not surprisingly, therefore, social, cultural and religious norms influence menstrual hygiene practices profoundly.

Menstrual Hygiene in the Industrialized World

Habits and practices: The use of disposable sanitary pads, panty liners, and tampons is ubiquitous in Western industrialized countries. The cultural acceptance of disposable external and internal protection in industrialized nations evolved over time. Although invented in 1896, disposable sanitary pads were not successfully introduced to the North American market until 1921. Perhaps for cultural and economic reasons, for two more decades, some women still employed cloth rags to absorb menstrual flow, boiling them for re-use after each menstrual period (47).

In 1936, commercial tampons were introduced in the United States as "a civilized solution to the problem of sanitary protection" (48). In reality, tampons have been used in many cultures since ancient times (47,49). As early as the 15th century BCE, Egyptian women used soft papyrus. Ancient Japanese women made tampons from paper and Roman women employed wool. Some nomadic Africans use absorbent material from indigenous mosses and plant seedpods and traditional Hawaiian women employ furry portions of native ferns. Prior to the commercial introduction of tampons, the more avant-garde women in American culture used natural sea sponges cut to size or made their own tampons from tightly rolled surgical cotton (50).

In Western societies, tampons were initially controversial. The medical and popular literature between 1936 and 1966 cites concerns about the presence of a foreign body in the vagina, the potential for sepsis, and the impact on virginity and sexuality (47). Beginning with women's entry into the workforce during World War II and through the Women's Liberation Movement of the 1970s, tampons became more widely accepted for their convenience and for the increased freedom they provide to participate fully in the workplace, sports, and social activities.

Although product sales figures are available, surprisingly little published information exists on the present-day menstrual hygiene practices in developed countries. Available data indicate that a sizable proportion of women use tampons or tampons and pads in combination. A 1996 survey of 193 women from urban southeast Texas (mean age, 23 years) found that 48% of respondents used tampons exclusively, 19% used sanitary pads, 18% used pads and tampons in combination, and 10% used panty liners (Table 1) (51). Tampons were used intermenstrually by 13% of respondents. Tampons and pads were changed at least every six hours by a majority of women. About 95% reported washing their hands after doing so at least some or most of the time.

A 1999 survey of middle-class Californian women ranging in age from 18 to 96 indicated that tampon use declined from 80% among women younger than 41 years to 72% among menstruating women between the ages of 48 and 57 (Table 2) (52). The frequency of pad and panty liner use was similar in those younger than 41 years (71% and 75%, respectively) and those over 48 (73% and 78%, respectively). For unexplained reasons, the usage prevalence of use of all product types was lowest in the age group of 41 to 47. In the Texas study, 43% of respondents limited bathing during their menstrual period; in the California study, the proportion of women who reported limiting bathing during menstruation declined from 11% in the under 41 age-group to 4%

Table 1 Menstrual Protection Practices Among 193 Texan Women, Aged 18 and Older (1996)

	Percent prevalence					
Products and practices	Never	Sometimes	Half of the time	Most of the time	Always	Not reported
Tampons	11	15.5	11	12	48	2.6
Sanitary pads	24	30	11	12	19	2.6
Tampon/pad combinations	40	24	7	5	18	6
Panty liners	22	44	9	11	10	3.6
Tampons/pads/liners between periods	82	9	1	0.5	2	5
Washing hands after use	2	4	3.6	14	74	2.6
Limiting bathing during menstruation	70	9	4	2	10	9

Source: From Ref. 51.

among women aged 48 to 57. About half reported handwashing before using sanitary pads and 70% reported doing so after changing them.

About a quarter of American women begin using sanitary protection before their period starts and about one-third continue use for several days after flow ends. Panty liners are the most common product choice for intermenstrual use, although all three forms of protection are reportedly employed before and after the menstrual period. Tampon use is prevalent among American adolescents

Table 2 Menstrual Protection Practices by Age Among 180 Middle-Class Californian Women (1999)

	Percent frequency		
Products and practices	<41 years old ($n = 180$)	41–47 years ($n = 171$)	48–57 years ($n = 83$)
Natural sea sponges	2	2	1
Reusable cotton pads	0	1	1
Tampons	81	63	72
Sanitary pads	71	61	73
Tampon/pad combinations	54	47	51
Panty liners	75	60	78
Tampons/pads/liners between periods	14	12	24
Wash hands after using	94	75	94
Limit bathing during menses	11	3	4

Source: From Ref. 52.

and young women. Surveys conducted in the 1990s indicate that 70% of adolescents and 81% of college students used tampons alone or in combination with pads (53,54). Mothers and friends were the most influential in determining the teenagers' choice of tampon use (54,55). Clinicians report that American girls are expressing an interest in tampons at an earlier age and that athletes are particularly eager to use tampons (56).

A Texas-based survey conducted in the late 1980s among Caucasian, African American, and Mexican American women indicated that significantly more Caucasian women used tampons alone (26%) or with pads (36%) than African American women (57). Proportionately, more African American women used tampons alone (16%) or with pads (27%) as compared to Mexican Americans, 11% of whom used tampons alone and 21% of whom used tampons with pads. In this study population, tampon use started in the teenage, but the highest usage frequency of tampon usage, either alone (26%) or with pads (33%), occurred in the age group of 20 to 29.

Published information on the number of menstrual products used annually is scarce. A toxicological risk assessment published by the Danish National Institute for Public Health and the Environment reported the average yearly consumption rates per user group as 325 menstrual sanitary pads, 598 panty liners, and 50 postpartum sanitary pads (58).

Health implications: The principal health concern related to tampon use is its association with menstrual toxic shock syndrome (TSS). TSS is a rare but recognizable and treatable disease (see Table 3 for signs and symptoms) (59). Women aged 15 to 24 are the highest risk group for menstrual TSS, with adolescents making up a significant proportion of cases (60,61). The reported incidence of menstrual TSS peaked in the early 1980s and has since declined significantly (60,62). All tampons are associated with a low risk for menstrual TSS; the risk is independent of chemical composition per se, but increases with tampon

Table 3 Signs and Symptoms of Toxic Shock Syndrome[a]

A sudden high fever (usually 102°F or higher)
Vomiting
Diarrhea
A rash that looks like sunburn
Dizziness
Muscle aches
Fainting or near fainting when standing up

[a]Five clinical criteria are fever, hypotension, rash, desquamation, and abnormalities in three or more organ systems. Desquamation may not be apparent with early treatment and discharge.
Source: From Ref. 59.

absorbency (63). Other hygiene practices, such as bathing frequency, douching, and the use of feminine deodorants, are not associated with menstrual TSS risk (64).

Although a full understanding of the pathogenesis of menstrual TSS is still being sought, one of the most important individual risk factors is whether a woman has serum antibodies to TSS toxin (65). Most women have substantial levels of antibody and are at low risk for the disease (60,66).

Today, millions of women use tampons safely. Physicians consider them a reasonable choice for girls and women who express a preference and are able to use them appropriately (50,56). Because young girls may be less aware of the risk factors for menstrual TSS, adolescent education is important. In the United States, statements on package inserts suggest that women use the lowest tampon absorbency required to absorb their level of flow; they may substitute tampons of lower absorbency or sanitary pads as their menstrual flow tapers. Beginners must remember to remove that last tampon: the forgotten tampon is the most common vaginal foreign body complaint in adolescents (67).

Tampons are regulated as medical devices by the U.S. Food and Drug Administration (FDA). The FDA recently promulgated revised nomenclature for tampon standardized absorbency labeling (Table 4) (68,69). The FDA recommends that tampons not be worn 24 hours a day, 7 days per week, but alternated with pad use (62). Although supporting scientific evidence is lacking, women are advised to change tampons often (every four to eight hours). Package inserts suggest that tampons can be used overnight up to eight hours.

In the European Union, where disposable tampons are regulated as "articles," the European Disposables and Nonwoven Association (EDANA) implemented a voluntary Code of Practice in 2001 that provides for a harmonized system of categorizing tampon absorbency throughout Europe and for package

Table 4 Tampon Absorbency Ratings (U.S. Food and Drug Administration)

Absorbency range in grams[a]	Descriptive term for absorbency
Less than 6	Light
6–9	Regular
9–12	Super
12–15	Super plus
15–18	Ultra absorbency
Above 18	None

[a]These ranges are defined, respectively, as follows: Less than or equal to 6 g; greater than 6 g up to and including 9 g; greater than 9 g up to and including 12 g; greater than 12 g up to and including 15 g; greater than 15 g up to and including 18 g; and greater than 18 g.
Source: From Refs. 68, 69.

inserts on TSS symptoms and safe tampon usage. The EDANA code of practice has been adopted by all major European tampon manufacturers.

Between 1977 and 1989, reports on vaginal ulcers associated with tampon use appeared in the medical literature (70–77). Most often associated with the prolonged use of superabsorbent tampons, these microlesions were typically asymptomatic and healed spontaneously. A more recent case involving prolonged use presented as intermenstrual bleeding (78). Ulceration can be avoided by choosing tampons with an appropriate absorbency and using the products as recommended (50).

In recent years, research on the health effects of sanitary pads has appeared in the medical literature. External sanitary protection is not generally associated with significant health concerns. An industry-sponsored series of prospective trials of pads and panty liners, conducted in North America and Europe between 1984 and 2003, found no evidence that modern products cause adverse gynecological effects, adverse dermatological effects on the vulva or perineum, or clinically meaningful changes in the isolation frequencies or cell densities of vaginal and vulvar microflora (79). The 12 separate trials included a cumulative total of 1600 adult and adolescent participants.

Anecdotal reports of contact dermatitis to pads exist (80–84). Such problems are usually transient, secondary to another condition such as a vulvar dermatosis or infection, or due to a preexisting sensitivity to perfume, raw materials, or adhesives (82–84). A woman who has a prior sensitivity to such materials may be unable to tolerate exposure from other sources; she should try an alternative version from the same product line or another brand.

Manufacturers avoid materials that induce contact sensitization by controlling the composition and quality of raw materials used in these products and by conducting toxicological risk assessments of the raw materials (85,86). Confirmatory, repeat insult patch testing prior to market introduction (87) and the use diagnostic patch tests both prior to marketing and in postmarket surveillance systems are important complements to the safety assurance process (79,88).

It has been suggested that pads may increase the risk of UTIs by transferring intestinal flora such as *Escherichia coli* to the vulva (50). No meaningful evidence exists for this hypothesis. Because enteric microbes often reside on the perineum and external labia majora in the absence of the introital or the urethral colonization, their mere presence is not a risk factor for infection (89–91). The most important risk factor for recurrent UTI in women of reproductive age is sexual intercourse (92,93), which promotes colonization of the introitus and the urethra with uropathogenic *E. coli* in susceptible women (94,95). Host factors play a major role in determining individual susceptibility to this disease (96–98). Clinical trials in women wearing pads under a variety of conditions have failed to show a clinically significant change in genital microbial populations associated with their use (79).

It is also postulated that external sanitary pads and liners, nylon underwear, pantyhose, and tight clothing may trap heat and moisture in the genital region, creating an environment for yeast to multiply. Several epidemiological studies assessed a possible link to vulvovaginal candidiasis (VVC), but the weight of the evidence fails to support the theory (99). For example, two retrospective case–control studies involving University students (one with 157 and the other with 1300 participants) found no association of VVC with tight-fitting clothing, synthetic fabric underwear, panty hose, type of menstrual protection, or pad use between periods (100,101). A prospective study of 163 sex workers found no link between recurrent VVC and tight clothing or synthetic underwear (102), and a survey of perianal colonization with *Candida* species, a potential reservoir for urogenital recolonization, found no correlation between recurrent VVC and the use of tight-fitting trousers or synthetic fabric underwear (103).

A recent study linked patient-reported and nonlaboratory confirmed cases of recurrent VVC in women on the maintenance antifungal therapy with wearing panty liners in the same week or in the week before an episode (104). Statistical associations suggesting a temporal link to panty liner use are fraught with confounding factors. For example, patient-reported diagnoses are unreliable and diagnoses based solely on signs and symptoms can be inaccurate in 50% to 70% of the time (105,106). Moreover, panty liner use may be temporally (though not causally) linked to urogenital infections, because absorption of vaginal discharge is a common reason for using these products. Moreover, panty liners are worn in anticipation of the onset of menses; because patients often report an exacerbation of VVC symptoms just prior to menstruation, this temporal coincidence could contribute to a spurious statistical association. Panty liner use to absorb postcoital discharge may also result in a noncausal association with VVC, because monthly intercourse frequency, intercourse frequency in the weeks preceding infection, and oral intercourse frequency in the month prior to infection have been associated with both episodic and recurrent cases (101,107,108).

Prospective, examiner-blind clinical trials in the general population failed to show a connection between panty liner use and an increased risk of vulvovaginal infection. An industry-sponsored, six-month, prospective clinical trial involving 204 women comparing daily panty liner users to nonusers found no increase in the prevalence of vaginal or vulvar colonization with *Candida* species and no evidence for symptomatic infection based on culture results (109). A trial comparing the microbiological effects of daily use of thick and ultrathin menstrual pads for two months led to the same conclusion (110).

Menstrual Hygiene in the Developing World

In the developing world, cloth and household absorbent materials (cotton wool, tissue, gauze) are often used for menstrual protection, particularly in the rural areas and among economically disadvantaged groups. Economic factors favor the use of reusable cloth. Moreover, in many cultures, girls are committed to the traditions and practices learned from their mothers and other female relatives.

Traditional beliefs also discourage the use of tampons. For example, the notion that unimpeded blood flow is related to good health permeates many indigenous cultures worldwide (41,42,111,112). Such traditions hold that the menstrual flow is necessary to rid the body of toxins and to dispel unclean substances introduced by intercourse.

Finally, pervasive taboos exist against revealing that one is menstruating. This can discourage the use of disposable pads or tampons, as well as participation in household and social activities. Some traditional religious cultures segregate women during the menstrual period and women undergo ritual cleansing after flow ceases.

Habits and practices: In Latin America, rural women typically use cloth for menstrual protection. Because the woman washes the cloth herself, she believes that she maintains good hygiene and gains control against revealing odor and infection. Cloth is both economical and reusable, an advantage for those with limited disposable income. Moreover, cultural taboos exist against disposing of blood-soaked materials; hence, discreet washing and reusing of cloth are the most acceptable practices. Less traditional women who choose disposable protection may choose cotton wool, tissue, or gauze instead of cloth, because they consider these materials more economical than commercial products and because they are readily available in the home.

Among schoolgirls in India, mothers, female relatives, textbooks, and magazines are principal sources of menstrual information (113–115). Schools are a source of information less frequently than in the United States (116). Rural Indian girls' understanding of menstrual physiology is quite rudimentary (113,114,116). The use of cloth as a menstrual absorbent predominates among urban and rural schoolgirls; urban girls cite lack of confidence as the main reason for not choosing commercial pads. Menstrual absorbents are typically washed or disposed of in the Dhoby (a pond or river bank used for public laundry) or in a canal. Girls take special baths to promote hygiene and may consume certain foods to promote menstrual flow and, therefore, good health.

It is impossible to generalize about African practices because traditional customs and attitudes vary among sub-Saharan communities (42). For example, traditional Nigerian culture does not encourage family discussions of sexuality. A study involving 352 schoolgirls found that a large proportion were inadequately informed about menstruation, although girls whose parents had at least secondary school education had received instruction on menstruation and hygiene from their parents (117). Half the girls used tissue paper as absorbent; 22% used sanitary pads, 12% used cloth, and 3% used tampons.

In traditional Zimbabwean society, menstruation is associated with desires of the flesh and is considered spiritually unhygienic (112). At menarche, a girl first informs her grandmother of the event, who then informs the mother. Cloth or cotton wool is used commonly to absorb menses, and it is the grandmother who teaches the girl how to prepare her pads and pleat them so they will not show. Women with higher levels of education understand menstrual cycle physiology; less educated women view menstruation as an occurrence that signals the ability to bear children, cleanses the system, and helps maintain a trim abdomen. Menstruating women refrain from intercourse.

In China, menstrual practices are influenced by the concept of Yin and Yang (118). Yin, the negative female force, represents darkness, coldness, and emptiness. Yang, the positive male force, promotes light, warmth, and fullness. These opposing forces must be balanced for health and harmony to prevail. The most symbolic blending of Yin and Yang is the union of wife and husband.

Because sexuality is a taboo subject in traditional Chinese culture, menstrual information is not discussed proactively. However, strict behavioral norms are imparted once girls reach menarche: "hot" Yang foods are eaten to strengthen the body and "cold" Yin foods are avoided. Similarly, hair should not be washed, as it induces cold.

Urban Chinese women typically use commercial sanitary pads for menstrual protection. Tampons are commercially available; however, some Chinese clinicians express a concern that tampons may promote cervical ectopy. In the Chinese medical paradigm, cervical ectopy is traditionally viewed as "chronic cervicitis," an ulceration or erosion of the ectocervix thought to predispose women to infection. Western culture considers cervical ectopy a physiologically normal, hormonally regulated phenomenon that regresses with age (119–121).

Cloth is used in rural parts of China (122). Women wash the cloth and reuse it repeatedly, but for traditional reasons, never dry the cloth in the sun. In poorer districts, women may resort to paper and unwashed cloth to meet their needs.

Health implications: Because data from the developing world are lacking, definitive statements cannot be made about the impact of indigenous menstrual hygiene practices on gynecological health. Inadequate menstrual hygiene has been implicated as a risk factor for genital tract infection, particularly when cloth rags are used and washed in contaminated water (123). A study in rural China (where cloth is typically used as menstrual absorbent) found a strong statistical link between menstrual hygiene, genital hygiene, and cervical cancer risk; the use of commercial sanitary pads was a protective factor (122).

Most statistics on gynecological morbidity in developing countries are derived from antenatal and family planning clinic patients or from studies on populations at risk for sexually transmitted diseases (STDs) (115,124–127). Population-based studies are rare and limited resources make the conduct of large, systematic studies difficult. Moreover, cultural barriers may inhibit women from discussing intimate problems or revealing symptoms that may be stigmatizing (128).

Menstrual Practices in Orthodox Judaism and Traditional Islamic Societies

In Orthodox Jewish society, ritual law regarding menstruation is defined in Leviticus (one of the five books of the Hebrew Torah) and further interpreted in the Mishnah (39,129). A menstruating woman becomes "niddah" and is considered spiritually unclean (tame'ah) just prior to the beginning of flow, during menstruation, and for seven days afterward (130). Standards for ritual practice vary among Orthodox sects. In the most conservative interpretations, the menstruating woman is segregated from her husband and forbidden contact with the synagogue and sacred objects. Some traditions uphold the custom that a menstruating woman may not prepare food or wine. After checking for the absence of flow for seven days after the menstrual period, the woman undergoes a ritual bath or immersion (Mikvah) to reinstate spiritual and marital cleanliness. Orthodox Jewish girls get menstrual information from mothers and girlfriends (129). In Israeli Orthodox schools, the wife of a rabbi may present lectures on sexual development, marriage, and motherhood.

In Islamic societies, menstrual practices depend on the degree of cultural and religious conservatism, which differs among countries and between urban and rural regions. In conservative cultures, menarche signals that the girl is becoming a young woman and must observe the tradition of modest dress (hijab) and separation of the sexes (131). The Quran dictates certain restrictions be placed on the menstruating woman (39,132). Sexual intercourse is prohibited during the menstrual period. The menstruating woman is considered spiritually unclean with regard to religious duties until she completes a ritual washing; therefore, while menstruating, she is exempt from entering a mosque, from ritual prayer and fasting, and from making the pilgrimage to Mecca (Hajj).

A Muslim girl learns about menstruation from her mother, her sisters, and religious books (131). In conservative societies, menstruation is strictly a woman's issue, never to be discussed in the presence of men. The mother informs the father privately of the girl's menarche. Sanitary napkins are the most commonly used menstrual protection product; a virgin woman, for fear of losing her virginity, does not use a tampon. Some girls refrain from exercise and many ordinary activities due to fear of pain or increased blood loss (133). Some believe that they should not bathe until the end of the menstrual period. In one study, Saudi girls reported refraining from changing their sanitary protection at school or work for up to eight hours, for fear of increasing blood loss or, paradoxically, of trapping menstrual flow within the body (131,133). A ritual wash is performed at the end of the menstrual period. Traditional beliefs hold that hot drinks, including indigenous herbs, will relieve pain and prevent blood clotting within the body, but that cold foods should be avoided.

Other Genital Hygiene Practices

Routine Perineal Cleansing

Perineal hygiene is part of routine bodily cleansing. In America, showers and baths are the norm, with showers being more common. Handheld showerheads are popular in Western Europe but are less popular in America: in a California study, they were used by a one-quarter to one-third of women (52). Sponge baths and the use of handheld showerheads become more prevalent with increasing age, when reduced mobility becomes a factor. The bidet, common in Europe, is used rarely in America (52).

Ethnic differences in genital hygiene may be related to cultural beliefs. For example, studies in the United Kingdom found that immigrants of the Afro-Caribbean descent were more likely than the Caucasian women to wash the vulva with bubble bath or antiseptic (134). This appears consistent with the traditional belief system that rigorous bodily cleanliness is essential to health and well-being (111). However, cleansing with harsh soaps, chemicals, and antiseptics may cause vulvar contact dermatitis (135,136). For example, such practices were reported by 68% of patients with persistent vulvar symptoms (137).

In some parts of the developing world, practices are adapted to the lack of running water. In rural China, for example, mothers teach their daughters to cleanse the genitalia using water from a basin. This is done everyday from an early age, in the evening before going to bed, or before sexual intercourse (122). Washing from a basin, sponge baths, and bathing in rivers and streams are practiced in other regions of the world lacking running water.

Wet Wipes

Wet wipes are gaining popularity in North America and Western Europe. In the California study cited previously, usage rose with age from 26% among women younger than age 41 to 40% among women older than age 48 (52). Such products are often used more than once a day. Baby wipes, premoistened toilet wipes, and feminine wipes are all common choices (Farage and Bramante, unpublished data, 2004). In the late 1980s, reports appeared of allergic contact dermatitis to preservatives in some European wipes (138). The preservative in question (methylchloroisothiazolinone) is now highly regulated. Moreover, quantitative sensitization risk assessments have progressed over the last 20 years, such that it is now possible to safely formulate consumer products containing such preservatives at levels so low that they pose no significant risk of inducing contact sensitization.

Feminine Hygiene Sprays

Scented feminine hygiene sprays were popular in the United States in the 1970s. They fell out of favor as anecdotal reports of inflammatory reactions ensued (139). Clinicians consider deodorant sprays unnecessary and generally recommend against their use (50). However, the sprays continue to appeal to women who have deep-rooted beliefs about the need to avoid odor.

Douching

Vaginal douching is the insertion of a device into the vagina for flushing liquid into the vaginal vault. A preponderance of evidence links the practice to serious adverse health effects, with limited evidence of benefits. Nevertheless, douching is a strongly held cultural norm and a difficult habit to change among those who practice it.

Douche preparations: Several types of douche preparations are used. Substances found in the home reportedly used as douches include vinegar and water, household bleach, Lysol® (Reckitt & Coleman, Wayne, NJ), baking soda, yogurt, and water (140). Commercial preparations include solutions of vinegar or other acidifying agents (e.g., sodium citrate, sodium lactate, diazolidinyl urea), antiseptics, antibacterial preparations, alcohol, surfactant solutions, and antimicrobials (povidone-iodine).

Prefilled disposable bottles, refillable hanging bags, or refillable expandable bags are employed to irrigate the vagina. Bag-type applicators deliver a significantly greater volume and an eight-fold higher exposure duration than do disposable bottles (141).

Prevalence: Twenty-seven percent of American women douche regularly (Table 5). Among ethnic groups, African American and Latino women are more likely to douche than Caucasians (142) and Afro-Caribbean immigrants to the United Kingdom are more likely to douche than Caucasian British women (134). Douching is also commonly practiced in Africa: 29% of South African women (143) and 97% of pregnant women in the Cote d'Ivoire (144) reported douching. Douching with a variety of substances (soap and water, shampoos, toothpaste, and commercial antiseptics) is a routine practice among sex workers in developing countries (145,146).

In the United States, douching is more prevalent among women who are less educated, living in poverty, or who have a higher risk of sexually transmitted infections (141,142,147). One survey found douching to be least frequent among adolescents aged 15 to 19 (16%) and most common among women aged 20 to 24 (28%) (142). A California survey among middle class white women found a higher prevalence of douching by those older than age 41 (27% to 30%)

Table 5 Percentage of North American Women Who Douche Regularly by Age and Ethnicity (U.S. National Survey of Family Growth, 1995)

Age range (years)	Total	Non-Hispanic black	Non-Hispanic white	Hispanic
15–44	26.9	55.3	20.8	33.4
15–19	15.5	36.8	10.8	16.4
20–24	27.8	60.4	20.4	32.5
25–29	30.0	58.7	23.9	38.0
30–34	30.6	60.4	24.5	35.1
35–39	28.9	62.5	21.9	41.2
40–44	26.9	53.1	21.1	38.5

Source: From Ref. 142.

compared to those younger than age 41 (19%) (52). The frequency of douching among the U.S. women ranges from daily to monthly.

Motivating factors: Women who douche do so primarily to feel clean and they consider douching to be a sound hygienic practice (147–149). Among African American women, douching is often initiated on the advice of the mother, family, or friends; Caucasian American women are more influenced by the media (150). The majority of practitioners begin douching at menarche.

The importance of feminine cleanliness is paramount among women who douche. It is a principal motivating factor among African Americans who favor this practice (148,150). This may be related to traditional belief systems, which maintain that cleanliness contributes to health and that the body should be kept clean inside and out (111). Women also douche to avoid odor and to be clean after menstruation and sexual activity; hence in both Europe and North America, early onset of douching is more prevalent among those who initiate sexual activity at an earlier age (151,152).

Strongly held cultural beliefs and the perceived lack of suitable alternatives make it difficult for women to give up douching (150). Warnings that douching may be harmful are not highly persuasive; women reason that commercial douche preparations would not be widely available if they were unsafe. Among African American women who douche, health-care providers are not viewed as credible sources of information when their advice conflicts with trusted sources such as family members (111,150). Caucasian women who douche are somewhat more likely to consider douching unhealthy and may be more readily influenced by health-care providers to give up the practice (149).

Health implications: Epidemiologically, douching is associated with an increased risk of bacterial vaginosis (BV), pelvic inflammatory disease (PID), ectopic pregnancy, preterm births, STDs, and cervical cancer (140). Potential confounding factors cloud the epidemiologic assessment of the health risks, making it difficult to assess whether douching is a causative factor or simply a more common behavior among demographic groups at risk for such health conditions (Table 6). The strength of the association varies widely among case–control studies; few prospective studies are available.

In laboratory studies, douching preparations were antimicrobial to vaginal organisms (153). Depending on their composition and antimicrobial properties, these preparations caused either a transient washout effect in the vagina or a decrease in the density of vaginal microbes beyond the washout effect (154). Microbial counts eventually recovered (155).

BV is associated with an anaerobic shift in the vaginal microbial ecology that causes a fishy, malodorous discharge. Several studies have demonstrated an increased risk of BV among women who douche. For example, African American and Afro-Caribbean women, groups who douche more often than Caucasians, also have a higher risk for BV (134,156). It is unclear whether the statistical link to douching reflects the fact that women with malodorous

Table 6 Health Conditions Epidemiologically Associated with Douching

Health condition	Hypotheses supporting a causative role for douching	Potential confounding factors
BV	Douching temporarily alters the microbial ecology of the vagina, which may facilitate disease acquisition	Women may douche in response to BV symptoms Women who douche share risk factors with women at risk for BV and sexually transmitted diseases
STDs	Douching temporarily alters the microbial ecology of the vagina, which may facilitate disease acquisition Douching with irritating substances may make the vaginal mucosa and cervix more susceptible to colonization by invading pathogens	Women douche to feel clean after sexual intercourse Douching is more prevalent among sexually active women Women who douche share demographic characteristics with women at risk for STDs Women may douche in response to symptoms of infection
PID	The physical pressure of douching may facilitate uterine colonization by ascending pathogens The risk of PID is linked to douching frequency	Early sexual debut, having multiple sex partners, exposure to STDs, and other demographic risk factors for PID are also common to women who douche
Ectopic pregnancy	Douching may promote upper and lower genital tract infections that increase the risk of ectopic pregnancy	Ectopic pregnancy is more common in women with a history of PID. Such women share common risk factors with women who douche
Preterm births	Douching may play a role in infection-related preterm births	Preterm birth and douching are more prevalent among certain demographic groups
Cervical cancer	Sexually transmitted infection with HPV is a risk factor for cervical cancer Cancer risk rises with douching frequency	Risk factors for STDs are shared by women who douche

Abbreviations: BV, bacterial vaginosis; HPV, human papilloma virus; PID, pelvic inflammatory disease; STDs, sexually transmitted diseases.

discharge are more likely to douche, or whether alterations in the vaginal flora caused by douching predispose women to acquiring BV. Douching is more common during menstruation and after intercourse, a time of instability in some vaginal microbial populations (157,158). In one study, douching after menstruation was the strongest predictor of BV (158). Others found that douching with commercial antiseptics was strongly associated with BV risk (134) and that the acquisition of BV was linked having a new sexual partner and douching for hygiene (159). Such findings support the theory that douching may alter the protective balance of vaginal flora and contribute to the acquisition of BV.

PID is a polymicrobial infection of the upper urogenital tract initiated by ascending pathogens. BV, non-Caucasian race, low socioeconomic status, multiple sexual partners, and exposure to sexually transmitted organisms, the major risk factors for PID, are also common in women who douche. A meta-analysis of research published between 1965 and 1995 concluded that douching increases the risk of PID by 73% and the risk of ectopic pregnancy by 76% (134). Although women who douche and women at risk for PID share many of the same characteristics, douching serves as a pressurized vehicle for ascending microbes, which may facilitate the acquisition of PID. PID is also a risk factor for ectopic pregnancy, which may explain the statistical link of the latter to douching.

Douching is more prevalent among women at risk for STDs and HIV. In a study of racial and ethnic differences in vaginal flora, douching more than once a month was associated with the vaginal colonization by sexually transmitted microbes, although the latter was associated more consistently with race than with behavioral factors (156). Most studies indicate a statistical association of douching with STDs and HIV infection; however, a few studies in developing countries among women at high risk for STDs suggest that the practice lowers the risk of HIV infection (160) and human papilloma virus (HPV) regression (161) in such populations.

Based on the weight of the evidence, the consensus remains that douching is unnecessary for genital hygiene and may have serious adverse consequences on reproductive health. Nevertheless, few professional organizations have explicit policies on the health consequences of douching. This may be due to the difficulty in drawing firm conclusions about causation from cross-sectional epidemiologic studies. A randomized controlled trial of douching intervention (B-WELL trial) will evaluate the efficacy of intervention in changing adolescent douching behavior (162). Successful intervention strategies may ultimately provide a tool for prospectively assessing the risks and benefits of vaginal douching.

Perineal Powders

In the United States, some women customarily apply talc powders to the perineum on a daily basis. Such women are more likely to be overweight and to douche, smoke, and drink alcohol (163). The average duration of exposure can exceed 20 years (164).

Since 1979, numerous retrospective epidemiological studies have linked perineal talc exposure to ovarian cancer. The increased risk is highest for invasive forms of the disease. Some studies among women who use perineal powders suggested that tubal ligation was protective (164,165).

The statistical link between perineal talc application and ovarian cancer is highly controversial because of weak odds ratios, the absence of a clear dose-response relationship, and the lack of a robust mechanistic hypothesis to explain how talc exposure may cause or promote ovarian cancer.

A 2003 meta-analysis of 16 studies with an aggregate of 11,933 subjects found a 33% increased risk of ovarian cancer in perineal talc users but no clear dose-response relationship (166). Conversely, analysis of a subset of hospital studies showed no relationship to talc use, suggesting that a spurious statistical association may account for population-based data.

These studies were all retrospective. By contrast, a long-term prospective study of 121,700 nurses found no overall association between perineal talc powder and ovarian cancer (167). There was a moderately increased association for invasive forms of the disease. The risk of epithelial ovarian cancer among talc users was no higher among women who had not had a tubal ligation.

Hence, the weight of the evidence among retrospective case-control studies, coupled with the results of the large, prospective study involving nurses, suggests that the statistical association between perineal talc exposure and ovarian cancer risk may be the result of selection bias or other confounding factors. Body mass index may be one such factor, as overweight women are more likely to use perineal powders and are at higher risk for ovarian cancer (168). Uncontrolled socioeconomic variables may also play a role in the observed association.

Hair Removal

In the West, pubic hair removal is practiced for esthetic reasons. Common methods include shaving, the use of chemical depilatories, wax epilation, electrolysis, and laser hair removal. All methods tend to cause occasional mild folliculitis. Rare instances of severe cases progressing to keloid scars have been reported on the legs (169). In the late 1990s, an epidemic of allergic contact dermatitis to colophonium in epilating wax occurred in Europe (170). Occupational allergy to colophonium was also reported in a beautician who handled epilating waxes (171).

Pubic hair removal is performed in some countries. In response to a survey of 635 Turkish women, 98% reported pubic hair removal on a regular basis (once a week, every few weeks, or once a month) (Farage, Unpublished data, 2000). Hair removal is performed before or after the menstrual period, either with a lemon–sugar paste or by shaving. Those who shaved reported a higher frequency of skin irritation than those who used a lemon–sugar paste.

GENITAL HYGIENE AMONG OLDER WOMEN

Hygiene Challenges Posed by Light Urinary Incontinence

Stress and urge urinary incontinence become more common with age. Stress incontinence is characterized by accidental spurts of urine following abdominal pressure (coughing, laughing, sneezing, lifting). Urge incontinence is characterized by an urge to urinate and the rapid loss of urine (sometimes in significant amounts) prior to controlled micturition. Sufferers may have a combination of stress and urge incontinence. Some women begin experiencing light incontinence after having delivered children; for others, the onset is postmenopausal.

In Western Europe, reported prevalence of stress incontinence ranges from 40% to 60%; urge incontinence ranges from 7% to 20%, and mixed stress and urge incontinence ranges from 20% to 50% (172–174). In North America and Western Europe, women cope with light incontinence in various ways. In a Swedish study of post menopausal women, 4% of respondents (18% of stress incontinence sufferers) had urine loss sufficient to necessitate either the wearing of a sanitary napkin or changes in underwear several times a day (175). In general, to address this challenge, women use panty liners, menstrual pads, or pads designed for incontinence protection; some resort to frequent changes in underwear. Thirty percent reported some degree of vulvar irritation associated with their condition. Pelvic muscle exercises or Kegel exercises are a conservative approach to treating mild stress incontinence.

Hygiene Challenges Posed by Irregular Uterine Bleeding

The perimenopause is a transitional time between the reproductive years and menopause. Ovarian steroid hormone production decreases in stages, beginning with a drop in progesterone, reduced levels of both estrogen and progesterone and, finally, a depletion of both hormones to postmenopausal levels. Irregular uterine bleeding and spotting can occur during this transition, necessitating anticipatory or daily use of sanitary pads or panty liners.

Approximately 30% of women over age 40 experience menorrhagia, i.e., abnormally heavy or prolonged menstrual bleeding. Benign uterine fibroid tumors are a common cause of this condition. Use of tampons and pads in combination, coupled with frequent changes, are often necessary to cope with excessive menstrual bleeding. The condition can be quite disruptive to everyday life and may pose particular problems for women in Orthodox religious traditions that consider a bleeding woman to be ritually unclean. Continuous use of oral contraceptives (omitting the placebo pills of the fourth week) is sometimes used to remedy the situation by eliminating menstrual cycling (131). Even in such cases, special dispensation may be needed from the Rabbi or Muslim cleric so that occasional breakthrough bleeding does not render the woman ritually unclean.

Perineal Hygiene Among Older Women

Genital hygiene is of particular importance to the health and well being of older women. The consequences of inadequate hygiene vary. Mild skin irritation and fungal or bacterial skin infections become more common in older people who have a diminished capacity to care for themselves. Atrophic vulvovaginitis is prevalent after menopause. Moreover, the risk of pressure ulcers and incontinence dermatitis can be significant when older women suffer impaired mobility and urinary or fecal incontinence. Health conditions linked to genital hygiene in older women are described in the following sections.

Intertrigo and vulvar folliculitis: Intertrigo is an inflammation of the genitocrural folds, the labia, and the perineum sometimes seen in older or morbidly obese women (176). It manifests with erythema and excessive moisture. Vulvar folliculitis presents as red, tender papules surrounding the hair follicles and may be associated with staphylococcal and streptococcal infection. Both conditions result from impaired ability to maintain adequate hygiene. Hygienic interventions and maintaining skin dryness are indicated treatments.

Tinea: Tinea is a fungal infection of the feet, nails, and vulvar skin folds. Though a rare condition, its prevalence rises in older women because of diminished cellular immune responses (177). The most characteristic presentation is a ring-shaped eruption with an actively advancing border and scaly, healing center. However, any pruritic, scaly eruption of the vulva is suspect: it should be scraped for microscopic examination and treated with antifungal therapy, if appropriate. Maintaining dry skin helps prevent this condition.

Incontinence dermatitis: Preventing and managing incontinence dermatitis are the principal hygiene challenges in people with severe incontinence. Incontinence dermatitis is sometimes referred to as perineal dermatitis, which is a broad term that encompasses inflammation and tissue damage to the vulva, perineum, perianal region, and buttocks. The condition creates much pain and discomfort in elderly sufferers.

Prevalence of incontinence. In North America and Europe, urinary incontinence is prevalent among people over the age of 65. A community-based survey of 1584 Caucasian and African American women in the United States aged 70 to 79, found a prevalence of 21% (178). Of these, 40% reported stress incontinence and 42% reported urge incontinence. The frequency of urinary incontinence was higher among Caucasian women (27%) than among African-American women (14%). Fifteen percent of Mexican American women aged 65 or older reported having urinary incontinence (179). A community-based survey of Italian women aged 65 or older found a 26% prevalence (180).

Pathogenesis of incontinence dermatitis. The etiology of incontinence dermatitis in elders (Fig. 3) is inferred from research on pediatric diaper

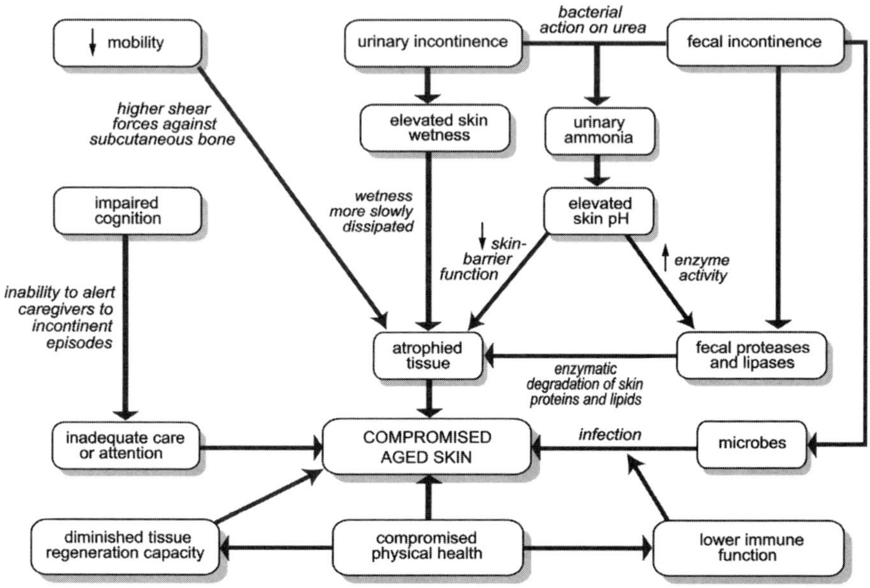

Figure 3 Factors that contribute to the morbidity of incontinence dermatitis in older people. *Source*: Adapted from Refs. 3, 181–183.

dermatitis. Elevated skin wetness, elevated pH, and the presence of fecal enzymes set the stage for skin damage. Hydrated skin is more susceptible to mechanical forces, whereas the elevated pH induced by urinary ammonia alters skin barrier function and activates fecal enzymes that compromise skin integrity. Moreover, several additional factors increase the risk of skin injury in older people (181,182). Skin atrophy makes the tissue inherently more fragile. Skin hydration following occlusion is significantly greater, and dissipated more slowly, in aged skin (183). Immobility increases the impact of mechanical forces; moving an immobile person across a chair or bed produces not only superficial friction but also generates shear forces in the underlying tissue because of pressure from the sacral bone (184). In those with impaired immune function, overgrowth of cutaneous pathogens or invasion of fecal bacteria is more likely to be a complication. Poor nutritional status can impede tissue recovery. Finally, impaired cognition can limit the person's ability to alert caregivers to incontinent episodes.

Incontinence dermatitis in older people begins with mild erythema of the skin, then progresses to an intense red appearance, often accompanied by blistering, erosion, and serous exudates. In darker skin, the initial inflammation reaction may be more difficult to detect. With urinary incontinence, dermatitis begins between the labial folds; dermatitis associated with fecal incontinence originates in the perianal area and progresses to the posterior aspect of the upper thighs. Secondary infection with *Candida albicans* causes erythematous, punctate vesicles that form a central confluence; satellite lesions may be visible on the border of the infection. Because of friction, vesicles may assume a macular appearance. The infected skin takes on a dark red color.

Hygiene measures. Examination and care of the genitalia should include gentle separation of the labia and exposure of the skin folds between the mons pubis and the inner aspect of the upper thigh. The buttocks should be separated and examined, as well as the crease between the buttocks and the posterior upper thigh. In women who are obese, skin folds of the lower abdomen must also be exposed and examined, particularly in women who are diabetic or immunocompromised (184).

Although no systematic trials exist on the impact of perineal hygiene on skin health, general guidelines have been developed for preventive care (184,185). The focus is on keeping the skin dry, maintaining a healthy skin pH, avoiding mechanical forces, and minimizing contact with urine and feces. The use of specially formulated perineal skin cleansers or disposable wipes is preferred over bar soap and a washcloth. The former avoid the high pH of most soap bars and the friction forces created by rubbing a washcloth against the skin (182). Powders are used to absorb excess moisture; cornstarch-based powders are sometimes favored because of the controversy regarding perineal talc. Moisture-barrier preparations are also employed. Superabsorbent incontinence pads or garments are used to absorb wetness and keep it away from the skin. Wet or soiled garments should be changed promptly.

Treatment of incontinence dermatitis. Prospective clinical trials are needed to study the effectiveness of preventive hygiene measures as well as the efficacy of therapeutic intervention. To our knowledge, the only published prospective study of preventive care was a preliminary trial of structured nursing intervention in 15 institutionalized patients with dementia (186). An equal number developed dermatitis (two in the structured care intervention group and three in the unstructured care group) regardless of whether cleansers, moisturizers, or moisture-barrier preparations were used. Dermatitis developed only in those with urofecal incontinence and followed more than four incontinent episodes in 24 hours. None of the patients was capable of informing caregivers of incontinent episodes. The small number of subjects and their poor mental health limit the conclusions that can be drawn from this study.

Case reports provide evidence for the effectiveness of barrier creams and hydrogel dressings in treating incontinence dermatitis (187,188). In one case report, applying a commercial barrier cream three times per day prevented dermatitis from postsurgical diarrhea (10–20 stools a day) during a one-month follow-up period (187). In another, a 68-year old woman, who presented with candidiasis secondary to urofecal incontinence and diarrhea, was treated with a regimen of skin cleansing followed by application of an antifungal powder and then a layer of barrier cream. Her dermatitis cleared within three days (187).

Case reports also support the efficacy of hydrogel dressings for treating excoriation (188). The first case involved a disabled woman with incontinence who suffered perianal excoriation unresponsive to a titanium-based barrier cream and paraffin wax. Resolution was achieved in three days by applying hydrogel every two hours and after every incontinent episode. Another case involved a man incontinent of urine who had perianal dermatitis and a sacral pressure ulcer. Application of hydrogel cream resulted in improvement after five days of treatment.

CONCLUSION

Genital hygiene needs change dramatically over a woman's lifetime. Menstrual hygiene practices vary by age, culture, and religious tradition. General hygiene practices may be constrained by family economics or the available infrastructure in different regions of the world. Some hygiene practices carry the potential for adverse health effects. Education is key to reducing these risks; however, resource limitations, cultural constraints, and the intimate nature of the subject matter can present barriers to effective intervention and the institution of more healthful hygiene practices.

REFERENCES

1. Berg RW, Buckingham KW, Stewart RL. Etiologic factors in diaper dermatitis: the role of urine. Pediatr Dermatol 1986; 3:102.
2. Buckingham KW, Berg RW. Etiologic factors in diaper dermatitis: the role of feces. Pediatr Dermatol 1986; 3:107.
3. Berg RW. Etiology and pathophysiology of diaper dermatitis. Adv Dermatol 1988; 3:75.
4. Berg RW, Milligan MC, Sarbaugh FC. Association of skin wetness and pH with diaper dermatitis. Pediatr Dermatol 1994; 11:18.
5. Andersen PH et al. Faecal enzymes: in vivo human skin irritation. Contact Dermatitis 1994; 30:152.
6. Grove GL et al. Assessment of skin hydration caused by diapers and incontinence articles. Curr Probl Dermatol 1998; 26:183.
7. Zimmerer RE, Lawson KD, Calvert CJ. The effects of wearing diapers on skin. Pediatr Dermatol 1986; 3:95.
8. Leyden JJ et al. Urinary ammonia and ammonia-producing microorganisms in infants with and without diaper dermatitis. Arch Dermatol 1977; 113:1678.
9. Fluhr JW, Elias PM. Stratum corneum pH: formation and function of the "acid mantle". Exog Dermatol 2002; 1:163.
10. Hachem JP et al. pH directly regulates epidermal permeability barrier homeostasis, and stratum corneum integrity/cohesion. J Invest Dermatol 2003; 121:345.
11. Benjamin L. Clinical correlates with diaper dermatitis. Pediatrician 1987; 14:21.
12. Atherton DJ. A review of the pathophysiology, prevention and treatment of irritant diaper dermatitis. Curr Med Res Opin 2004; 20:645.

13. Lund C. Prevention and management of infant skin breakdown. Nurs Clin North Am 1999; 34:907.
14. Wong DL et al. Diapering choices: a critical review of the issues. Pediatr Nurs 1992; 18:41.
15. Odio M, Friedlander SF. Diaper dermatitis and advances in diaper technology. Curr Opin Pediatr 2000; 12:342.
16. Putet G. Effect of Bepanthen ointment in the prevention and treatment of diaper rash on premature and full-term babies. Realites Pediatriques 2001; 63:33.
17. Baldwin S et al. Skin benefits from continuous topical administration of a zinc oxide/petrolatum formulation by a novel disposable diaper. J Eur Acad Dermatol Venereol 2001; 15:5.
18. Odio MR et al. Continuous topical administration of a petrolatum formulation by a novel disposable diaper. 1. Effect on skin surface microtopography. Dermatology 2000; 200:232.
19. Odio MR et al. Continuous topical administration of a petrolatum formulation by a novel disposable diaper. 2. Effect on skin condition. Dermatology 2000; 200:238.
20. Davis JA et al. Comparison of disposable diapers with fluff absorbent and fluff plus absorbent polymers: effects on skin hydration, skin pH, and diaper dermatitis. Pediatr Dermatol 1989; 6:102.
21. Campbell RL et al. Effects of diaper types on diaper dermatitis associated with diarrhea and antibiotic use in children in day-care centers. Pediatr Dermatol 1988; 5:83.
22. Campbell RL et al. Clinical studies with disposable diapers containing absorbent gelling materials: evaluation of effects on infant skin condition. J Am Acad Dermatol 1987; 17:978.
23. Campbell RL. Clinical tests with improved disposable diapers. Pediatrician 1987;14:34.
24. Keswick BH, Seymour JL, Milligan MC. Diaper area skin microflora of normal children and children with atopic dermatitis. J Clin Microbiol 1987; 25:216.
25. Paradise JE et al. Vulvovaginitis in premenarcheal girls: clinical features and diagnostic evaluation. Pediatrics 1982; 70:193.
26. Jaquiery A et al. Vulvovaginitis: clinical features, aetiology, and microbiology of the genital tract. Arch Dis Child 1999; 81:64.
27. Fischer G, Rogers M. Vulvar disease in children: a clinical audit of 130 cases. Pediatr Dermatol 2000; 17:1.
28. Fischer G, Margesson LJ. Vulvar itching in prepubertal girls: let's be specific. J Am Acad Dermatol 2003; 48:986.
29. Mazzola BL et al. Behavioral and functional abnormalities linked with recurrent urinary tract infections in girls. J Nephrol 2003; 16:133.
30. Elvik SL. Vaginal discharge in the prepubertal girl. J Pediatr Health Care 1990; 4:181.
31. Song HJ et al. Prevalence and risk factors for enterobiasis among preschool children in a metropolitan city in Korea. Parasitol Res 2003; 91:46.
32. Acosta M et al. Enterobiasis among school children in a rural population from Estado Falcon, Venezuela, and its relation with socioeconomic level. Invest Clin 2002; 43:173.
33. Sung JF et al. Pinworm control and risk factors of pinworm infection among primary-school children in Taiwan. Am J Trop Med Hyg 2001; 65:558.

34. Markin AV, Terekhova TV, Strugova AA. Effects of school environment factors on enterobiasis morbidity among students. Gig Sanit 1997; 5:16.
35. Grebniak NP, Agarkova LD. Sanitary-epidemiological characteristics of preschool institutions. Gig Sanit 2000; 6:46.
36. Williams TS, Callen JP, Owen LG. Vulvar disorders in the prepubertal female. Pediatr Ann 1986; 15:588.
37. Herman-Giddens ME, Berson NL. Harmful genital care practices in children. A type of child abuse. JAMA 1989; 261:577.
38. Hornor G, Ryan-Wenger NA. Aberrant genital practices: an unrecognized form of child sexual abuse. J Pediatr Health Care 1999; 13:12.
39. Whelan EM. Attitudes toward menstruation. International Committee on Applied Research in Population. Stud Fam Plann 1975; 6:106.
40. Olesen VL, Woods NF. Culture, society and menstruation. Health Care Women Int 1986; 7:1.
41. Skidmore M. Menstrual madness: women's health and well-being in urban Burma. Women Health 2002; 35:81.
42. Wambua LT. African perceptions and myths about menopause. East Afr Med J 1997; 74:645.
43. Ford CS. A Comparative Study on Human Reproduction, New York, NY: New York University Press, 1945.
44. Smith OW, Smith GV. A fibrinolytic enzyme in menstruation and late pregnancy toxemia. Science 1945; 102:253.
45. Zondek B. Does menstrual blood contain a specific toxin? Am J Obstet Gynecol 1953; 65:1065.
46. Abraham S et al. Menstruation, menstrual protection and menstrual cycle problems. The knowledge, attitudes and practices of young Australian women. Med J Aust 1985; 142:247.
47. Friedman N. "Invented by a doctor:" a medical and social history of tampons. In: Wolner R, ed. Everything You Must Know About Tampons. New York, NY: Berkley Publishing Group, 1981:33.
48. Thornton MJ. Use of vaginal tampons for absorption of menstrual discharges. Am J Obstet Gynecol 1943; 46:259.
49. McCalman I. Menstrual practices of the Amandebele people in the Essexvale area. Cent Afr J Med 1968; 14:111.
50. Stewart EG, Spencer P. The V Book. A Doctor's Guide to Complete Vulvovaginal Health, New York, NY: Bantam Books, 2002.
51. Czerwinski BS. Adult feminine hygiene practices. Appl Nurs Res 1996; 9:123.
52. Czerwinski BS. Variation in feminine hygiene practices as a function of age. J Obstet Gynecol Neonatal Nurs 2000; 29:625.
53. Buchta RM. Adolescent tampon usage: incidence and initiation of usage. Adolesc Pediatr Gynecol 1995; 8:17.
54. Omar HA, Aggarwal S, Perkins KC. Tampon use in young women. J Pediatr Adolesc Gynecol 1998; 11:143.
55. Emans SJ et al. Hymenal findings in adolescent women: impact of tampon use and consensual sexual activity. J Pediatr 1994; 125:153.
56. Adams Hillard PJ. Menstruation in young girls: a clinical perspective. Obstet Gynecol 2002; 99:655.

57. Finkelstein JW, von Eye A. Sanitary product use by white, black, and Mexican American women. Public Health Rep 1990; 105:491.
58. Janssen PJCM, Van Veen MP, Speijers GJA. Danish National Institute for Public Health and the Environment (RIVM). Health risk assessment for organotin in textiles, Report No. RIVM Report 613350 002, 2000.
59. Reingold AL et al. Toxic shock syndrome surveillance in the United States, 1980 to 1981. Ann Intern Med 1982; 96:875.
60. Hajjeh RA et al. Toxic shock syndrome in the United States: surveillance update, 1979 1996. Emerg Infect Dis 1999; 5:807.
61. Litt IF. Toxic shock syndrome—an adolescent disease. J Adolesc Health Care 1983; 4:270.
62. Centers for Disease Control and Prevention. Reduced incidence of menstrual toxic shock syndrome—United States, 1980 – 1990. MMWR Morb Mortal Wkly Rep 1990; 39:421.
63. Berkley SF et al. The relationship of tampon characteristics to menstrual toxic shock syndrome. JAMA 1987; 258:917.
64. Osterholm MT et al. Toxic shock syndrome: relation to catamenial products, personal health and hygiene, and sexual practices. Ann Intern Med 1982; 96:954.
65. Christensson B, Johansson PJ, Oxelius VA. Imbalanced serum IgG subclass pattern in toxic shock syndrome patients: deficiency of specific IgG1 and IgG4 subclass antibodies to toxic shock syndrome toxin 1. Clin Exp Immunol 1986; 66:443.
66. Schroder E et al. Prevalence of serum antibodies to toxic-shock-syndrome-toxin-1 and to staphylococcal enterotoxins A, B and C in West-Germany. Zentralbl Bakteriol Mikrobiol Hyg 1988; 270:110.
67. Altchek A. Vulvovaginitis, vulvar skin disease, and pelvic inflammatory disease. Pediatr Clin North Am 1981; 28:397.
68. Dotzel MM. Medical devices; labeling for menstrual tampon for the "ultra" absorbency, U.S. Food and Drug Administration, HHS, Final rule. Fed Regist 2000; 65:62282.
69. Shuren J. Medical devices; labeling for menstrual tampons; ranges of absorbency, change from "junior" to "light", U.S. Food and Drug Administration, HHS, Final rule. Fed Regist 2004; 69:52170.
70. Barrett KF et al. Tampon-induced vaginal or cervical ulceration. Am J Obstet Gynecol 1997; 127:332.
71. Berkeley AS et al. The potential of digitally inserted tampons to induce vaginal lesions. Obstet Gynecol 1985; 66:31.
72. Danielson RW. Vaginal ulcers caused by tampons. Am J Obstet Gynecol 1983; 146:547.
73. Friedrich EG, Jr, Siegesmund KA. Tampon-associated vaginal ulcerations. Obstet Gynecol 1980; 55:149.
74. Friedrich EG, Jr. Tampon effects on vaginal health. Clin Obstet Gynecol 1981; 24:395.
75. Jimerson SD, Becker JD. Vaginal ulcers associated with tampon usage. Obstet Gynecol 1980; 56:97.
76. Weissberg SM, Dodson MG. Recurrent vaginal and cervical ulcers associated with tampon use. JAMA 1983; 250:1430.

77. Raudrant D et al. Study of the vaginal mucous membrane following tampon utilisation; aspect on colposcopy, scanning electron microscopy and transmission electron microscopy. Eur J Obstet Gynecol Reprod Biol 1989; 31:53.
78. Nordin AJ, Bates RG. Tampon-induced vaginal bleeding presenting as intermenstrual bleeding. Int J Gynaecol Obstet 1995; 51:261.
79. Farage MA et al. Safety evaluation of modern feminine hygiene pads: two decades of use. Female Patient 2004; 29:23.
80. Eason EL, Feldman P. Contact dermatitis associated with the use of Always sanitary napkins. CMAJ 1996; 154:1173.
81. Harris NL. Always sanitary napkins: further reports and manufacturer response. CMAJ 1996; 155:1035.
82. Larsen WG. Sanitary napkin dermatitis due to the perfume. Arch Dermatol 1979; 115:363.
83. Kanerva L et al. Colophonium in sanitary pads. Contact Dermatitis 2001; 44:59.
84. Rademaker M. Allergic contact dermatitis to a sanitary pad. Australas J Dermatol 2004; 45:234.
85. Gerberick GF et al. Understanding fragrance allergy using an exposure-based risk assessment approach. Contact Dermatitis 2001; 45:333.
86. Felter SP et al. Application of the risk assessment paradigm to the induction of allergic contact dermatitis. Regul Toxicol Pharmacol 2003; 37:1.
87. Farage MA et al. A modified human repeat insult patch test for extended mucosal tissue exposure. Contact Dermatitis 2003; 49:214.
88. Farage MA et al. A clinical method for testing the safety of catamenial pads. Gynecol Obstet Invest 1997; 44:260.
89. Schlager TA et al. Effect of periurethral colonization on the risk of urinary tract infection in healthy girls after their first urinary tract infection. Pediatr Infect Dis J 1993; 12:988.
90. Stamey TA. Periurethral or perineal bacteria in urinary tract infections? JAMA 1981; 245:127.
91. Stapleton A et al. Effect of secretor status on vaginal and rectal colonization with fimbriated Escherichia coli in women with and without recurrent urinary tract infection. J Infect Dis 1995; 171:717.
92. Scholes D et al. Risk factors for recurrent urinary tract infection in young women. J Infect Dis 2000; 182:1177.
93. Hooton TM et al. A prospective study of risk factors for symptomatic urinary tract infection in young women. N Engl J Med 1996; 335:468.
94. Russo TA et al. Chromosomal restriction fragment length polymorphism analysis of Escherichia coli strains causing recurrent urinary tract infections in young women. J Infect Dis 1995; 172:440.
95. Stamey TA, Sexton CC. The role of vaginal colonization with enterobacteriaceae in recurrent urinary infections. J Urol 1975; 113:214.
96. Mulvey MA et al. Bad bugs and beleaguered bladders: interplay between uropathogenic Escherichia coli and innate host defenses. Proc Natl Acad Sci USA 2000; 97:8829.
97. Madersbacher S, Thalhammer F, Marberger M. Pathogenesis and management of recurrent urinary tract infection in women. Curr Opin Urol 2000; 10:29.
98. Funfstuck R et al. Pathogenetic aspects of uncomplicated urinary tract infection: recent advances. Clin Nephrol 1997; 47:13.

99. Mardh PA et al. Facts and myths on recurrent vulvovaginal candidosis—a review on epidemiology, clinical manifestations, diagnosis, pathogenesis and therapy. Int J STD AIDS 2002; 13:522.
100. Geiger AM, Foxman B. Risk factors for vulvovaginal candidiasis: a case–control study among university students. Epidemiology 1996; 7:182.
101. Foxman B. The epidemiology of vulvovaginal candidiasis: risk factors. Am J Public Health 1990; 80:329.
102. Otero L et al. Vulvovaginal candidiasis in female sex workers. Int J STD AIDS 1998; 9:526–530.
103. Mardh PA, Novikova N, Stukalova E. Colonisation of extragenital sites by Candida in women with recurrent vulvovaginal candidosis. BJOG 2003; 110:934.
104. Patel DA et al. Risk factors for recurrent vulvovaginal candidiasis in women receiving maintenance antifungal therapy: results of a prospective cohort study. Am J Obstet Gynecol 2004; 190:644.
105. Berg AO et al. Establishing the cause of genitourinary symptoms in women in a family practice. Comparison of clinical examination and comprehensive microbiology. JAMA 1984; 251:620.
106. Eckert LO et al. Vulvovaginal candidiasis: clinical manifestations, risk factors, management algorithm. Obstet Gynecol 1998; 92:757.
107. Hellberg D et al. Sexual behavior of women with repeated episodes of vulvovaginal candidiasis. Eur J Epidemiol 1995; 11:575.
108. Spinillo A et al. Epidemiologic characteristics of women with idiopathic recurrent vulvovaginal candidiasis. Obstet Gynecol 1993; 81:721.
109. Farage MA et al. Labial and vaginal microbiology: effects of extended panty liner use. Infect Dis Obstet Gynecol 1997; 5:252.
110. Voss A et al. [Quantitative study of vaginal flora during the menstrual cycle], Geburtshilfe Frauenheilkd 1993; 53:543.
111. Snow LF. Traditional health beliefs and practices among lower class black Americans. West J Med 1983; 139:820.
112. McMaster J, Cormie K, Pitts M. Menstrual and premenstrual experiences of women in a developing country. Health Care Women Int 1997; 18:533.
113. Drakshayani Devi K, Venkata Ramaiah P. A study on menstrual hygiene among rural adolescent girls. Indian J Med Sci 1994; 48:139.
114. James A. Menstrual hygiene. A study of knowledge and practices. Nurs J India 1997; 88:221.
115. Joseph GA et al. General and reproductive health of adolescent girls in rural south India. Indian Pediatr 1997; 34:242.
116. Hoerster KD, Chrisler JC, Rose JG. Attitudes toward and experience with menstruation in the U.S. and India. Women Health 2003; 38:77.
117. Abioye-Kuteyi EA. Menstrual knowledge and practices amongst secondary school girls in Ile Ife, Nigeria. J R Soc Health 2000; 120:23.
118. Ellis D, Ho MS. Attitudes of Chinese women towards sexuality and birth control. Can Nurse 1982; 78:28.
119. Chang AR, 'Erosion' of the uterine cervix; an anachronism. Aust N Z J Obstet Gynaecol 1991; 31:358.
120. Critchlow CW et al. Determinants of cervical ectopia and of cervicitis: age, oral contraception, specific cervical infection, smoking, and douching. Am J Obstet Gynecol 1995; 173:534.

121. Jacobson DL et al. Histologic development of cervical ectopy: relationship to reproductive hormones. Sex Transm Dis 2000; 27:252.
122. Zhang ZF et al. Risk factors for cancer of the cervix in a rural Chinese population. Int J Cancer 1989; 43:762.
123. Wasserheit JN et al. Reproductive tract infections in a family planning population in rural Bangladesh. Stud Fam Plann 1989; 20:69.
124. Bang RA et al. High prevalence of gynaecological diseases in rural Indian women. Lancet 1:85.
125. Bhatia JC et al. Levels and determinants of gynecological morbidity in a district of south India. Stud Fam Plann 1997; 28:95.
126. Wasserheit JN. The significance and scope of reproductive tract infections among Third World women. Suppl Int J Gynecol Obstet 1989; 3:145.
127. Younis N et al. A community study of gynecological and related morbidities in rural Egypt. Stud Fam Plann 1993; 24:175.
128. Zurayk H et al. Comparing women's reports with medical diagnoses of reproductive morbidity conditions in rural Egypt. Stud Fam Plann 1995; 26:14.
129. Brooks MH. Beliefs of orthodox Jewish girls about menstruation. Fam Pract 1984; 1:113.
130. Siegel SJ. The effect of culture on how women experience menstruation: Jewish women and Mikvah. Women Health 1985; 10:63.
131. Kridli SA. Health beliefs and practices among Arab women. MCN Am J Matern Child Nurs 2002; 27:178.
132. Dhami S, Sheikh A. The Muslim family: predicament and promise. West J Med 2000; 173:352.
133. Moawed S. Indigenous practices of Saudi girls in Riyadh during their menstrual period. East Mediterr Health J 2001; 7:197.
134. Rajamanoharan S et al. Bacterial vaginosis, ethnicity, and the use of genital cleaning agents: a case control study. Sex Transm Dis 1999; 26:404.
135. Marren P, Wojnarowska F. Dermatitis of the vulva. Semi Dermatol 1996; 15:36.
136. Lee JY, Wang BJ. Contact dermatitis caused by cetrimide in antiseptics. Contact Dermatitis 1995; 33:168.
137. Marin MG et al. Adverse behavioral and sexual factors in chronic vulvar disease. Am J Obstet Gynecol 2000; 183:34.
138. Minet A et al. Allergic contact dermatitis from Kathon CG in moist toilet paper. Contact Dermatitis 1989; 21:107.
139. Feminine hygiene deodorant sprays. Med Lett Drugs Ther 1970; 12:88.
140. Martino JL, Vermund SH. Vaginal douching: evidence for risks or benefits to women's health. Epidemiol Rev 2002; 24:109.
141. Cottrell BH. Vaginal douching. J Obstet Gynecol Neonatal Nurs 2003; 32:12.
142. Abma JC et al. Fertility, family planning, and women's health: new data from the 1995 National Survey of Family Growth. Vital Health Stat 1997; 23:1.
143. Myer L et al. Intravaginal practices, HIV and other sexually transmitted diseases among South African women. Sex Transm Dis 2004; 31:174.
144. La Ruche G et al. Vaginal douching: association with lower genital tract infections in African pregnant women. Sex Transm Dis 1999; 26:191.
145. Reed BD, Ford K, Wirawan DN. The Bali STD/AIDS study: association between vaginal hygiene practices and STDs among sex workers. Sex Transm Infect 2001; 77:46.

146. Fonck K et al. Sexually transmitted infections and vaginal douching in a population of female sex workers in Nairobi, Kenya. Sex Transm Infect 2001; 77:271.
147. Lichtenstein B, Nansel TR. Women's douching practices and related attitudes: findings from four focus groups. Women Health 2000; 31:117.
148. Funkhouser E et al. Douching beliefs and practices among black and white women. J Womens Health Gend Based Med 2002; 11:29.
149. Ness RB et al. Why women douche and why they may or may not stop. Sex Transm Dis 2003; 30:71.
150. Gazmararian JA et al. Why do women douche? Results from a qualitative study. Matern Child Health J 2001; 5:153.
151. Mardh PA et al. Correlation between an early sexual debut, and reproductive health and behavioral factors: a multinational European study. Eur J Contracept Reprod Health Care 2000; 5:177.
152. Oh MK et al. Early onset of vaginal douching is associated with false beliefs and high-risk behavior. Sex Transm Dis 2003; 30:689.
153. Pavlova SI, Tao L. In vitro inhibition of commercial douche products against vaginal microflora. Infect Dis Obstet Gynecol 2000; 8:99.
154. Onderdonk AB et al. Quantitative and qualitative effects of douche preparations on vaginal microflora. Obstet Gynecol 1992; 80:333.
155. Monif GR et al. Quantitative and qualitative effects of povidone-iodine liquid and gel on the aerobic and anaerobic flora of the female genital tract. Am J Obstet Gynecol 1980; 137:432.
156. Newton ER et al. Predictors of the vaginal microflora. Am J Obstet Gynecol 2001; 184:845.
157. Eschenbach DA et al. Influence of the normal menstrual cycle on vaginal tissue, discharge, and microflora. Clin Infect Dis 2000; 30:901.
158. Schwebke JR, Richey CM, Weiss HL. Correlation of behaviors with microbiological changes in vaginal flora. J Infect Dis 1999; 180:1632.
159. Hawes SE et al. Hydrogen peroxide-producing lactobacilli and acquisition of vaginal infections. J Infect Dis 1996; 174:1058.
160. Gresenguet G et al. HIV infection and vaginal douching in central Africa. Aids 1997; 11:101.
161. Romney SL et al. Effects of beta-carotene and other factors on outcome of cervical dysplasia and human papillomavirus infection. Gynecol Oncol 1997; 65:483.
162. Simpson T et al. Vaginal douching among adolescent and young women: more challenges than progress. J Pediatr Adolesc Gynecol 2004; 17:249.
163. Rosenblatt KA et al. Characteristics of women who use perineal powders. Obstet Gynecol 1998; 92:753.
164. Cramer D et al. Genital talc exposure and risk of ovarian cancer. Int J Cancer 1999; 81:351.
165. Mills PK et al. Perineal talc exposure and epithelial ovarian cancer risk in the Central Valley of California. Int J Cancer 2004; 112:458.
166. Huncharek M, Geschwind JF, Kupelnick B. Perineal application of cosmetic talc and risk of invasive epithelial ovarian cancer: a meta-analysis of 11,933 subjects from sixteen observational studies. Anticancer Res 2003; 23:1955.
167. Gertig DM et al. Prospective study of talc use and ovarian cancer. J Natl Cancer Inst 2000; 92:249.

168. Weiss NS et al. Ovarian cancer. In: Schoettenfeld D, Fraumeni JF, eds. Cancer Epidemiology and Prevention, New York: Oxford University Press, 1996:1040.
169. Mimouni-Bloch A, Metzker A, Mimouni M. Severe folliculitis with keloid scars induced by wax epilation in adolescents. Cutis 1997; 59:41.
170. Goossens A et al. An epidemic of allergic contact dermatitis due to epilating products. Contact Dermatitis 2002; 47:67.
171. de Argila D, Ortiz-Frutos J, Iglesias L. Occupational allergic contact dermatitis from colophony in depilatory wax. Contact Dermatitis 1996; 34:369.
172. Hampel C et al. Prevalence and natural history of female incontinence. Eur Urol 1997; 32:3.
173. Hannestad YS et al. A community-based epidemiological survey of female urinary incontinence: the Norwegian EPINCONT study. Epidemiology of Incontinence in the County of Nord-Trondelag. J Clin Epidemiol 2000; 53:1150.
174. Temml C et al. Urinary incontinence in both sexes: prevalence rates and impact on quality of life and sexual life. Neurourol Urodyn 2000; 19:259.
175. Iosif CS, Bekassy Z. Prevalence of genito-urinary symptoms in the late menopause. Acta Obstet Gynecol Scand 1984; 63:257.
176. Nathan L. Vulvovaginal disorders in the elderly woman. Clin Obstet Gynecol 1996; 39:933.
177. Shenefelt PD, Fenske NA. Aging and the skin: recognizing and managing common disorders. Geriatrics 1990; 45:57.
178. Jackson RA et al. Urinary incontinence in elderly women: findings from the Health, Aging, and Body Composition Study. Obstet Gynecol 2004; 104:301.
179. Espino DV et al. Prevalence and severity of urinary incontinence in elderly Mexican-American women. J Am Geriatr Soc 2003; 51:1580.
180. Maggi S et al. Prevalence rate of urinary incontinence in community-dwelling elderly individuals: the Veneto study. J Gerontol A Biol Sci Med Sci 2001; 56:M14.
181. Faria DT, Shwayder T, Krull EA. Perineal skin injury: extrinsic environmental risk factors. Ostomy Wound Manage 1996; 42:28.
182. Fiers SA. Breaking the cycle: the etiology of incontinence dermatitis and evaluating and using skin care products. Ostomy Wound Manage 1996; 42:32.
183. Roskos KV, Guy RH. Assessment of skin barrier function using transepidermal water loss: effect of age. Pharm Res 1989; 6:949.
184. Gray M. Preventing and managing perineal dermatitis: a shared goal for wound and continence care. J Wound Ostomy Continence Nurs 2004; 31:S2.
185. Fiers S, Thayer D. Management of intractable incontinence. In: Urinary and Fecal Incontinence: Nursing Management, 2nd ed., Doughty, D. B. Mosby, St Louis, 2000.
186. Lyder CH et al. Structured skin care regimen to prevent perineal dermatitis in the elderly. J ET Nurs 1992; 19:12.
187. Haugen V. Perineal skin care for patients with frequent diarrhea or fecal incontinence. Gastroenterol Nurs 1997; 20:87.
188. Vernon T. Managing excoriation. Nurs Times 2000; 96:12.
189. Berg RW. Etiologic factors in diaper dermatitis: a model for development of improved diapers. Pediatrician 1987; 14:27.

13

Products for Vulvar Hygiene

Miranda A. Farage
Feminine Care Clinical Sciences, The Procter & Gamble Company, Cincinnati, Ohio, U.S.A.

Lisa Lennon
The Procter & Gamble Company, Cincinnati, Ohio, U.S.A.

INTRODUCTION

Women use a wide variety of products for vulvar hygiene. These include products for cleanliness and odor control, such as soaps and body washes, premoistened wipes and towelettes, douches, deodorant sprays, body splashes, and other fragrances. However, it is impossible to discuss vulvar hygiene without including menstrual products, such as tampons, pads, and panty liners. Cleanliness and odor control during the menstrual period is often of primary concern to a woman and the products used for menstrual protection are an integral part of this process. Moisturizers, lubricants, and hair-removal products are also important to a woman's overall hygiene regimen. In addition, some subgroups of women may have special needs for products to control incontinence or for over-the-counter (OTC) medications. This chapter discusses the products women use for vulvar hygiene, perceived or real benefits, and potential health effects of these products.

CLEANLINESS AND ODOR-CONTROL PRODUCTS

Soaps, Body Washes, and Bubble Bath

Soaps are water-soluble sodium or potassium salts of fatty acids, produced by saponification or basic hydrolysis of a fat or oil with a strong alkali (Fig. 1A) (1). Evidence exists that several ancient civilizations knew of soap making and

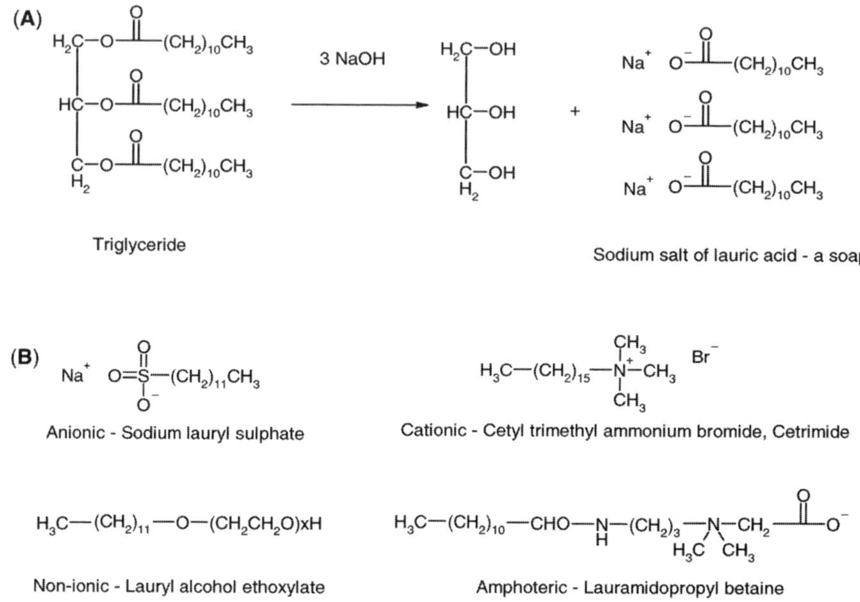

Figure 1 (**A**) Basic hydrolysis: a fat or oil with a strong alkali to form soap. (**B**) Structures of common surfactants.

used the resulting material as hair styling aids, to treat skin diseases, and for washing (2). However, it is likely that soap was not used routinely for personal cleansing until about the second century A.D. During the time of the Roman Empire, bathing was extremely popular, but its popularity declined with the fall of Rome in 467 A.D. During the Middle Ages, bathing fell out of fashion in Europe until the 17th century. However, there were regions of the medieval world where personal cleanliness remained important throughout the Middle Ages. Daily bathing was a common custom in Japan during the time, and in Iceland, pools warmed with water from hot springs were popular gathering places on Saturday evenings.

Soap making remained largely a household chore until the mid-19th century. At about this time, high-yield methods were developed for making soda ash or sodium carbonate out of common table salt, thereby improving the quality and yield of soap products, lowering the cost, and facilitating a move toward the commercial manufacturing of soap. These discoveries, along with the development of power to operate factories, made soapmaking one of America's fastest-growing industries by 1850 and changed soap from a luxury item to an everyday necessity. Investigation into the use of synthetic detergents began in the early 1900s and, with the end of World War II, synthetics starting replacing soaps for some cleaning chores, such as laundry and houschold cleaning (Fig. 1B). As surfactant chemistry became more and more sophisticated, these synthetic detergents began to replace soap in many of the bars and liquids used for personal cleansing.

Synthetic detergents are "synthesized" or put together chemically from a variety of raw materials. They have a major advantage over soaps in that they do not combine as readily with mineral salts to form soap curd (bathtub ring) (1). In addition, detergents offer excellent performance over a wide range of temperatures and water hardness, and greater skin mildness (2).

Whether a fatty acid soap or a synthetic detergent, the function of "soaps" is to reduce the surface tension of water and to solubilize materials such as grease and oils that cannot be removed easily by water alone (3). Materials used for personal cleansing, such as bar soaps, body washes, bubble bath, and feminine washes consist of mixtures of surfactants. Many of these products incorporate additional ingredients to provide added consumer benefits, such as fragrances, deodorant protection, antibacterial components, and skin moisturizers or softeners (4,5).

Most large manufacturers of personal cleansing products have rigorous approaches to evaluate the products for adverse skin effects (6,7). A number of test methods have been developed. Many test protocols include exaggerated use testing, or patch testing, on sensitive body sites. Extended use testing by volunteer participants using the products at home is sometimes part of the safety assessment.

The medical community generally assumes that soaps and other personal cleansing agents can contribute to vulvitis (8). However, given the broad use of these products, there are relatively few specific case reports of adverse reactions of the vulva as a result of using personal cleansing products. It is likely that consumers who experience mild irritant reactions that they perceive to be related to the use of a specific product simply switch products.

Douches

Douching has a long and ancient history, reaching as far back as 1500 B.C., when an Egyptian papyrus recommended a garlic and wine douche for the treatment of menstrual disorders. In the days of Hippocrates, vaginal rinsing was thought to be the only method of curing vaginal infections. Different ethnic groups have used douching off and on throughout history, but in America, douching had its heyday beginning in the early 1920s and carried on through the 1950s, when women's magazines regularly featured advertisements for douche brands such as Lysol® (Lehn and Fink Products Company, Montvale, New Jersey, U.S.A.), Sterizol® (Sterizol Company, Ossining, New York, U.S.A.), and Zonite® (Lee Pharmaceuticals, El Monte, California, U.S.A.). As recently as the early 20th century, the medical community recommended douching for the treatment of specific gynecological conditions (9).

Douching is a common practice in the United States and the sale of commercial douche products has tripled since 1974 (10). Some of the studies that have been conducted on the prevalence of douching are summarized in

Table 1 Summary of Selected Studies on the Prevalence of Douching

Type of study	Findings	References
United States		
Summarized from the 1995 National Survey of Family Growth	55% of African American women, 33% of Hispanic women, and 21% of Caucasian women douche.	(10)
Telephone survey of 535 adult women in the southeastern U.S.	59% of African American women and 36.5 % of Caucasian women responded that they engage in this practice.	(11)
Summarized from the 1988 National Survey of Family Growth	36.7% of women overall engage in this practice (66.5% of African American women and 32% of Caucasian women).	(12)
Survey of 169 adolescents attending a family planning clinic in a small southern town.	69% of those surveyed (75% of African American women and 64% of Caucasian women) reported a history of douching	(13)
Other Countries		
Survey of 552 women in an antenatal clinic in the Ivory Coast.	98% reported vaginal douching as a common practice.	(14)
Survey of 543 female sex workers in Nairobi.	72% douche regularly.	(15)
Indonesian study among 599 pregnant women.	91% had douched at least once in the month prior to the survey.	(16)

Table 1. In the United States, the practice is generally more prevalent among African American women than Caucasian women (17,18).

Differences in the estimated occurrence of this practice in the United States may be related to geographic location and socioeconomic status. Geographic differences exist, with the highest overall percentage in the south (35–48%), followed by the midwest (24–32%), northeast (23–31%), and the west (20–28%) (10,12). Education, income levels, and age at first intercourse were inversely related to douching (12). Sixty-nine percent of adolescent females attending a family planning clinic in a small southern town reported douching (13).

Compared to the United States, vaginal douching is less common in Europe and the United Kingdom (about 7% of women, overall) (19). Studies in African nations indicated that the percentage of women who engage in this practice is extremely high (Table 1).

Gazmararian, et al. (10), found that douching starts at a young age in the United States and its practice is reinforced by family, friends, and the media. There are a number of reasons women give for douching, including the perception that the practice kills germs, prevents pregnancy (20), prevents sexually transmitted disease (21), and helps ameliorate vaginal itching and discharge (11). Some women douche after menstruation and/or intercourse for cleanliness and odor control (17). In some cultures, there are additional perceived benefits to douching. In sub-Saharan Africa, it is perceived that the astringent properties of vaginal douches enhance sexual pleasure (15).

The composition of douches can range from homemade solutions of salt, vinegar and water, or water alone, to purchased douches marketed expressly for the purpose. In the United States, of women who reported current douching, about one-third use a homemade product (11). In a study conducted in the United States by Oh et al., in 2002 (20), a majority of adolescent women surveyed used commercially marketed products. However, baking soda, Betadine® (Purdue Frederick Company, Norwalk, Connecticut, U.S.A.), Pine-Sol® (The Clorox Company, Oakland, California, U.S.A.), and Lysol were also used. In the Nairobi study, Fonck, et al. (15) found that water with soap was used most commonly (81%) followed by salty water (18%), water alone (9%), and a commercial antiseptic (5%). In Indonesia, soap and water (63%), water (19%), betel leaf (8%), and a commercial agent (2%) were used (16). Betel leaf is a traditional plant used for medicine. It contains antiseptic and irritant properties and is often used for cleaning the vagina in the postpartum period.

It is now recognized that douching is associated with a host of negative consequences. Douching kills beneficial bacteria that live in the vagina (Lactobacilli). Stripped of Lactobacilli, the pH balance of the vagina is altered, creating a risk for infection and a variety of adverse health effects. The adverse effects that have been associated with douching are outlined in Table 2 and have been reviewed in additional publications (27,28). Effects include adverse reproductive

Table 2 Negative Health Consequences Associated with Douching

Consequence	References
Impaired fertility	(9)
Preterm birth	(18)
Low birth weight	(22)
Ectopic pregnancy	(23)
Bacterial vaginosis	(15)
Pelvic inflammatory disease	(24)
Upper genital tract infection	(24)
Endometritis	(24)
Vulvovaginal candidiasis, STDs	(17)
Cervical cancer	(25)
HIV infection	(26)

Abbreviation: STDs, sexually transmitted diseases.

effects, an increase in the occurrence of sexually transmitted diseases (STDs) and pelvic inflammatory disease, and an increase in risk for HIV and cervical cancer. Rajamanoharan, et al. (19) found that any douching agent (proprietary products, vinegar and water, soap, bubble bath, or antiseptics) was associated strongly with bacterial vaginitis. Baird, et al. (9) showed that regular douching with water only, water and vinegar, or commercial solutions was associated with reductions in fertility.

Premoistened Wipes and Towelettes

These products are relatively recent additions to the consumer market. Baby wipes were the first premoistened wipes to penetrate the market significantly. Now, this range of products includes flushable personal cleansing cloths and products targeted specifically for women. The formulations of these products vary, but consist mainly of water with mild surfactant, preservatives, antimicrobials, and fragrance. Some brands include skin treatment agents, such as lotions with vitamin E or aloe.

Major manufacturers have developed means for testing premoistened wipes for potential skin irritant effects. These include long-term use testing as well as exaggerated exposure methods designed specifically for these products, such as the modified forearm-controlled application test designed by The Procter & Gamble Company for Wipes™ (29). There are very few reports in the literature of adverse reactions to these products.

Dusting Powder

Some women apply talcum powder either directly to the vulva or indirectly through application to menstrual pads, diaphragms, or condoms for odor control. It has been suggested that application of talcum powder to the genital area may be associated with an increased risk of ovarian cancer (30). Several epidemiological studies have been conducted in an attempt to verify this association and some suggest a slight increase in the risk of ovarian cancer with talcum powder use. However, other studies show no association at all. A confounding factor in many of these studies is that, prior to 1973, low levels of asbestos were sometimes present in talcum powders. All powder products marketed after 1973 have been required by law to be free of asbestos.

Although the association between talcum powder and ovarian cancer is still unresolved, modern products marketed specifically for feminine hygiene use have replaced talcum powder with cornstarch.

Other Products for Cleanliness and Odor Control

A variety of other products are available for use by women to control odor. These include feminine deodorant sprays, body splashes, fragrances, and feminine suppositories.

Feminine deodorant sprays first entered the market in 1962 in Europe and in 1966 in the United States. Typically, these products are packaged in an aerosol or pump spray for external use, primarily to be applied on or adjacent to the female genitalia to absorb moisture, deodorize, neutralize, or otherwise control odor (31). These products may contain antimicrobial agents, astringents, and perfumes (32). In their early days, some of these products contained talcum powder to absorb moisture, but the modern products have replaced talcum with cornstarch or baking soda. The aerosol products also contain propellants.

There are few reports in the scientific literature of adverse reactions of modern feminine deodorant sprays. A careful choice of ingredients and safety testing prior to marketing minimize any risks of irritation or sensitization.

Other products available for odor control are feminine suppositories containing antimicrobials, such as benzalkonium chloride. Such products are often used after small surgical procedures. However, some brands are advertised as deodorants and sold for routine use.

MENSTRUAL PROTECTION PRODUCTS

Many products are used for menstrual protection, although disposable pads, tampons, and panty liners are the most common (Fig. 2). However, some

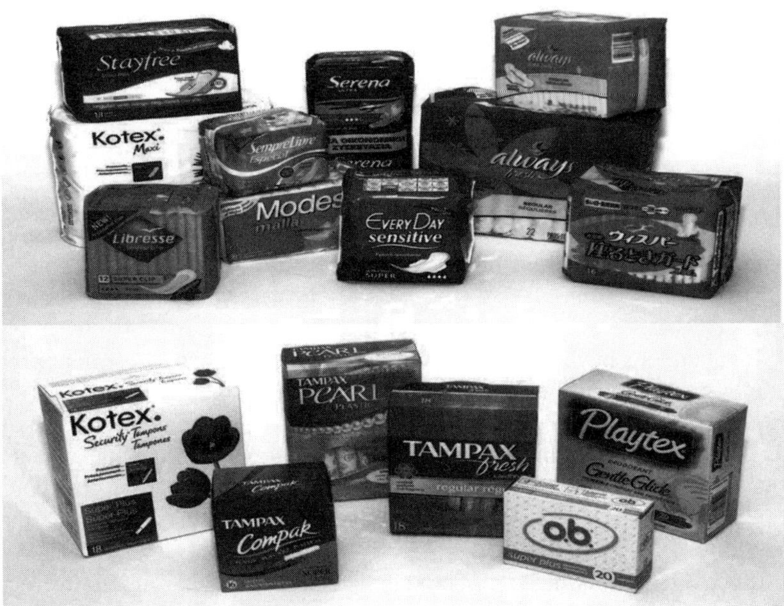

Figure 2 Examples of common menstrual protection products. (*See color insert p. 8.*)

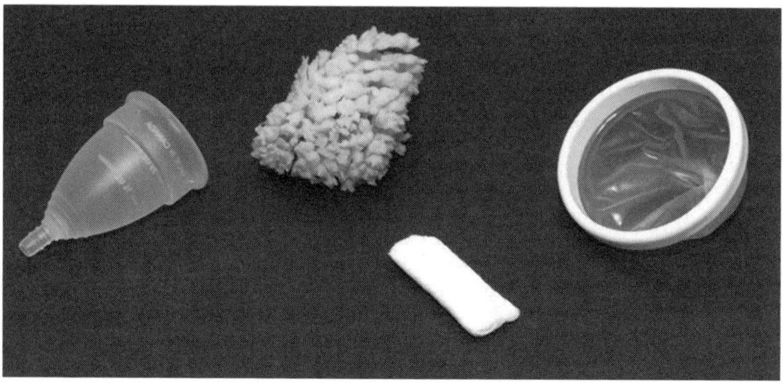

Figure 3 Examples of alternative menstrual protection (such as Diva Cup, sea sponges, and Padette interlabial pad). (*See color insert p. 8.*)

women use alternative protection, such as menstrual cups, internally worn sponges, and washable pads made from fabric (Fig. 3).

Tampons

The forerunners of the modern tampon were homemade from various materials, such as papyrus (ancient Egypt), wool (ancient Rome), paper (ancient Japan), plant materials (Hawaii, Asia, Africa), linen vinegar-dipped cloth (France, 18th century), cotton, wool, or linen with a string attached. Modern tampons began with cotton tampons from the Tampax® brand (Procter & Gamble Company, Cincinnati, Ohio, U.S.A.) in 1936 (33). Today's mainstream market offers a large selection of tampon products of varying absorbencies made of cotton, rayon, or a combination of these two materials. They are typically about two inches in length and with a diameter of about a half inch, with a cotton string attached securely to one end for removal after use. Tampons are available with or without applicators (the applicators can be made of cardboard or plastic) and with or without perfumes (i.e., scented or unscented).

Modern tampons have been used safely for many years as convenient products for menstrual protection. Tampons are classified by the FDA as Class 2 medical devices and are, therefore, subject to testing requirements by the FDA (34). In addition, major manufacturers have developed detailed testing plans to ensure the safety of tampons prior to marketing (35). Menstrual tampons require specific labeling to clearly identify the degree of absorbency for the tampon (36).

There are no safety issues if modern tampons are used according to instructions. However, historically, tampon use has been associated with some adverse health consequences and misperceptions about potential health effects.

Table 3 Standardized Tampon Absorbencies

Absorbency range	Terminology of absorbency
<6 g	Junior absorbency
6–9 g	Regular absorbency
9–12 g	Super absorbency
12–15 g	Superplus absorbency
15–18 g	Ultra absorbency
>18 g	No term

Source: From Ref. 36.

Toxic Shock Syndrome

Toxic shock syndrome (TSS) is a rare but treatable disease that can be life threatening in some individuals. TSS is caused by the release of superantigens (usually TSST-1) from certain strains of *Staphylococcus aureus* that are present in the body. These superantigens have systemic effects on the host (37). In the 1980s, contracting TSS was associated with using highly absorbent tampons (38,39). Since that time, such superabsorbent products have largely disappeared from the market. Standardized absorbency ratings have been developed (Table 3) and are a required part of labeling for tampon products (36).

Shifts in Vaginal Microflora

The use of tampons does not significantly alter the normal changes that occur in the vaginal microflora during menses, as demonstrated by Onderdonk, et al. (40). These authors evaluated the qualitative and quantitative changes in vaginal microflora during the course of the menstrual cycle. They found no difference in the results from volunteers using tampons composed of different fibers (100% cotton, 70% cotton and 30% viscose rayon, and 100% polyacrylate rayon).

Vaginal Ulcers

With normal, recommended use of tampons, vaginal ulcers do not occur. In some cases, improper insertion of tampons can cause mechanical irritations to the vaginal wall (33). In addition, tampons can cause minor vaginal dryness and irritation if they are too absorbent for the menstrual flow or worn at times other than active menstruation.

Endometriosis

There is no evidence that tampons can lead to or aggravate endometriosis. Endometriosis is a disease in which the tissue lining the uterus, the endometrium, grows outside the uterus in the form of implants, nodules, and cysts. The cause is unknown, but some researchers have speculated that endometriosis may be caused by a backward flow of endometrial cells during menstruation, leading some to speculate that tampons may play a role in the development of this disease. However, this theory has been discounted (33).

Compromising Virginity

Tampons do not compromise virginity. Tampons are used by an estimated 70% of women in the United States, Canada, and much of Western Europe. However, tampon usage in Japan and the rest of the Asia/Pacific region, Latin America, and Africa is estimated at less than 15% (41,42). In some regions, the reasons for the low percentage of women using tampons may include a fear that tampons will compromise virginity. However, there is no evidence that tampon usage significantly alters the size of the opening in the hymen.

Dioxin Exposure

Modern tampons do not contain dioxin. Dioxin is a general term that describes a group of about 30 chemicals that are highly persistent in the environment and have been associated with cancer. They can be produced by a variety of processes, including combustion (as a result of cooking or internal combustion engines) and chlorine bleaching of paper pulp. The United States Environmental Protection Agency has estimated that most dioxin exposure (>95%) occurs through the diet (43). Modern tampons are made of cotton, rayon, or blends of cotton and rayon. The rayon is made from cellulose fibers derived from wood pulp that is bleached to increase the absorbency of the material and to make the product more aesthetically pleasing. However, modern bleaching methods do not involve chlorine bleaching and are dioxin free (44).

Disposable Pads and Panty Liners

For many years, women used rags to contain menstrual flow. These were not very reliable and had to be soaked and laundered after use. The first disposable sanitary pad was created in 1896 by Johnson & Johnson (New Brunswick, New Jersey, U.S.A.) (Lister's Towels) but failed to catch on. In World War I, nurses found bandages to be an excellent absorbing material for menstrual flow. Soon thereafter, Kimberly-Clark introduced Kotex® in 1921, and Johnson & Johnson introduced Modess®, the first successful disposable pads. Disposable pads were definitely more effective and convenient than rags. However, they were a long way from current products. They had to be held in place with pins or special belts worn around the waist and a range of protective gear were available to compensate when the pads failed, such as special panties or "sanitary aprons" (made of cloth-coated rubber, and worn backwards over the buttocks) (33,45).

The first major improvement in disposable pads came about 50 years after their initial introduction, when adhesive backing was introduced, enabling use of the pads without pins or special belts. The quality and effectiveness of pads have continued to improve in the last few decades. Performance improved substantially with the development of superabsorbent materials, i.e., polymeric gelling compounds developed to lock the moisture in the core of the pad and not release it under pressure. Procter & Gamble introduced ultrathin pads based on superabsorbent materials, which were seven times thinner than the early pads, making them more comfortable and less noticeable in tighter-fitting fashions. In addition, many modern pads incorporate a top sheet designed to wick moisture into the core and away from the wearer's skin for a drier feeling.

Modern pads offer women a wide variety of products designed specifically to meet their needs. Procter & Gamble introduced "wings" or flexible side extensions of the pad that wrap over the edge of the panty to prevent panty soiling and to hold the pad securely in place. Pads are available in a number of sizes and lengths, ranging from small, thin panty liners for managing discharges between periods or to use in combination with tampons, to larger, longer pads that offer maximum protection overnight. Most brands come in scented or unscented varieties. Some are packaged with wrappers for discrete disposal (46).

Major manufacturers of pads and panty liners have developed and published methods of evaluating the safety of these products. In-use clinical assessments of irritation and the impact of product use on the microflora of the vulva are important parts of this evaluation (47–49). However, new protocols have been developed that are designed specifically to evaluate the contribution of both the chemical composition of these products and the potential for mechanical irritation through friction (50,51).

Alternative Menstrual Products

Several alternative forms of menstrual protection are available from specialty shops or the internet. Examples are shown in Figure 3. Menstrual cups are flexible, nonabsorbent containers made of natural gum rubber or medical silicon inserted in the vagina that can collect about one ounce of menstrual fluid. They can then be emptied, washed, and reused. Sea sponges can also be used, but they must be cleaned thoroughly and sanitized by boiling before reuse. Disposable interlabial pads are composed of materials similar to modern tampons. These are worn externally and held in place by the labia. They are most suited for light menstrual flow.

PRODUCTS FOR INCONTINENCE CONTROL

Urinary incontinence or the accidental release of urine is a fairly common problem among women (52). The most common type is stress incontinence, which occurs when pressure is put on the bladder by coughing, laughing, sneezing, or physical activity. It occurs when the pelvic floor muscles no longer support the bladder properly. The resulting drop in the bladder can cause it to push against the vagina and prevent the tightening of the muscles that ordinarily close off the urethra. Stress incontinence can be caused by childbirth, weight gain, or other conditions that stretch the pelvic floor muscles.

Urge incontinence, also called overactive bladder, is an urgent sensation to urinate even when the bladder may not be full. In many cases, the cause of urge incontinence is unknown. However, it can be caused by emotional stress, irritation of the bladder, or neurological conditions such as Parkinson's disease or stroke. Some women suffer from a combination of stress and urge incontinence.

Typically, urinary incontinence does not cause major health problems but it can be embarrassing and can affect a woman's self-esteem and confidence. There are a range of products available to control incontinence, including adjustable briefs (a diaper-style garment), pull-up briefs or undergarments, and pads held in place with belts or adhesive strips. These products have benefited greatly from the development of super absorbent materials such as the types used in menstrual pads and baby diapers. Irritation and rashes are important potential health effects that can occur with extended use of these products, especially in individuals who are bedridden. However, advances in materials and technology have reduced the likelihood of these effects.

OTHER PRODUCTS USED ON THE VULVA

Some products are used on the vulva for greater comfort during intercourse or for aesthetic purposes. These products include lubricants and moisturizers, products for hair removal, and products to dye pubic hair.

Lubricants and Moisturizers

Vaginal dryness can occur as estrogen levels fluctuate. Dryness occurs commonly with aging. However, in some women, vaginal dryness can occur during pregnancy, while nursing, or at certain times in the menstrual cycle. In addition, some disease states can cause vaginal dryness, such as Sjögren's syndrome, an autoimmune disease, which affects the body's moisture-producing glands.

A number of commercial products are available to counteract vaginal dryness, such as K-Y Jelly® (McNeil-PPC, Inc., Round Rock, Texas, U.S.A.) and Astroglide® (BioFilm, In., Vista, California, U.S.A.). These are water-soluble, glycerin-based products. Vegetable and olive oils are also used by some women, although these tend to be messy. Petroleum-based lubricants, such as petroleum jelly, can harbor bacteria and cause damage to latex condoms, rendering them ineffective against unplanned pregnancy and STDs.

Hair Removal Products

Hair removal methods include trimming with scissors or a hair clipper, shaving, depilation, waxing, electrolysis, and laser hair removal. Trimming and clipping have few adverse effects as long as they are done carefully to avoid cutting the delicate skin of the vulva. Shaving is easy to do at home but can sometimes leave bumps on the skin. A number of depilatories are formulated specifically for use on the "bikini line." Use on areas outside the bikini line, such as the vulva, can lead to irritation.

Waxing plucks the hair from the root, therefore, the results last longer. Home products contain combinations of waxes and a resin that makes the wax adhere to skin (33). At-home products are formulated for use on the bikini line, and not on other areas of the genitalia.

Electrolysis uses an electric current to destroy the hair root. Each hair is treated individually with either a needle epilator or a tweezers epilator. Home electrolysis devices are available but it may be difficult to apply the device accurately to an area that cannot be seen very easily. Therefore, professional electrolysis is preferable. Adverse effects of electrolysis can include pain during treatment and swelling and inflammation after treatment. Electrolysis can cause scarring and changes in skin color in some people (52).

Laser hair removal is relatively new. As the laser is moved over the skin, the light passes through and is absorbed by the melanin (pigment) in the hair follicles. It is believed that the heat generated by the laser breaks apart the follicle and the hair falls out over a period of approximately two months. The treatment is best suited for fair-skinned people with dark hair. In darker skinned people, the skin pigment can absorb the laser before it reaches the hair follicle, making the treatment less effective. Light-colored hair may not contain enough melanin. Multiple treatments are required to achieve a meaningful reduction in the amount of hair on the area. Adverse effects of laser hair removal include an extreme sensitivity of the treated skin. Rarely, peeling, blistering, and burning of the skin may occur, as well as brown spots or a slight loss of pigment in areas where the laser has been used.

Dyes

As pubic hair tends to be darker than hair color and grays with age, some women resort to dyeing. Home hair coloring products are not formulated for use on the vulva and would likely cause irritation if used for that purpose. A professional colorist and a dye formulated for facial hair are the best choices. However, irritation may still occur.

MEDICATIONS

Vaginal Creams

Medicated or anti-itch creams are marketed for the relief of external feminine itching. Mainly, these consist of the active ingredient present in other products available to treat itching on the skin, that is, hydrocortisone. The main risk associated with the use of these products is that they treat the symptoms without identifying and treating the underlying cause of the itching.

Antifungal Preparations

In the early 1990s, manufacturers began to make drugs for the treatment of Candidal vaginitis available without prescription (OTC). The basis for this switch, as for any prescription drug, was that:

1. The drugs are safe and effective without the supervision of a licensed practitioner.
2. The drugs have a low potential for misuse and abuse.
3. The drugs treat a common, benign, and self-diagnosable condition.
4. The labeling instructions can be understood by the average person (53).

As a result of this switch, a number of antifungal medications are now available without a prescription, including clotrimazole, miconazole nitrate, and butoconazole nitrate.

The primary advantages of the OTC status to the consumer are patient autonomy, convenience, more rapid relief of symptoms, and cost savings by reducing the number of physician visits and reduction in the costs of the drug. The potential disadvantages are misdiagnosis, with resulting overuse of the antifungal drugs and the potential for developing drug resistance, and possible delays in the diagnosis and treatment of the actual underlying medical condition causing the symptoms (54). If the underlying condition is serious, such as an STD, the patient runs the risks of increased morbidity and/or inadvertently transmitting the disease to a partner. The debate around the wisdom of the switch to the OTC status for antifungals remains very active in the medical literature.

CONCLUSION

Women use a wide variety of products for cleanliness and odor control of the external genitalia. When produced by a reputable manufacturer with careful safety testing programs, most of these products have minimal or no adverse health effects. However, most members of the medical community agree that many of these products are not necessary. Nevertheless, many women feel a need to use extra care and attention in order to feel confident about genital hygiene.

Products for menstrual protection and the control of incontinence have developed dramatically in recent years. The development of products based on superabsorbent materials has given women a wide range of choices for discreet protection.

REFERENCES

1. Soap and Detergent Association. Chemistry. Available at: http://www.cleaning101.com/chemistry. Accessed August 11, 2005.
2. Soap and Detergent Association. History. Available at: http://www.cleaning101.com/history. Accessed August 11, 2005.

3. Virtual Chembook. http://www.elmhurst.edu/~chm/vchembook/554soap.html. Accessed August 11, 2005.
4. Ertel K. Modern skin cleansers. Dermatol Clin 2000; 18:561.
5. Abbas S, Goldberg JW, Masaro M. Personal cleanser technology and clinical performance. Dermatol Ther 2004; 17:35.
6. Barel AO et al. A comparative study of the affects on the skin of a classical bar soap and a syndet cleansing bar in normal use conditions and in the soap chamber test. Skin Res Technol 2001; 7:98.
7. Robinson MK, Perkins MA. A strategy for skin irritation testing. Am J Contact Dermat 2002; 13:21.
8. MedLine Plus. Vulvitis definition. Available at: http://www.nlm.nih.gov/medlineplus/ency/article/001445.htm. Accessed August 11, 2005.
9. Baird DD et al. Vaginal douching and reduced fertility. Am J Public Health 1996; 86:844.
10. Gazmararian JA et al. Why do women douche? Results from a qualitative study. Matern Child Health J 2001; 5:153.
11. Funkhouser E et al. Douching beliefs and practices among black and white women. J Womens Health Gend Based Med 2002; 11:29.
12. Aral SO, Mosher WD, Cates W, Jr. Vaginal Douching among women of reproductive age in the United States: 1988. Am J Public Health 1992; 82:210.
13. Foch BJ, McDaniel ND, Chacko MR. Racial differences in vaginal douching knowledge, attitude, and practices among sexually active adolescents. J Pediatr, Adolesc Gynecol 2001; 14:29.
14. La Ruche G et al. Vaginal douching: association with lower genital tract infections in African pregnant women. Sex Transm Dis 1999; 26:191.
15. Fonck K et al. Sexually transmitted infections and vaginal douching in a population of female sex workers in Nairobi, Kenya. Sex Transm Infect 2001; 77:271.
16. Joesoef MR et al. Douching and sexually transmitted diseases in pregnant women in Surabaya, Indonesia. Am J Obstet Gynecol 1996; 174:115.
17. Lichtenstein B, Nansel TR. Women's douching practices and related findings: findings from four focus groups. Women Health 2000; 31:117.
18. Bruce FC, Fiscella K, Kendrick JS. Vaginal douching and preterm birth: an intriguing hypothesis. Med Hypotheses 2000; 54:448 [Erratum: Med Hypotheses 2000; 54:859.
19. Rajamanoharan S et al. Bacterial vaginosis, ethnicity, and the use of genital cleaning agents: a case control study. Sex Transm Dis 1999; 26:404.
20. Oh MK et al. Early onset of vaginal douching is associated with false beliefs and high-risk behavior. Sex Transm Dis 2003; 30:689.
21. Wilson TE et al. A case-control study of beliefs and behaviors associated with sexually transmitted disease occurrence in Estonia. Sex Transm Dis 2001; 28:624.
22. Fiscella E et al. The risk of low birth weight associated with vaginal douching. Obstet Gynecol 1998; 92:913.
23. Zhang J, Thomas AG, Leybovich E. Vaginal douching and adverse health effects: a meta-analysis. Am J Public Health 1997; 87:1207.
24. Ness RB et al. Douching and endometritis: results from the PIDevaluation and clinical health (PEACH) study. Sex Transm Dis 2001; 28:240.
25. Bayo S et al. Risk factors of invasive cervical cancer in Mali. Int J Epidemiol 2002; 31:202.

26. Myer L et al. Intravaginal practices, HIV and other sexually transmitted diseases among South African women. Sex Transm Dis 2004; 31:174.
27. Cottrell BH. Vaginal douching. J Obstet Gynecol Neonatal Nurs 2003; 32:12.
28. Simpson T et al. Vaginal douching among adolescent and young women: more challenges than progress. J Pediatr Adolesc Gynecol 2004; 17:249.
29. Farage MA. Development of a modified forearm controlled application test method for evaluating the skin mildness of disposable wipe products. J Cosmet Sci 2000; 51:153.
30. American Cancer Society. Cancer recurrence information. Available at: http://www.cancer.org/docroot/CRI/content/CRI_2_6x_Talcum_Powder_and_Cancer.asp?sitearea = . Accessed August 11, 2005.
31. Feminine hygiene sprays remain controversial despite FDA action. JAMA 1972; 219:449.
32. Feminine hygiene deodorant sprays. Med Lett Drugs Ther 1970; 12:88.
33. Smarts V. Everyday habits that make a difference. In: Stewart E, Spencer P, eds. The V Book: A Doctor's Complete Guide to Vulvovaginal Health. New York: Bantam Books, 2002:81.
34. U.S. Food and Drug Administration. Premarket Notification [510(k)]. Available at: http://www.fda.gov/cdrh/devadvice/314.html. Accessed August 11, 2005.
35. Shein SE et al. Clinical safety-in-use of a new tampon design. Infect Dis Obstet Gynecol 2003; 11:89.
36. Code of Federal Regulations, Title 21, Volume 8, revised as of April 1, 2004 (21CFR801.430).
37. Schlievert PM, Tripp TJ, Peterson ML. Reemergence of Staphylococcal toxic shock syndrome in Minneapolis-St.Paul, Minnesota, during the 2000–2003 surveillance period. J Clin Microbiol 2004; 42:2875.
38. Berkley SF et al. The relationship of tampon characteristics to menstrual toxic shock syndrome. JAMA 1987; 258:917.
39. Osterholm MT et al. Toxic shock syndrome: relation to catamenial products, personal health and hygiene, and sexual practices. Ann Intern Med 1982; 96:954.
40. Onderdonk AB et al. Qualitative assessment of vaginal microflora during use of tampons of various compositions. Appl Environ Microbiol 1987; 53:2779.
41. HighBeam Research. A worldwide overview of the sanitary protection market, 1993.
42. HighBeam Research. Feminine hygiene products: a market overview (Part 2), 1999.
43. U.S. EPA National Center for Environmental Assessment. Dioxin Reassessment, NAS Review Draft, April 29, 2005. Available at: http://cfpub.epa.gov/ncea/cfm/recordisplay.cfm?deid=87843. Accessed August 11, 2005.
44. U.S. FDA Center for Devices and Radiological Health. Tampons and asbestos, dioxin, and toxic shock syndrome, 7/23/1999. Available at: http://www.fda.gov/cdrh/consumer/tamponsabs.html. Accessed August 11, 2005.
45. Museum of menstruation. Available at: http://www.mum.org/formfit.htm. Accessed August 11, 2005.
46. The Procter & Gamble Company. Available at: http://www.pg.com/product_card/prod_card_fem_protection.html. Accessed April 10, 2006.
47. Farage M et al. A clinical method for testing the safety of catamenial pads. Gynecol Obstet Invest 1997; 44:260.
48. Farage M et al. Labial and vaginal microbiology: effects of extended panty liner use. Infect Dis Obstet Gynecol 1997; 5:252.

49. Farage MA et al. Safety evaluation of modern hygiene pads: two decades of use. Female Patient 2004; 29:23.
50. Farage MA et al. Development of a new test for mechanical irritation: behind the knee as a test site. Skin Res Technol 2001; 7:193.
51. Farage MA, Meyer SJ, Walter D. Development of a sensitive test method to evaluate mechanical irritation potential on mucosal skin. Skin Res Technol 2004; 10:85.
52. Web MD. Available at: http://www.my.webmd.com/webmd_today/home/default, htm. Accessed August 11, 2005.
53. Rheinstein PH. FDA perspective: prescription to over-the-counter drug switches. Am Fam Physician 1997; 56:1211.
54. Lipsky MS, Waters T. The "prescription-to-OTC switch" movement: its effects on antifungal vaginitis preparations. Arch Fam Med 1999; 8:297.

14

Vulva Ethnic Differences: An Overview

Marina Goldovsky and Howard I. Maibach
Department of Dermatology, University of California School of Medicine, San Francisco, California, U.S.A.

INTRODUCTION

Are there differences in the vulva according to ethnicity? Reasonable evidence suggests that there are some differences in vulvar skin properties and function between ethnic (racial) groups. Previous studies have demonstrated equally thick stratum corneum in black and white skin, although black skin contains more cell layers (1). Black skin has a higher transepidermal water loss (TEWL), variable blood vessel reactivity, decreased skin surface pH, and larger mast cell granules than white skin (2). Such differences in skin properties could account for racial disparities with regard to diagnosis of vulvar dermatologic conditions.

We searched MD Consult; Science Citations Index; PubMed; Cochrane Database; the Melvyl Catalogue in the CDL-Hosted Database of University of California, San Francisco; Google; Yahoo; dermatology textbooks; as well as the University of California, San Francisco, Surge Building library files for relevant literature published between 1967 and December 2004. The following key words were searched: race, ethnicity, black, African, white, Caucasian, Hispanic, Asian, vulva, skin of vulva, and skin physiology.

We found that there were few studies of vulvar ethic differences and that the few existing studies often had inconclusive results and findings that conflicted with other studies. This chapter presents a compilation of results of the studies of the vulvar ethnic differences with regard to TEWL, water content, corneocyte variability, blood vessel reactivity, skin elastic recovery, skin extensibility, pH gradient, lipid content, and skin surface microflora.

ASSESSMENTS OF VARIABLE CHARACTERISTICS OF ETHNICALLY/RACIALLY DIFFERENT SKIN

Transepidermal Water Loss

Table 1 (3–12) quantifies our knowledge of ethnic differences in skin for TEWL. Most studies assessed the TEWL on the forearm, back, and inner thigh.

Berardesca and Maibach (4) supported the findings that TEWL is higher in blacks in their 1988 study. The investigators determined the difference in irritation between young black and white patients by applying the irritant 0.5% sodium lauryl sulfate (SLS) to untreated, pre-occluded skin. They found a statistically significant difference in the TEWL, with blacks having 2.7 times higher TEWL levels than whites ($P < 0.04$), suggesting that black skin in the pre-occluded state is more susceptible to irritation (Table 1). Hispanics were found to have higher TEWL values compared to whites, but this was not statistically significant (5). At baseline, Sugino et al. found TEWL to be blacks > Caucasians ≥ Hispanics ≥ Asians. After tape stripping, Berardesca and Maibach (4) found that TEWL is 1.2 times higher in black women than in Caucasian women on the midvolar forearm. Data from the studies in Table 1 are conflicting, possibly due to testing on different anatomic sites.

All the evidence supports that blacks have higher TEWL than whites, except for Berardesca et al. (6), who found no significant difference and Warrier et al., who found TEWL blacks < whites. TEWL measurements of Asian skin are inconclusive, as they have been found to be equal to black skin and greater than Caucasian skin (7), and less than all the other ethnic groups (8). Future research should include more races and larger sample sizes.

Water Content

Various researchers studied ethic differences in water content (hydration) of the skin on multiple body sites using various techniques (in vivo resistance, capacitance, conductance, and impedance) (Table 2) (4–6,8,10,13,14). The results of the stratum corneum water content of the various studies are difficult to interpret, as other factors (e.g., sweat production, hair on the site of measurement) might impair the quality of the electrode contact with the skin. Overall, the studies indicate that racial differences in water content measured by resistance, capacitance, conductance, and impedance are inconclusive.

Corneocyte Variability

Three studies investigated corneocyte desquamation in black, white, and Asian subjects (Table 3) (10,14,15). All the studies had statistically significant—yet

Table 1 Transepidermal Water Loss

References	Technique	Subjects	Site	Results
(3)	In vitro	Blacks 10 (mean age 38.6); Caucasians 12 (mean age 41.1)	Inner thigh	• TEWL blacks 1.1× > Caucasians (mean corrected log TEWL 2.79 and 2.61 $\mu g/cm^2/hr$, respectively) ($P < 0.01$, for both values)
(4)	In vivo with topical application of SLS (irritant)	Black men 10 (age 29.9 ± 7.2); white men 9 (age 30.6 ± 8.8)	Back	• No significant difference in TEWL between blacks and whites at baseline *After SLS stress*: • TEWL blacks (untreated, pre-occluded, and predelipidized) > whites but only statistically significant (2.7× greater) for the 0.5% SLS applied in the pre-occluded area ($P < 0.04$)
(5)	In vivo with topical application of SLS (irritant)	Hispanic men 7 (age 27.8 ± 4.5); white men 9 (age 30.6 ± 8.8)	Upper back	• No significant differences in TEWL between Hispanics and whites at baseline *After SLS stress*: • TEWL Hispanics (untreated, pre-occluded, and predelipidized) > whites, but not statistically significant
(6)	In vivo	Blacks 15 (mean age 46.7 ± 2.4); whites 12 (mean age 49.8 ± 2); Hispanics 12 (mean age 48.8 ± 2)	Volar and dorsal forearm	• No significant difference in TEWL between sites or races at baseline
(7)	In vivo with topical application of MN—vasodilator	Blacks 7; Caucasians 8; Asians 6 (ages 23 to 32)	Volar forearm	*Vasodilator given*: • Before tape stripping: TEWL blacks and Asians 1.3× > Caucasians ($P < 0.01$); no difference between blacks and Asians

(Continued)

Table 1 Transepidermal Water Loss (*Continued*)

References	Technique	Subjects	Site	Results
				After eight and twelve tape strips: • TEWL Asians > blacks > Caucasians ($P < 0.05$) (Asians 1.7× > Caucasians)
(8)	In vivo	Blacks, Caucasians, Hispanics, Asians (number of subjects, ages not specified)	Not documented	• Baseline TEWL blacks > Caucasians ≥ Hispanics ≥ Asians
(9)	In vivo	Skin type V/VI: African American 4 Filipino 2 Hispanic 1 Skin type II/III: Asian 6; Caucasian 8 (ages 22 to 38)	Volar forearm	• Skin type V/VI required more tape strippings (66.7 ± 6.9) compared to skin type II/III (29.6 ± 2.4) to achieve the same TEWL, i.e., skin type V/VI had increased water barrier strength (integrity) • Barrier function in skin type V/VI recovered more quickly
(10)	In vivo	Black women 30; Caucasian women 30 (ages 18 to 45)	Left and right medial cheeks, midvolar forearms, lateral mid-lower legs	• TEWL blacks < whites on cheeks (20% less) & legs (17% less) at baseline ($P < 0.05$); also lower on forearm but not statistically significant
(11)	In vivo	Black women 8; Caucasian women 10; (mean age 42.3 ± 5, both)	Midvolar forearm	*After tape stripping*: • TEWL blacks 1.2×> Caucasians after 3 ($P < 0.05$) & 6 tape strips ($P < 0.03$)

Note: Ages reported in years.
Abbreviations: TEWL, transepidermal water loss; SLS, sodium lauryl sulfate; MN, methyl nicotinate.
Source: Adapted from Ref. 2.

Table 2 Water Content

References	Technique	Subjects	Site	Results
(13)	In vivo—resistance	St. Louis (ages 83 to 92 mo): black boys (22), black girls (32); white boys (65), white girls (55) San Diego (mean age 23 yr): black men (16), black women (5); white men (16), white women (5)	First and third fingers of right hand	• Skin resistance blacks > whites at baseline ($P < 0.01$); i.e., blacks have lower water content
(4)	In vivo with topical application of SLS (irritant)—capacitance	Black men (10) (age 29.9 ± 7.2); white men (9); (age 30.6 ± 8.8)	Back	• No significant differences between blacks and whites at baseline or after SLS stress
(5)	In vivo with topical application of SLS (irritant)—capacitance	Hispanic men (7); (age 27.8 ± 4.5); white men (9); (age 30.6 ± 8.8)	Upper back	• No significant differences between Hispanics and whites at baseline *After SLS stress*: • Hispanics > whites when negative visual score was given for irritation ($P < 0.01$) (large standard deviations)
(6)	In vivo—conductance	Blacks (15) (mean age 46.7 ± 2.4); whites (12) (mean age 49.8 ± 2); Hispanics (12) (mean age 48.8 ± 2)	Volar and dorsal forearm	• Blacks (13% less) volar < dorsal forearm ($P < 0.02$) Whites (22% less) dorsal < volar forearm ($P < 0.001$) Hispanics (11% less) dorsal < volar forearm ($P < 0.05$)

(*Continued*)

Table 2 Water Content (*Continued*)

References	Technique	Subjects	Site	Results
				• Black and Hispanics > whites on dorsal forearm at baseline • Hispanics > blacks and whites on volar forearm at baseline
(8)	In vivo—impedance	Blacks, Caucasians, Hispanics, Asians (number of subjects, ages not specified)	Not documented	• Asians > Caucasians, blacks and Hispanics
(10)	In vivo—capacitance	Black women (30); white women (30) (ages 18 to 45)	Left and right medial cheeks, midvolar forearms, lateral midlower legs	• Blacks > whites on cheeks at baseline ($P < 0.05$) • No significant difference between races on the forearms and legs
(14)	In vivo-capacitance	Black women (7), white women (5) (mean age 25.8 ± 4.2, both); black women (5), white women (5) (mean age 64.7 ± 3.8, both)	Preauricle, post neck, dorsal upper arm, dorsal forearm, volar forearm, lower back, abdomen, thigh, lower leg	• No significant differences between blacks and whites at baseline

Note: Ages reported in years unless specified otherwise.
Abbreviation: SLS, sodium lauryl sulfate.
Source: Adapted from Ref. 2.

Table 3 Corneocyte Variability

References	Subjects	Site	Results
(15)	Black (mean age[a] 33.5 ± 7.5); Caucasian (mean age 31 ± 7); Asian (mean age 26.5 ± 7.5) (18 to 25 subjects per group)	Upper outer arm	• No difference in corneocyte surface area • Spontaneous desquamation (corneocyte count) blacks 2.5× > Caucasians and Asians ($P < 0.001$)
(10)	Black women (30); white women (30) (ages 18 to 45)	Left and right medial cheeks, midvolar forearms, lateral midlower legs	• Desquamation index blacks < whites on cheeks (18% less) and forearms (20% less) ($P < 0.05$); but no significant differences on the legs
(14)	Black women (7), white women (5) (mean age 25.8 ± 4.2, both); black women (5), white women (5), (mean age 64.7 ± 3.8, both)	Preauricle, post neck, dorsal upper arm, dorsal forearm, volar forearm, lower back, abdomen, thigh, lower leg	• No difference in desquamation index between blacks and whites except at preauricular area ($P = 0.02$) (which race greater is not specified)

[a]Ages reported in years.
Source: Adapted from Ref. 2.

conflicting—results. Corcuff et al. (15) reported that spontaneous desquamation measured on the upper outer arm was 2.5 times greater in blacks than in whites and Asians ($P < 0.001$); Warrier et al. (10) found desquamation to be less in blacks and Manuskiatti et al. (14) detected a difference only at the preauricular measurement site. Again, variation in the anatomic site may cause variable results, as well as the environmental conditions when the tests were conducted. Racial differences in corneocyte desquamation are inconclusive. The most clinically provocative observation is that of Corcuff, et al. who found a 2.5 times greater spontaneous desquamation rate in blacks compared to Caucasians and Asians.

Blood Vessel Reactivity

Several studies have investigated racial blood vessel reactivity as an assessment of skin physiology, irritation, evaluation of dermatologic pathology/treatments, effects and delivery of drugs, and wound healing. Earlier evaluation of cutaneous microcirculation depended on visual scoring to assess erythema or pallor (blanching), which has been proven to be unreliable. Two techniques, laser Doppler velocimetry (LDV) and photoplethysmography (PPG), can measure cutaneous blood flow. LDV has been utilized in skin physiology research, diagnostics, predictive testing of irritancy of substances (cosmetics, cleansing agents, topical medications, etc.), and cutaneous effects of drugs. PPG has been applied to skin physiology studies, dermatological disorders, and systemic diseases (16,17).

Table 4 summarizes the findings of six studies of blood vessel reactivity in blacks, whites, Hispanics, and Asians (4,5,7,17–19). Each study involved the administration of different vasodilating or vasoconstricting substances, thus, the results cannot be compared. However, each study, except for Berardesca et al. (5), found some variation in blood vessel reactivity when comparing Hispanics and whites. These findings are indicative of disparities in irritation, dermatotoxicology, and dermatopharmacology among different ethnic groups.

Skin Elastic Recovery and Extensibility

Racial differences in skin elastic recovery (Table 5) and extensibility (Table 6) were recorded by Berardesca et al. (6) and Warrier et al. (10). Extensibility is measured by applying torque parallel to the skin and measuring the amount of stretch; elastic recovery is the time the skin takes to return to its original state after the torque is released.

These data vary by anatomic site of testing and by race, and age of study participants may affect the results, as well. Therefore, conclusions cannot be drawn from these data and further investigation, involving larger populations of participants and controlling for age differences, is necessary.

Table 4 Blood Vessel Reactivity

References	Technique	Subjects	Site	Results
(17)	Topically administered MN (vasodilator); LDV and PPG	Blacks (6) (age 20 to 30); whites (6) (age 20 to 30); whites (6) (age 63 to 80)	Volar forearm	*Vasodilator given*: • No significant difference in time to peak response, area under response-time curve, or time for response to decay to 75% of its maximum value • PPG maximum response young black (40% less) < young white ($P < 0.05$)
(4)	Topically administered SLS (irritant); LDV	Black men (10) (age 29.9 ± 7.2); white men (9) (age 30.6 ± 8.8)	Back	*SLS stress*: • No significant difference between blacks and whites • Blood vessel reactivity minimal in blacks from baseline to application of 0.5% SLS on untreated skin (see text for details)
(5)	Topically administered SLS (irritant); LDV	Hispanic men (7) (age 27.8 ± 4.5); white men (9) (age 30.6 ± 8.8);	Upper back	*SLS stress*: • Similar LDV response in Hispanics and whites

(*Continued*)

Table 4 Blood Vessel Reactivity (*Continued*)

References	Technique	Subjects	Site	Results
(18)	Topically administered corticoid[a] (vasoconstrictor); DV	Black men (6); Caucasian men (8) (mean age 27 ± 3, both)	Forearm	*After vasoconstrictor given*: • 40% decreased area under the curve response blacks compared to whites ($P < 0.04$) • 50% decreased peak response in blacks compared to whites ($P < 0.01$) • Decreased decay slope after peak blood flow in blacks compared to Caucasians; in blacks, $y = 3.3672 - 0.0737\times$ before treatment compared to $y = 2.5347 - 0.0367\times$ after treatment ($P < 0.04$) $\Rightarrow$ i.e., less blood vessel reactivity in blacks
(19)	Topically administered MN (vasodilator); LDV	Blacks (5); Caucasians (5); Asians (5) (ages 20 to 35)	Upper 1/3 volar forearm	*Vasodilator given*: • Area under the curve for LDV response versus time blacks > Caucasians for all MN concentrations ($P < 0.05$)

				• Area under the curve for LDV response versus time Asians > Caucasians for higher dose levels of MN ($P < 0.05$)
(7)	Topically administered MN (vasodilator); LDV	Blacks (7); Caucasians (8); Asians (6) (ages 23 to 32)	Volar forearm	*Vasodilator given*: • *Before tape stripping*: no difference between the groups in basal perfusion flow, but lag time before vasodilatation was blacks > Caucasians > Asians ($P < 0.05$) • *After 8 and 12 tape strips*: lag time before vasodilatation decreased in all three groups, but significantly decreased in Asians > Caucasians > blacks ($P < 0.05$)

[a]Corticoid, clobetasol propionate 0.05% ointment.
Abbreviations: MN, methyl nicotinate; LDV, laser Doppler velocimetry; PPG, photoplethysmography; SLS, sodium lauryl sulfate.
Source: Adapted from Ref. 2.

Table 5 Skin Elastic Recovery

Reference	Technique	Subjects	Site	Results
(6)	In vivo	Blacks (15) (mean age 46.7 ± 2.4); whites (12) (mean age 49.8 ± 2); Hispanics (12) (mean age 48.8 ± 2)	Volar and dorsal forearm	• No significant difference between races on dorsal forearm • Elastic recovery blacks (26% less) < whites on volar forearm ($P < 0.001$)
(10)	In vivo	Black women (30); white women (30) (ages 18 to 45)	Left and right medial cheeks, midvolar forearms, lateral midlower legs	• No significant difference between races on the legs • Elastic recovery blacks 1.5× > whites on cheeks ($P < 0.05$)

Source: Adapted from Ref. 2.

pH Gradient

Berardesca et al. (11) and Warrier et al. (10) (Table 7) also explored the differences in pH between the skin of Caucasian and black women. At baseline, no significant differences were found. After tape stripping, a lower pH in black

Table 6 Skin Extensibility

Reference	Technique	Subjects	Site	Results
(6)	In vivo	Blacks (15) (mean age 46.7 ± 2.4); whites (12) (mean age 49.8 ± 2); Hispanics (12) (mean age 48.8 ± 2)	Volar and dorsal forearm	• Significant dorsal < volar extensibility within whites and Hispanics ($P < 0.001$ and $P < 0.002$, respectively) • Black > white extensibility dorsal forearm ($P < 0.01$) • Black < white extensibility volar forearm ($P < 0.01$)

Source: Adapted from Ref. 2.

Table 7 pH Gradient

Reference	Subjects	Site	Results
(11)	Black women (8); Caucasian women (10) (mean age 42.3 ± 5, both)	Midvolar forearm	• No significant difference in pH at baseline *After tape stripping*: • pH significantly decreased in blacks after three tape strips, i.e., superficial SC layers • No differences between races after 9, 12, and 15 tape strips, i.e., deeper SC layers
(10)	Black women (30); white women (30) (ages 18 to 45)	Left and right medial cheeks, midvolar forearms, lateral midlower legs	• pH blacks (pH = 5.15) < whites (pH = 5.52) on cheeks at baseline ($P < 0.05$) • No significant difference in pH on the legs at baseline

Abbreviation: SC, stratum corneum.
Source: Adapted from Ref. 2.

skin compared to white skin was recorded in the superficial layers of the stratum corneum, but not in the deeper layers.

However, the studies differed in anatomic testing sites and one study did not test after tape stripping. Although the results suggest that there may be some difference in the pH of stratum corneum between these races, the factors responsible for this remain unknown.

LIPID CONTENT

Three studies evaluated lipid content (Table 8) (8,20,21). Again, the studies were variable in the anatomic sites tested, and one early study also evaluated the skin of black male cadavers. Sugino et al. (8) found increased lipids in blacks as compared to whites; Reinertson and Wheatley (20) found higher lipid levels in blacks, and Harding et al. (21) found no difference between participants from the United Kingdom and Thailand.

Surface Microflora

Researchers inoculated forearm skin of 10 black and 10 white men with *Candida albicans* and visually scored the severity of dermatitis by the severity

Table 8 Lipid Content

Reference	Subjects	Site	Results
(20)	*Cadavers*: Black man (1); white men (3) *Living*: Black man (1); white man (1) (ages 49–68)	*Cadavers*: Abdomen *Living*: Back and thigh	• Lipid and sterol content in total epidermis blacks > whites
(8)	Black, white, Hispanic, and Asian (number of subjects, age not specified)	not documented	• Ceramide levels blacks (50% less) < whites and Hispanics ($P < 0.05$)
(21)	U.K. (41); Thai (dry season) (31); Thai (humid season) (31) (ages 20 to 40)	Scalp	• U.K. and Thai subjects demonstrated similar levels of total lipids

Source: Adapted from Ref. 2.

of pustules (Table 9) (10,22). They also assessed microflora population after aerobic incubation. Another study evaluated facial skin microflora in black and white women. Both studies found that blacks had more skin microflora than whites, but the results differed with regard to the density of

Table 9 Skin Surface Microflora

Reference	Subjects	Site	Results
(22)	Black men (10); white men (10) (ages 21–59)	Forearm	• *Candida albicans* blacks (150% greater) > whites ($P < 0.025$) • Aerobes blacks (650% greater) > whites ($P < 0.025$)
(10)	Black women (30); white women (30); (ages 18 to 45)	Left and right medial cheeks, midvolar forearms, lateral midlower legs	• Density of *Propionibacterium acnes* blacks > whites, but not statistically significant • No significant difference in aerobes

Source: Adapted from Ref. 2.

aerobes. Thus, further investigation will be necessary before conclusions can be drawn.

Mast Cell Granules

Sueki et al. (23) used electron microscopy to study punch biopsies of normal skin from black and white men. The study revealed statistically significant structural differences between the mast cells of black versus white skin (Table 10); black skin had larger mast cell granules, increased parallel-linear striations, and increased tryptase localized to parallel-linear striation. Further research should focus on investigating pro-inflammatory mediators and involve a larger participant pool.

CLINICAL OBSERVATIONS

Clinically, acute contact dermatitis occurs more commonly in whites than in blacks (1). Blacks, however, develop disorders of pigmentation and lichenification more often than whites. Hyperpigmentation is thought to occur more readily in black patients after contact with mild irritants. These data suggest that there are ethnic/racial predispositions to certain skin conditions.

Qualitatively, it has been noted that vulvar appearance in dark-skinned blacks and Hispanics is somewhat different from fair-skinned patients with atopic dermatitis and neurodermatitis (7). The erythema is masked by the dark skin color, leading examiners to underestimate the severity of the inflammatory process. Lichenification is often exaggerated and postinflammatory hyperpigmentation is always present (24). Wesley and Maibach (2) concluded that differences exist, but that much remains to be done to clarify extent, mechanisms, and clinical relevance.

Racial (ethnic) differences in the skin of the vulva are likely to exist, considering such differences in other areas of the body. Given reasonable evidence of objective studies supporting differences in the skin function and physiology among ethnicities/races in general, it is likely that such difference also exists in regard to the skin of vulva, in particular. Racial hair differences are dramatic and unquestioned (25).

CONCLUSION

Evidence supports black skin having a higher TEWL, greater variable blood vessel reactivity, decreased skin surface pH, and larger mast cell granules than white skin. Although differences exist in water content, corneocyte desquamation, elastic recovery/extensibility, lipid content, and skin microflora, they are inconclusive (Table 11). Further evaluation of Asians and Hispanics is needed for a better understanding and less conflicting results.

It is known that the vulva is more permeable than the exposed skin due to its structure, hydration, occlusion, and susceptibility to friction. Future studies in

Table 10 Mast Cell Granules

Reference	Technique	Subjects	Site	Results
(23)	EM of biopsy specimen	Black men 4 (mean age 29.2 ± 3); Caucasian men (4) (mean age 29.4 ± 1.2)	Medial-lateral buttock	• Mast cells contain 1.5× larger granules in black skin compared to white skin ($P < 0.0001$) • Mast cells contain 15% more PLS in blacks compared to whites ($P < 0.05$) • Mast cells contain 30% less curved lamellae in blacks compared to whites ($P < 0.05$) • Tryptase immunoreactivity localized to PLS regions in black skin, compared to curved lamellae regions in white skin ($P < 0.0001$) • Cathepsin G localized to electron-dense amorphous subregions in both black and white skin

Abbreviations: EM, electron microscopy; PLS, parallel-linear striations.
Source: Adapted from Ref. 2.

Table 11 Conclusions

Evidence supports	Insufficient evidence for	Inconclusive
• TEWL black > white skin • Variable racial blood vessel reactivity • pH black < white skin • Larger mast cell granules, increased PLS, and increased tryptase localized to PLS in black compared to white skin	• Deductions regarding Asian and Hispanic skin Racial differences in: • Skin elastic recovery/extensibility • Skin microflora	Racial differences in: • Water content • Corneocyte desquamation • Lipid content

Abbreviations: TEWL, transepidermal water loss; PLS, parallel-linear striations.
Source: Adapted from Ref. 2.

Table 12 Considerations for Future Research of Racial Skin Differences

- Baseline versus "stress" test differences
- Anatomic site examined
- Open versus occluded stresses
- Ethnic groups in the same versus varying geography
- Comparable climatic conditions
- Presentation of hard data and statistical analysis
- Larger sample sizes
- Relationship of study parameters to degree of pigmentation
- Definition of ethnicity/race
- Comparable diets (e.g., controlled diets)
- Socioeconomic factors
- Prior dermatologic disease
- Skin care prior to study
- Body mass relationship

Source: Adapted from Ref. 2.

dermatology should address such differences by studying vulvar skin directly (Table 12). We suggest using objective techniques similar to those listed in Table 1 when studying the vulva. Such studies will be more challenging to perform given the potential difficulty accessing the vulva and collecting objective data, and the potential difficulty in recruiting sufficient numbers of participants to achieve statistical power. A greater understanding of these ethnic/racial differences should lead clinicians to a more effective path toward management.

REFERENCES

1. Berardesca E, Maibach HI. Ethnic skin: overview of structure and function. J Am Acad Dermatol 2003; 48:S139.
2. Wesley NO, Maibach HI. Racial (ethnic) differences in skin properties: the objective data. Am J Clin Dermatol 2003; 4:843.
3. Wilson D, Berardesca E, Maibach HI. In vitro transepidermal water loss: differences between Black and white human skin. Br J Dermatol 1988; 199:647.
4. Berardesca E, Maibach HI. Racial differences in sodium lauryl sulphate induced cutaneous irritation: black and white. Contact Dermatitis 1988; 18(2):65–70.
5. Berardesca E, Maibach HI. Sodium-lauryl-sulphate-induced cutaneous irritation. Comparison of white and Hispanic subjects. Contact Dermatitis 1988; 19:136.
6. Berardesca E et al. In vivo biophysical characterization of skin physiological differences in races. Dermatologica 1991; 182:89.
7. Kompaore F, Marly JP, Dupont C. In vivo evaluation of the stratum corneum barrier function in Blacks, Caucasian, and Asians with two noninvasive methods. Skin Pharmacol 1993; 6:200.

8. Sugino K, Imokawa G, Maibach HI. Ethnic difference of stratum corneum lipid in relation to stratum corneum function [abstract]. J Invest Dermatol 1993; 100:587.
9. Reed JT, Ghadially R, Elilas PM. Skin type, but neither race nor gender, influence epidermal permeability function. Arch Dermatol 1995; 131:1134.
10. Warrier AG et al. A comparison of Black and white skin using noninvasive methods. J Soc Cosmet Chem 1996; 47:229.
11. Berardesca E et al. Differences in stratm corneum pH gradient when comparing white Caucasian and Black African-American skin. Br J Dermatol 1998; 139:855.
12. Aramaki J et al. Differences of skin irritation between Japanese and European women. Br J Dermatol 2002; 146:1054.
13. Johnson LC, Corah NL. Racial differences in skin resistance. Science 1962; 139:766.
14. Manuskiatti W, Schwindt DA, Maibach HI. Influence of age, anatomic site and race on skin oughness and scaliness. Dermatology 1998; 196:401.
15. Corcuff P et al. Racial differences in Corneocytes: a comparison between black, white, and oriental skin. Acta Derm Veneral 1991; 71:146.
16. Wahlberg JE, Lindberg M. Assessment of skin blood flow: an overview. In: Berardesca E, Elsner P, Maibach HI, eds. Bioengineering of the Skin: Cutaneous Blood Flow and Erythema. Boca Raton: CRC Press, Inc., 1995:23.
17. Berardesca E, Maibach HI. Cutaneous reactive hyperemia: racial differences induced by corticoid application. Br J Dermatol 1989; 129:787.
18. Guy RH et al. Are there age and racial differences to methyl nicotinate-induced vasodilatation in human skin? J Am Acad Dermatol 1985; 12:1001.
19. Gean CJ et al. Cutaneous responses to topical methyl nicotinate in Black, Oriental, and Caucasian subjects. Arch Dermatol Res 1989; 281:95.
20. Reinertson RP, Wheatley VR. Studies on the chemical composition of human epidermal lipids. J Invest Dermatol 1959; 32:49.
21. Harding CR et al. Dandruff: a condition characterized by decreased levels of intercellular lipids in scalp stratum corneum and impaired barrier function. Arch Dermatol Res 2002; 294:221.
22. Rebora A, Guarrera M. Racial differences in experimental skin infection with candida albicans. Acta Derm Venereol 1988; 68:165.
23. Sueki H, Whitaker-Menezes D, Kligman AM. Structural diversity of mast cell granules in Black and white skin. Br J Dermatol 2001; 144:85.
24. Lynch PJ, Edwards L. Genital Dermatology. New York: Churchill Livingstone, 1994.
25. Olsen E. In disorders of hair and scalp. Body and facial hair.

15

Female Genital Alterations: A Sociological Perspective

Samar A. Farage
Department of Sociology, Pennsylvania State University, State College, Pennsylvania, U.S.A.

INTRODUCTION

In the last 30 years, female genital mutilation has become the topic of worldwide discussion and debate both as a health issue and a human rights violation (1–5). In 1996, the World Health Organization estimated that approximately 100 million women undergo different forms of genital alterations in over 60 developing countries (6). Three types of such alterations are recognized widely by authorities as constituting genital mutilation. The first type, called Sunna circumcision, involves the removal of the prepuce with or without the excision of part or all of the clitoris. The second type of mutilation involves partial or total removal of the clitoris as well as scraping off the labia majora and minora. The third type, the most extreme form, consists of infibulation or pharaonic circumcision, which removes the clitoris, adjacent labia, and then sews the scraped sides of the vulva leaving a small opening for urine and menstrual blood (6).

Calling these forms of alteration "mutilation" has become a political issue. Some researchers have argued that using the term mutilation to refer to the traditional forms of female cuttings is a value-laden approach that condemns the cultural context of these practices. They also question the appropriateness of the use of the term "female circumcision" on the grounds that the severity of the harm done to women is underplayed by such comparison to male circumcision

(5,7). Thus, this chapter avoids using these value-laden terms and uses the neutral phrase "female genital alterations" (8). This terminology permits the exploration of practices of genital alteration regardless of country, rationale, or even degree of technological sophistication. In addition, because of the political connotations of "female genital mutilation," the sociological and medical literature on the topic has focused on practices in Africa and Asia and almost entirely overlooked the history and current prevalence of female genital alterations in the West.

Female genital alterations began in the Western countries around the 1820s and were mainly justified as a cure for the "diseases" caused by excessive masturbation and nymphomania. The advent of such surgical alterations was linked to a transformation of masturbation from a sin, condemned by the Church for centuries, into a medical condition. This chapter discusses the distinct forces that converged to create a new illness called "postmasturbatory disease," which comprised such different manifestations as epilepsy, syphilis, fatigue, and dementia thought to be caused by masturbation. The extraordinary obsession with masturbation during the 19th century that led to female genital surgeries cannot be understood without considering the strange confluence of economic, cultural, religious, and medical ideas.

The Masturbation Scare

Masturbation was not an object for prescientific or Galenic medicine, which reigned supreme from the 2nd century AD until the late Middle Ages. For 1500 years until the 17th century of Western history, the precepts guiding medical practices were based on the Galenic conception of the body as a flux of fluid humors: black bile, yellow bile, blood, and phlegm. Maintaining good health required the balance of these humors in their correct proportions; disease was signaled by either an excess or deficiency in these fluids (9). Hence, masturbation was considered quite therapeutic in certain cases, because it led to the evacuation of excessive seed in the body (10). Therefore, medieval physicians such as Avicenna, Albert the Great, and Riverius recommended the "friction of the genitals" for health purposes (11,12). This understanding of masturbation implied that it was not a moral issue within premodern medical thought. Even though some premodern physicians such as Boorde and Boerhaave in the 17th century warned of the debilitating psychological and physical effects of masturbation, they did not speak of it as a moral issue (13).[a] However, this would change profoundly in the modern period as a consequence of the influence of church edicts against masturbation.

[a]E. H. Hare (1962) documents the debilitating effects ascribed by Boerhaave in his *Institutes of Medicine* (1701): "the semen discharged too lavishly occasions a weariness, weakness, indisposition of motion, convulsions, leanness, dryness, heats and pains in the membranes of the brain, with a dullness of the senses, more especially of the sight, a tabes dorsalis, foolishness and disorder of the kinds." However, we can see no specific mention of masturbation per se (although it was included under sexual activity) until the beginning of the 18th century, and no belief that it was specifically harmful.

Masturbation was always a subject of discussion in religious circles; the church had condemned it as a minor variant of illicit sexual activities that were explicitly outside the realm of procreation and, therefore, were against nature (11,14,15). The church doctrine on masturbation was unequivocal: any kind of masturbation was forbidden and the physician who recommended it for health was no less a sinner than the person who engaged in it.[b] From the beginning of the Middle Ages, the position of the church evolved from a complex argument based on a stridently debated distinction between nocturnal emissions and voluntary pollutions. Its most vehement interdictions were aimed at the latter rather than the former, which were classified as a mere venial sin. In contrast, voluntary pollution was considered a mortal sin or sin against nature because it provoked sexual pleasure without carnal union (15). This claim was backed by the authority of two Biblical texts. The first from Genesis invoked the crime of Onan, who was punished by God for "spilling his seed" (Gen: 38; 6–10). The second is found in the first letter of St. Paul to the Corinthians (6; 9–10), who insisted that those guilty of "mollities" would be banned along with fornicators and sodomites from the Kingdom of God. The condemnation of the Church was not restricted to the bare act itself but extended to the lascivious thoughts that accompanied it. Thus, for example, thinking of the Virgin Mary aggravated the mortal sin into a "horrendum sacriligium" and imagining oneself in the company of a married woman was equivalent to adultery (14).

Hence, before the 18th century, the medieval physician and the medieval priest viewed masturbation differently. Before the second half of the 18th century, none among the theologians and jurists who condemned masturbation as a sin against nature based his verdict on medical grounds. On the other hand, few if any medieval doctors spoke of masturbation as a sin, much less as a mortal one (16).

The publication in 1710 in England of *Onania, or The Heinous Sin of Self Pollution and its Frightful Consequences in Both Sexes Considered, with Spiritual and Physical Advice to Those Who Have Already Been Injured by This Abominable Practice and Seasonal Admonition to the Youth of the Nation of Both Sexes*, was a signal event in the West.[c] Though written from within the Christian perspective (11,17), it marked the merger between the once distinct medical and religious positions on masturbation. By insisting that masturbation had reached epidemic proportions, the author aimed at fostering "Virtue and Christian Purity and to Discourage Vice and Uncleanliness." The book was extremely popular; it began as a 60-page pamphlet, and by the 16th edition had

[b]In the fourth Lateran council of 1215 under Innocent III, it was stated, "since the soul is much more precious than the body, we forbid any physician under pain of anathema, to prescribe anything for bodily health of sick persons that may endanger their souls."

[c]Authorship and date of publication are still subject to dispute according to most commentators, though the scholarly consensus seems to vacillate between John Marten and the priest Becker.

grown to 194 pages accompanied by a 142-page supplement comprising letters from sufferers, repented sinners, and supporters.

The book is divided into three sections: causes, consequences, and diseases caused by self-pollution. Masturbation was not only condemned as a sin, but by tracing its consequence upon both the body and the soul, the author inserted the moral consequences into the medical outcomes. For example, masturbation was linked to stunted growth, phimosis and paraphimosis, strangury, priapism, gonorrhea, ulcers, thin and waterish seed, fainting fits, epilepsy, consumption, loss of erection, premature ejaculation, and infertility. The book is notable for not only raising the specter of masturbation as a medical, moral issue but for describing the ill effects of masturbation on women. Hence, masturbation was believed to cause the relaxation of private parts and "retentive faculty" leading to infertility, because male semen could no longer be held within the woman. Moreover, according to the author of *Onania*, women who masturbated were prone to hysterical fits, barrenness, imbecility, fluor albis (leucorrhea), multiple miscarriages, and infertility. In addition, masturbators suffered physical transformations: "meager jaws, pale looks, feeble hams, legs without calves, their generative faculties weakened if not destroyed... dryness, emaciation, spirit sunk, body wasted, strength decayed" (14). Moreover, their entire progeny and the very future of the human race apparently lay in the balance: "from the wretches that survive, children may be expected so sick and weakly that they are a misery to themselves, a dishonor to the Human race and a scandal their parents" (18).

The remedies for this "heinous sin" were both physical and moral. While the recommendations of marriage repentance and renunciation were the usual fare of moral injunctions, the author distinguished himself as a clever marketer by hawking 10-shilling "strengthening tinctures," 12-shilling "prolific powders," and "Aromatik Snuff" (18). After the publication of *Onania*, the term "onanism" made its appearance for the first time in the encyclopedia, defined roughly as the involuntary efflux of semen (synonyms were "mastupratio, manstupratio, and manustupratio"). By tying together the medical and moral reflections on masturbation, *Onania* provided a fecund frame for the proliferation of moral anxieties and the multiplication of medical interventions around "nature's handmaiden."

The repercussions of this pamphlet were felt on the European continent and absorbed within the burgeoning spirit of the French Enlightenment. However, it was the book written in 1758 by the Swiss physician Samuel August Tissot that raised masturbation to the position of a "colossal boogey" (13). In this book, published in Latin as *Tentamen de Morbis ex Manustrupatione* and translated into French in 1760 as *L'Onanisme ou Dissertation Physique sur les Maladies Produites par la Masturbation*, Tissot departs from the English *Onania* and its moral-theological overtones (19). Instead, Tissot makes much of his scientific grounding by asserting that 1 oz of sperm is equal to exactly 40 oz of blood. Hence, at this purported ratio of exchange, it was not surprising that Tissot considered sperm a very valuable fluid, calling it a "precious liquid." This idea was echoed almost 100 years later by Dr. George Calhoun of the United States, who stated, "the production of semen takes place much more slowly than that of any other secretion in the human body. This is owing to the route that semen has to take. If all seminal canals were extended in one line, it would be about 5208 ft long . . . the immense length shows that it is difficult for the semen to reproduce but that its excessive loss must be attended with disastrous consequences on the whole organism" (14).

Tissot's scientific aims extended to the mental effects of masturbation. Following the third law of Newton on action and reciprocal reaction, Tissot theorized that orgasms were spasms of extreme nervous activity that necessitated an equal and opposing depression of the nerves. This dampening of the nervous activity caused permanent derangement when it occurred too frequently, making the individual more susceptible to apoplexy, paralysis, insanity, and other nervous diseases (17). This idea contributed to the 19th century notion of "masturbatory insanity" caused by permanent brain damage due to constant irritation.

Therefore, according to Tissot, masturbation denuded the body of blood and, thus, gave rise to grave physical and mental consequences. Included among these were weakening of the digestive system, loss of or excessive appetite, vomiting, indigestion, breakdown of the respiratory system, general debility and lassitude, as well as damages to the faculties and memory. The consequences to women were even more grave, because masturbation led to hysteria, "vapeurs affreuses," incurable jaundice, stomach cramps, prophase and ulceration of the womb, and clitoral rashes, for example. The young were particularly vulnerable, as the loss of "precious liquid" stunted their natural physical development and contributed to feeblemindedness (14,17).

By providing a pathological model of masturbation rooted in the seemingly scientific and secular domain, Tissot's book sparked the 19th century medico-scientific masturbation phobia in the United States. Masturbation was transformed from one of the many forms of seminal and excretory loss into a sexual practice potentially fatal to individuals and society alike (20,21).

THE MANAGEMENT OF SEXUALITY AS A PROBLEM: POSTMASTURBATION DISEASE

The drastic cures and genital alterations that were developed for the first time in the 19th century emerged as a response to the masturbation scare. However, this development cannot be understood fully without understanding how sex became an object of political intervention (22). Historians of the 19th century have pointed out that the health of the nation-state depended on a micro-regulation of individual bodies as well as the management of populations (23–27). As evidenced by the medical journal *The Lancet* in 1819, doctors thought of themselves as being "... responsible for the employment of (their) peculiar authority in promoting the purification and well being of human society" (28).

This political regulation of sexuality as a paradigmatic instance of health management emerged at the confluence of five distinct (yet related) forces:

1. Changes in medical authority
2. Changes in body perception
3. The invention of childhood sexuality
4. The new demands of the industrialized economy
5. A renewal of religious fervor and Victorian cultural ideals

Changes in Medical Authority: The Physician/Priest and the New Body

It is now well known that since the beginning of the 19th century, the moral authority of the physician in the United States grew to encompass that of the priest. As noted by the social historian Englehardt, "the cycle of sin, confession, penance, and redemption was transferred from the confessional to the consulting room" (29) (also see Ref. 30). In this new role of physician/priest, doctors not only attempted to cure diseases but also enforced the standards of a puritanical sexual morality well into the middle of the 20th century (31). By being able to tie the scientifically established consequences of masturbation to morally freighted proscriptions against it, doctors were able to give a new legitimacy to the idea of postmasturbatory diseases. From then on, such diseases would constitute the locus for the definition of normal sexuality and the massive political efforts to control people. Although the moral injunction against masturbation was venerable, the addition of the scientific standing of medicine in the early 19th century provided decisive weight to the political management of sexuality. For example, the nerve theory of Haller and Cullen; the discovery of tissues as the site of disease by Bichat and Broussais; the confirmation of the mechanical nature of respiration and circulation first suggested by Harvey; and the entitative nature of disease agents established by Mortgagni constituted some of the diverse strands that led the emergence of scientific medicine (32).

Changes in Body Perception

The explanations offered for postmasturbatory diseases since the early 19th century under the lights of scientific medicine were based on a new concept of the human body as being analogous to a machine (33,34). The older understanding of the body as composed of fluid humors was replaced by a structural and functional view, which implied that the body was reducible to a machine composed of nerves, fibers, muscles, and glands. This conception of the body was not only promulgated by the physicians but adopted by their patients, who would routinely speak of themselves using terminology such as "depleted energy," "nervous excitations," and "muscular fatigue" (32). A substantial current within the new scientific medicine was the belief that sexual excess threatened the loss of vital energy. This theme, which drew from the theories of energy conservation in physics of the mid-19th century, entailed that each person was invested with a finite quantity of energy and its misuse would lead to physical degeneration and mental depravity (35). This energy model of the body would be instrumental in the creation of a new "spermatic economy," in which sperm—like money and labor force—had to be used optimally (36).

The Invention of Childhood Sexuality

The idea of childhood sexuality did not exist before 1700. Neither priest nor physician paid any attention to the sexual behaviors of children. In the beginning of the 18th century, both the moralist and the medic began to censure childhood sexual activity as both sinful and/or pathological. By the 19th century, masturbation among children was considered a social evil and a threat to the polity as a whole; it became the first building block in the invention of childhood sexuality (37–39). Just as sexuality in general was considered a problem to be managed, childhood sexuality in particular would give rise to the concerted and institutionalized effort to control children. For example, whether through schools, churches, or new forms of parental supervision, the child was thought of as a distinct social entity in need of specialized attention (40). This belief gave rise to the vast industry of child-rearing techniques premised on regulating childhood sexual behavior and instilling childlike obedience to authority (26,38,41). As the flow of semen coincided with the onset of puberty, it was widely believed that any loss of semen at this age would stunt development and growth (20). As the well-being of a child became linked to his or her sexual propensities and behaviors, parents became willing agents to the nostrums of the 19th century medical establishment that recommended chastity belts, toothed rings on the penis, strait jackets, surgeries, and other such procedures (42,43).

The Demands of an Industrialized Economy

The onset of widespread industrialization in the United States beginning in the mid-19th century led to a heightened attention to the idea of labor force. The requirement of a hard-working pool of labor for the emerging factories promoted the ideas of labor productivity, work ethic, and the bourgeois character, who exercised financial thrift and sexual continence. The capitalist economy based on maximizing efficiency in the use of resources demanded maximum productivity with minimum waste. Furthermore, the fruits of industrialization were well understood to be the consequence of the interdependence arising from the division of labor. In this sense, economic strength and political order of a nation depended crucially on the self-discipline of people imbued by a strong sense of civic responsibility (16,20,44). This generalized schema had its counterpart in the "spermatic economy"; sperm, like money, had to be invested fruitfully. Therefore, such acts as masturbation and frequenting prostitutes were seen as wasting the potential to accumulate precious capital. As masturbation was a solitary vice performed alone, it was condemned as antisocial and narcissistic. The self-absorbed masturbator was considered the exemplar of those who refused to contribute to the well-being of the nation (20,44,45). The idea of climbing the social and economic ladder that was held as ideal in the 19th century American society required the laboring classes to mimic the sexual self-control or sublimation that contributed to the success of the middle classes (46,47). The professional and gentlemanly class differentiated itself by adhering to the repressive demands of continence to fuel their economic prowess. In a similar vein, the moral-medical attacks on prostitution and nymphomania were justified by the argument that such practices were unproductive and bore no useful fruit (15). Thus, prostitution and the regulation of women's sexuality received major impetus from the consideration of sexuality in economic terms (48). The wastefulness inherent in the commerce with oneself or others thus became a major front in the creation of sexuality as a problem to be managed. It was precisely this mentality that would later fuel the eugenic movement in the Anglo-American world.

Victorian Ideals and Religious Fervor

The division of labor required by the new industrial economy redefined the ideals of masculinity and femininity (33). The separation of work from home life cemented the division between the roles of men and women, mainly in the middle classes (49). In this newly defined role, women were confined to the home and thought to be frail, passive, and passionless (50–52). By the middle of the 19th century, men were thought of as producers whereas women were considered to be reproducers. This growing sexual division of labor was underscored by medico-scientific theories that posited the naturalness of this divide by arguing that women's passive nature left them ill-equipped for the competitive world of education, work, and politics. Women's delicate nervous system, monthly "illness," smaller brain, and specific reproductive organs all made them unhealthy to vote, work, go to college, or participate in the public arena (53). The Victorian ideal of a woman as nurturing, affectionate, intuitive, moral, domesticated, and dependent was assumed to have a biological basis in smaller and, therefore more sensitive, nerves that made women more prone to anxiety, neurasthenia, hysteria, and irrationalities (54–57). Medical prejudice considered women prisoners of their reproductive organs and thought that a woman's uterus and ovaries controlled her body and behavior from puberty to menopause. So deep was this medical idea rooted in the Victorian ideal that even as late as 1870, a physician is on record as stating, "It was as if the Almighty, in creating the female sex, had taken the uterus and built up a woman around it" (47). Thus, any exposure to sexual excesses was considered detrimental to their sexual purity and effectiveness as mothers (47,54). Indeed, a curious reversal of sexual identity was ascribed to masturbation. It was believed that men would become more effeminate while women would become more masculine (as agitating the clitoris would render it more penis-like) if either engaged in acts of "self-help" (33).

Another current feeding the Victorian ideal of the passionless woman was the rise of the Evangelical movement in the United States between 1790s and 1900s. Within this movement, rooted in Protestantism, there was no distinction between mortal and venial sins. Accordingly, all sexual acts were sins per se, unless for the purpose of procreation. Promoting of Christian values and virtues contributed to the transformation of women from sexual to moral beings responsible for the upbringing of future generations (51). In this role, churchmen such as Rev. John Todd (1800–1873) used their pulpits to bully women into exercising sexual restraint as proof of their moral and noble character. Pulpits—no less than manuals, pamphlets, and exhortations—were used to spread the masturbation phobia throughout the 19th century (36,58).

This combination of moral, economic, and medical factors that gave rise to sexuality as a problem created the conditions for an intensive and unprecedented investigation into techniques and methods to control the sexual behavior of men, women, and children (37,59). Notably, women were the principal experimental guinea pigs for the rash of surgical techniques, instruments, and devices aimed at controlling sexual energies (60–62).

TYPES OF FEMALE GENITAL ALTERATIONS

The application of surgical procedures to the genitalia of men, women, and children is a predominantly 19th century phenomenon in the West. Male circumcision has an ancient and largely religiously inspired history (60,63). However, genital surgeries on females and children are almost exclusively a product of the 19th century. Moreover, the use of instruments and devices to restrain sexual activity in the general population (as opposed to monks) gains much in inventiveness and intensity of pain during this period. While the above-mentioned factors contributed to the acceptance of genital surgeries and related devices, three rationales were given during the 19th century for their specific use (64–69).

First, as masturbation was linked to a wide and seemingly limitless range of diseases from epilepsy to rheumatism and insanity, the medical establishment focused much of its curative efforts on the genitalia. This therapeutic rationale was foremost among the justifications for genital surgical interventions and the invention of new methods for sexual restraint (70). For example, according to the 1848 report on the Massachusetts Lunatic Asylum, approximately 32% of admissions were for self-pollution (71). Further, it was a routine matter to castrate such inmates in droves to prevent masturbation and, thus, to cure them of insanity. Women in particular were "castrated" by removing their ovaries to cure them of psychological disorders (72,73).

The second dominant rationale was that of public health or sanitary injunctions. According to this line of reasoning, both doctors and public health officials were concerned with maintaining the general health of the population; they were involved in cleaning up pollution whether caused by industry or self (74). This large-scale effort to sanitize cities and bodies would also encourage putting self-polluters into insane asylums and then using them as a captive population for experimenting with advances in genital surgeries and devices of restraint. Even private entrepreneurs got into the sanitary game. Wellness centers sprung up all over the country, a good example of which is the Kellogg Center for Clean and Healthy Living (75). Not only were Kellogg's corn flakes sold as a healthy non-stimulant designed to dampen all sexual passions, but his centers were the hotbed for restraining techniques (41,76). Sylvester Graham, a Presbyterian minister, invented the Graham cracker, which, together with a mild vegetarian diet, was intended to reduce sexual cravings, while C.W. Post marketed his Postum cereal as the "Monk's Brew."

Lastly, a general rationale often mentioned was the need to eradicate childhood sexuality. It is notable that a vast proportion of the surgical interventions and instruments were applied to the bodies of young children, both boys and girls. For example, the antimasturbation school bench was designed to force students to keep their legs apart and avoid rubbing their genitals; long coats were forbidden and strenuous gymnastics, boxing, and other vigorous sports were recommended to channel the energy of the young into productive activities (43).

PROCEDURES OF THE 19TH AND 20TH CENTURIES

Methods to control female sexuality included relatively pain-free interventions such as hydrotherapy, dietary prescriptions, and educational exhortations. However, the use of inventive restraints of various kinds flourished during this period as a preferred method of controlling women's bodies (48). For instance, the Moody Girdle of Chastity of the mid-19th century is exemplary. It "... consisted of a cushion made out of rubber or some other soft material and suitably covered with silk, linen, or soft leather. This cushion or pad formed the base into which was fixed a kind of grating and this part of the apparatus rested upon the vulva, the pad being large enough to press upon the mons veneris ..." (43).

Dietary measures, hydrotherapy, educational exhortations, and even physical restraints seemed too slow in their effects on stopping masturbation. Surgery was a much quicker procedure and was often described as affording immediate relief and preventing the further development of illnesses and deterioration of patients (77).

The onset of surgical genital procedures can be attributed to the medical work of Dr. Marion Sims, the "father of gynecology" and the "architect of the vagina." By the mid-19th century, the traditional art of obstetrics expanded to include the new science of gynecology (36). Procedures that explored the interior of female anatomy were the brainchild of Dr. Sims in the United States. It was he who invented the vaginal speculum and systematized the use of uterine sound and curette, and cervical dilators. Around this time, the first specialized medical journal in the United States was devoted to obstetrics. Descriptions of ovariotomies, hysterectomies, and the repair of vesicovaginal fistulas conducted under the most primitive conditions were featured routinely in its pages. Dr. Sims performed surgery to repair vesicovaginal fistulas and applied his techniques, without the use of anesthesia, first on slave women in Alabama. Later, during the mid-19th century, he exported these techniques to upper-class women in New York.

While Dr. Sims was engaged in his surgical experiments in the United States, Dr. Isaac Baker Brown introduced clitoridectomies in England as a cure for epilepsy, syphilis, insomnia, unhappy marriages, and even insanity. He was the president of the Medical Society of London and considered an authority on the nervous diseases of women. As a consequence, his work on scissoring the clitoris became the model for this surgical intervention. Dr. Brown believed that all feminine weaknesses could be cured by the excision of the clitoris. According to him, the peripheral excitement of the pubic nerve, which ends in the clitoris, led to disease that could be divided into eight progressive stages of degeneration: hysteria, spinal irritation, hysterical epilepsy, cataleptic fits, epileptic fits, idiocy, mania, and death. Hence, restlessness, loss of appetite, back pain, and distaste for marital intercourse were considered signs that demanded clitoridectomy (78–80). In cases in which he avoided excising the clitoris, he would damage the vulva and the clitoris by applying caustic substances to cause painful sores.

It is interesting to note that by the 1860s, the work of Dr. Brown was castigated by the medical community in England and he was removed from his position in the obstetrical society. In England, the practice of clitoridectomies declined rapidly in the face of the vociferous criticism that centered on its brutality. Nevertheless, Dr. Brown's inventiveness found a fertile home in the United States. The evangelical impulse that gained ground quickly gave his techniques a moral legitimacy. What was then viewed with disfavor in England became the procedure of choice for the moral correction of women and girls in the United States.

By the 1880s, with the increasing association of masturbation and insanity, female castration or oophorectomy became widespread (81). This procedure was the 1882 invention of Dr. Robert Batty of Georgia and was called normal ovariotomy (73,82). The vogue of female castration received encouragement under the eugenic movement and lasted well into the 1940s. Indeed, the eugenic movement inspired not only castration but also the rampant use of sterilization as a cure for insanity and general debility (13,83).

The prevalence of genital surgeries as a legitimate medical procedure can be gauged by the establishment of the Chicago-based Orificial Surgery Society in the late 1880s (43,65). During its uninterrupted and popular run until the 1920s, the Society, which was composed of prominent medical experts, oversaw the regular publication of a professional journal and textbooks. The Society was anchored by the belief that the lower orifices were responsible for moral, religious, and emotional well-being. For example, as a disorder in the sphincters could cause nervous irritation, the Society recommended dilation, amputation, and related operations on women and men. Between approximately 1850 and 1950, the United States was the site for a sustained rash of surgical procedures perfomed on the genitalia of men, women, and children (60,84). Whereas the last recorded castration was performed in 1946, the last medically justified clitoridectomy occurred in Kentucky in 1953 in a 12-year-old girl (58). The call for developing new and better, improved techniques still was voiced in the late 1950s (85). In retrospect, it can be seen that the advent and flourishing of genital surgeries for over a century was a complex response to the masturbation scare.

CONTEMPORARY FEMALE GENITAL ALTERATIONS IN NORTH AMERICA

Even though the scare died down after the Kinsey Report of 1948, which normalized masturbation and even considered it a healthy release or an expression of self-love, genital surgeries for medical reasons did not end completely (15). Female circumcision was continued to be encouraged in the postwar years for cleanliness, hygiene (18), frigidity, cancer, urinary tract infections, prevention of sexually transmitted diseases such as AIDS and HIV (35), and genital anomalies. One gauge of the latter is that approximately 2% or approximately 80,000 live births in the United States annually are subjected to modifications of genitalia to define the sexuality (7,86,87). These operations (sex reassignment surgeries) are performed on infants whom the medical literature calls intersex children (88,89). In general, these rationales for female genital surgeries are less prominent than those of the preceding century.

Cosmetic Genital Surgery

Recently, a different rationale for female genital surgeries has begun to emerge. Triggered by standards of genital beauty established by the pornographic industry, fearing the aging of genitalia, and seeking the ultimate orgasm, women are both demanding and being tempted to undergo surgical alterations for cosmetic reasons (90,91). This practice seems to have escaped the scholarly literature, although the medical establishment has begun to enjoy its financial benefits. As documented in the popular press, genital plastic surgery appears as a growth area within the field of cosmetic surgery (92). Procedures once aimed at therapeutic interventions to correct incontinence, congenital malformations, and injuries sustained during childbirth are now sold as elements in the architectural redesigning of the vulva (93). The old procedures now carry new names, such as elective vaginal enhancement, vaginal rejuvenation, female genital aesthetics, vaginoplasty (tightening of the vagina), hoodectomy (unhooding of the clitoris), labiaplasty (reduction of the labia minora or labia majora), reduction of the mons pubis, hymenaplasty (reconstruction of the hymen), and raising the aging pubis (94).[d]

CONCLUSION

This chapter has examined the different rationales that were offered to legitimize female genital surgeries or alterations. These procedures, which began in the early 19th century, were rooted in the great terror associated with masturbation. The sustained effort for more than 100 years to control the bodies of women and children gave rise to a vast array of devices and techniques to surgically alter their genitalia. In retrospect, the therapeutic rationales offered since the early 1800s are clearly specious. Given the World Health Organization's definition of female genital mutilation ("all procedures that involve partial or total removal of female external genitalia and/or injury to the female genital organs for cultural or any other nontherapeutic reasons"), then the conclusion that the Western history of female genital surgery should be considered genital mutilation is compelling. More troubling is the realization that the procedures now conducted in the name of elective genital enhancements in Western countries are no less a form of mutilation. Thus, genital mutilation is not a practice peculiar to far-away developing countries.

REFERENCES

1. Amnesty International USA. Female Genital Mutilation: A Human Rights Info Pack. New York: Amnesty International, 1997.
2. Dorkenoo E. Cutting the Rose: Female Genital Mutilation: the Practice and Its Prevention. London: Minority Rights Group, 1995.
3. Hosken FP. Female Genital Mutilation: Women Speak: Facts and Actions. Lexington, MA: Women's International Network News, 1975.
4. Lightfoot-Klein H. Prisoners of Ritual: An Odyssey into Female Genital Circumcision in Africa. New York: Haworth Press, 1989.
5. Walley CJ. Searching for "voices": feminism, anthropology, and the global debate over female genital operations. Cult Anthropol 1997; 12:405.
6. World Health Organization. Female Genital Mutilation: Report of a WHO Technical Working Group. Geneva: World Health Organization, 1996.
7. James SM, Robertson CC. Genital Cutting and Transitional Sisterhood. Urbana/ Chicago: University of Illinois Press, 2002.
8. Gruenbaum E. The Female Circumcision Controversy. Philadelphia: University of Pennsylvania Press, 2001.
9. Farage SA. Galenic medicine. In: Mitcham C, ed. Encyclopedia of Science, Technology and Ethics. New York: MacMillian Press, 2005.
10. Galen C. On the Affected Parts. In: Siegel R, ed. Basel: Karger, 1976.

---

[d]See the compilation of recent media articles documenting this new fashion of genital cosmetic surgeries in Media Articles on Designer Vaginas (2001).

11. Singy P. Friction of the genitals and secularization of morality. J Hist Sexuality 2003; 12:345–365.
12. Burton R. Anatomy of Melancholia. New York: Vintage Books, 1977.
13. Hare EH. Masturbatory insanity: the history of the idea. J Mental Sci 1962; 108:1.
14. Stenghers J, Van Neck A. Masturbation: The History of a Great Terror. London: Palgrave, 2001.
15. Laqueur T. Solitary Sex: A Cultural History of Masturbation. New York: Zone Books, 2003.
16. Bennett P, Rosario V. The politics of solitary pleasures. In: Bennett P, Rosario V, eds. Solitary Pleasures. New York: Routledge, 1999:1.
17. Wong M. Because it's there: morals and medicine and masturbation in the 19th century. Historical Rev 2002; 79:263.
18. MacDonald R. The frightful consequences of onanism: notes on the history of a delusion. J Hist Ideas 1967; 28:423.
19. Stolberg M. Self pollution, moral reform and venereal trade: notes on the source and historical context of Onania 1716. J Hist Sexuality 2000; 9:37.
20. Rosario V. Phantastical pollutions: the public threat of private vice in France. In: Bennett P, Rosario V, eds. Solitary Pleasures. New York: Routledge, 1999:101.
21. Spitz R. Authority and masturbation: some remarks on a biographical investigation. Psychoanalyt Quarterly 1952; 21:493.
22. Caplan P, ed. The Cultural Construction of Sexuality. London: Tavistock, 1987.
23. Foucault M. History of Sexuality. New York: Vintage Books, 1980.
24. Foucault M. The battle for chastity. In: Foucault M, ed. Ethics, Subjectivity and Truth. New York: Routledge, 2002:192.
25. Weeks J. Sexuality and Its Discontents. London: Routledge, 1985.
26. Davidson A. The Emergence of Sexuality. Cambridge: Harvard University Press, 2001.
27. Brain D. From the history of science to the sociology of the normal. Contemp Sociol 1990; 19:902.
28. Smith FB. The People's Health 1830–1910. Canberra: Australian National University Press, 1979.
29. Engelhardt T. The disease of masturbation: values and the concept of disease. BHM 1974; 48:244.
30. Haller J, Haller R. The Physician and Sexuality in Victorian America. Urbana: University of Illinois Press, 1974.
31. Hamowy R. Medicine and the criminalization of sin: self-abuse in 19th century America. J Libertar Studies 1977; 1:229.
32. Porter R. The 18th century. In: Lawrence Conrad, ed. The Western Medical Tradition: 800–1800. Cambridge: Cambridge University Press, 1995:371.
33. Stolberg M. An unmanly vice: self pollution. Social Hist Med 2000; 1:1.
34. Duden B. The Woman Beneath the Skin: A Doctor's Patient in Eighteenth Century Germany. Cambridge: Cambridge University Press, 1991.
35. Hodges F. A short history of the institutionalization of involuntary sexual mutilations in the US. In: Denniston G, Milos M, eds. Sexual Mutilations: a Human Tragedy. New York: Plenum, 1997:17.
36. Barker-Benfield GJ. The Horrors of the Half-Known Life. New York: Harper Row, 1976.

37. Fishman S. The history of childhood sexuality. J Contemp His 1982; 17:269.
38. Aries P. Centuries of Childhood. London: Cape, 1973.
39. Neuman RP. Masturbation, madness and the modern concepts of childhood and adolescence. J Social Hist 1975; 8:8.
40. Shorter E. The Making of the Modern Family. New York: Basic Books, 1975.
41. Demos J. The American family in past time. Am Scholar 1974; 43:422.
42. Stone L. The Family, Sex, and Marriage in England, 1500–1800. New York: Harpers and Row, 1977.
43. Comfort A. The Anxiety Makers. New York: Dell Publishing Co., 1967.
44. Mosse G. Nationalism and respectability: normal and abnormal sexuality in the 19th century. J Contemp Hist 1982; 17:221.
45. Gilbert A. Doctor–patient/onanist diseases in the 19th century. J Hist Med Allied Sci 1975; 30:217.
46. Cominos P. The Victorian sexual respectability and the social system. Int Rev Soc Hist 1963; 8:18;216.
47. Rosenberg C, Smith-Rosenberg C. The female animal: medicine and biological views of women and her role in 19th century America. J Am Hist 1973; 60:332.
48. Daly M. Gynecology. Boston: Beacon Press, 1990.
49. Tilly L, Scott J. Women's work and the family in 19th century Europe. Compar Studies Society Hist 1975; 17:36.
50. Gronemen C. Nymphomania: A History. New York: W.W. Norton, 2000.
51. Cott N. Passionless: an interpretation of Victorian sexual ideology 1790–1850. Signs 1978; 4:219.
52. Walter R, ed. Primers for Prudery: Sexual Advice to Victorian America. Prentice Hall: Englewood Cliffs, 1974.
53. Stage S. Out of the attic: studies in Victorian sexuality. Am Quarterly 1975; 27:480.
54. Freedman E. Sexuality in nineteenth century America: behavior, ideology and politics. Rev Am Hist 1982; 10:196.
55. Vicinus M. Suffer and Be Still. Bloomington: Indiana University Press, 1972.
56. Thierot N. Gender and medicine in 19th century America. NWSA J 2000; 15:144.
57. Helmstadler RJ. Suffer and be still: women in the Victorian age: a review article. Am Hist Rev 1973; 78:693.
58. Ehrenreich B. For Her Own Good: 150 Years of Expert Advice to Women. New York: Anchor Books, 1978.
59. Hart G, Wellings K. Sexual behavior and its medicalization in sickness and health. Br Med J 2002; 324:896.
60. Remondino CP. History of Circumcision from the Earliest Times to the Present: Moral and Physical Reasons for Its Performance. New York: AMS Press, 1891 (reprint 2001).
61. Kandela P. Clitoridectomy. Lancet 1999; 353:1453.
62. Wright J. Female genital mutilation: an overview. J Advanced Nurs 1996; 24:251.
63. Webber S. Cutting history, cutting culture. Am J Bioeth 2003; 3:65.
64. Hutchinson J. On the Influence of circumcision in preventing syphilis. Med Times Gazette 1855; 2:542.
65. Bergman N. Report of a few cases of circumcision. J Orificial Surg 1898; 7:249.
66. Moses MJ. The value of circumcision as a hygienic and therapeutic measure. NY Med J 1871; 10:368.

67. Sayre L. Spinal anemia with partial paralysis and want of coordination from irritation of the genital organs. Trans Am Med Assoc 1875; 26:255.
68. Ricketts M. Circumcision: the last fifty of two hundred circumcisions. NY Med J 1894; 59:431.
69. Taylor W. Circumcision—its moral and physical necessities and advantages. Med Record 1899; 56:174.
70. Szasz T. The therapeutic state: remembering masturbatory insanity. Ideas Liberty 2000; 50:35.
71. Duffy J. Masturbation and clitoridectomy. JAMA 1963; 186:246.
72. Battey R. Castration in mental and nervous diseases. Am J Med Sci 1886; 92:483.
73. Battey R. Normal ovariotomy. Atlanta Med Surg J 1872; 10:32.
74. Wolbarst AL. Universal circumcision as a sanitary measure. JAMA 1914; 62:92.
75. Kellogg JH. Plain Facts for Old and Young: Embracing the Natural History and Hygiene of Organic Life. Burlington, IA: I.F. Senger & Co., 1877.
76. Darby R. The masturbation taboo and the rise of routine male circumcision. J Soc Hist 2003; 36:737.
77. Wallerstein E. Circumcision: An American Health Fallacy. New York: Springer, 1980.
78. Sheehan E. Victorian clitoridectomy: Isaac Baker Brown and his harmless operative procedure. In: Lancaster RN, di Leonardo M, eds. The Gender Sexuality Reader: Culture, History, Political Economy. New York: Routledge, 1997:325.
79. Coventry M. Making the cut. Ms Magazine, Oct/Nov 2000. Available at: http://www.msmagazine.com/oct00/makingthecut.asp. Accessed Sept 9, 2005.
80. Baker Brown I. On the Curability of Certain Forms of Insanity, Epilepsy, Catalepsy. London: Robert Hardwicke, 1866.
81. Pratt EH. Circumcision of girls. J Orifical Soc 1898; 6:385.
82. Thiery M. Battey's operation: an exercise in surgical frustration. Eur J Obstet Gynecol Reprod Biol 1998; 81:243.
83. Reilly PR. Involuntary sterilization in the US: a surgical solution. Q Rev Biol 1987; 69:153.
84. Paige-Ericken K. The ritual of circumcision. Human Nature 1978; May, 40.
85. Rathmann WG. Female circumcision: indications and a new technique. Gen Pract 1959; 20:115.
86. Creighton SM. Feminizing genital surgery: what should be done and when? J Pediatr Adolesc Gynecol 2005; 18:63.
87. Conway L. Vaginoplasty: male to female sex reassignment surgery. Available at www://ai.eecs. umich.edu/people/conway/conway.html. Accessed Sept 9, 2005.
88. Chase C. What is the agenda of the intersex patient advocacy movement? Endocrinologist 2003; 13:240.
89. Turner S. Intersex identities. Gender Societies 1999; 13:457.
90. Kellison C. $100 surgery for a million-dollar sex life. Playgirl 1975; May, 62.
91. Kellison C. Circumcision for women. Playgirl 1973; Oct 124.
92. Kinsey, Alfred. (The Kinsey Report) Sexual Behavior in The Human Male. Philadelphia: W.B. Saunders, 1948.
93. Navarro M. The most private of makeovers. New York Times 2004; Nov 28.
94. Wilding F. Vulvas with a difference. Available at: C-Theory.net. Accessed Sept 5, 2001.
95. www.labiaplastysurgeon.com. Accessed Sept 9, 2005.

PART V. INVESTIGATIONAL METHODS

16

Bioengineering Methods for the Vulva

Sibylle Schliemann, Britta Opper, and Peter Elsner
Department of Dermatology and Allergology, Friedrich-Schiller University, Jena, Germany

INTRODUCTION

Noninvasive bioengineering methods permit sophisticated detection and quantification of subclinical changes in skin physiology. Some methods have become standard in specialized fields such as skin pharmacology, cosmetology, and dermatological research. However, their application also can be beneficial when studying the female genital area. Human vulvar skin is an example of specialized skin, comprising keratinized epithelium and nonkeratinized mucosa, accompanied by considerable underlying age- and hormone-related changes throughout life. Exposure to humidity, occlusion, friction, and a particular microbial environment, coupled with the lack of UV exposure, contribute to unique functional skin characteristics, such as a less-complete water barrier function as compared to other body regions (1–3). Garments, shower gels, soaps, moisturizers, deodorants, sanitary pads, as well as condoms may induce subclinical skin irritation or even apparent contact dermatitis (4).

Therefore, enhanced susceptibility of the vulva to irritants might be assumed but, surprisingly, this has not been ascertained in general by bioengineering clinical studies (2,5). In contrast to apparent conditions such as acute allergic contact dermatitis, lichen sclerosus, or psoriasis, clinical assessment of low-grade vulvar irritation is often difficult due to considerable interindividual variability of normal vulvar skin, which can often include some degree of erythema even in unaffected women. In addition to simple clinical scoring systems such as that of Frosch and Kligman [which has been used for a long time for quantification of inflammatory responses and irritation in many experimental settings (2,6–8), noninvasive bioengineering methods allow researchers to monitor subclinical changes, for example, the inflammatory state and skin blood flow, the barrier function, and stratum corneum hydration.

In general, when applying bioengineering methods to female genital skin, a convenient measuring environment free of disturbance is a prerequisite. A trusting relationship between the patient and the investigator must be established in order to minimize artifacts caused by emotional stress. Indeed, even "training" of volunteers may be necessary to achieve reproducible measurements (9). In order to avoid typical pitfalls, it is necessary to become familiar with the technical background of the devices used and perform the procedures in a standardized manner (10). Area recognition is a problem in all noninvasive measurements used on genital skin. Dansyl chloride 1% in petrolatum as a fluorescent marker can be helpful in this regard (7).

COMMON BIOENGINEERING TECHNIQUES

Erythema Quantification—Skin Color Reflectance

The color of the skin, and of any object, depends on the wavelength of the light and the optical characteristics of the surface. Different chromophores, mainly hemoglobin and melanin in healthy skin, absorb different wavelengths of light. Detailed insight into the complex optical principles of the skin and chromophores is provided by Pierard and by Kollias (11,12). Measurement of skin color reflectance is a suitable method for erythema quantification in addition to clinical assessment. It has been applied frequently in the grading of contact dermatitis and irritant and allergic patch-test reactions (13). Its value has also been proven in studies on the vulvar skin with respect to erythema quantification in irritant contact dermatitis (7). Skin color reflectance is especially suitable for serial measurements and also can be used for ethnic skin (14,15). However, the sensitivity of an experienced dermatologist's eye may still be superior to instrumental erythema quantification (12).

In contrast to the spectrophotometric method, which uses broadband (scanning) or selected wavelengths, the Minolta Chroma Meter (Minolta Chroma-Meter CR-300®, Minolta, Osaka, Japan) is a tristimulus colorimeter, which refers to the recommendations of the Commission Internationale de l'Eclairage. Color is expressed in a three-dimensional coordinate system, in terms of three units: L^* (luminance/brightness) (white–black), a^* (red–green), and b^* (yellow–blue) (Fig. 1). a^* represents the red–green axis with +100 expressing full red and −100 expressing full green (13). The Chroma Meter is equipped with a polychromatic xenon flashlight for the illumination of the skin area and is easy to handle. Prior to the measurements, the instrument must be calibrated. As the genital skin color is influenced by the modulations of cutaneous blood flow, caused by temperature, orthostatic effects, the emotional

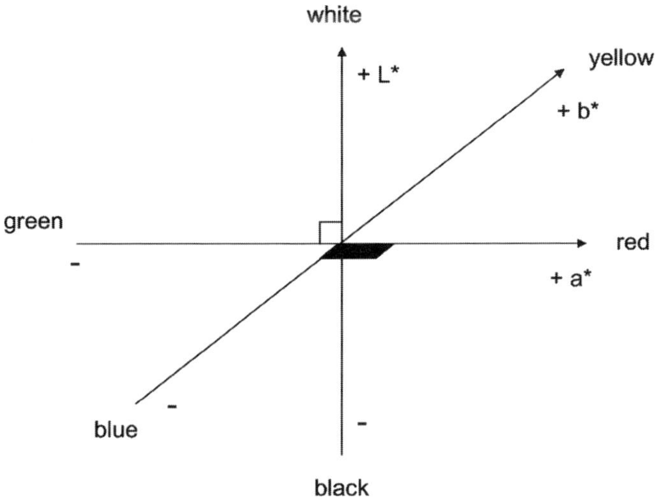

Figure 1 The Commission Internationale de l'Eclairage system: Guideline for the measurement of skin color and erythema. *Source*: Adapted from Ref. 13.

status as well as the intake of drugs or caffeine, measurements should always be performed in a standardized and reproducible setting, following the guidelines thoroughly (13,16). In order to obtain reliable results, the probe should be held to the skin without exerting pressure. Taking the arithmetic means of repeated measurements for analysis is advisable. Baseline L^*-values of healthy, unaffected vulvar skin were shown to be significantly lower, indicating a higher absorption of light, whereas a^*-values were significantly higher compared to forearm skin, due to higher basal blood flow on the vulva. After induction of experimental irritant contact dermatitis, a^* increased significantly in both sites, but less on the vulva, whereas the L^*-values remained unchanged on the vulva, but decreased at the forearm (7).

Cutaneous Blood Perfusion—Laser Doppler Flowmetry

The laser Doppler flowmetry (LDF) is an excellent noninvasive technique for monitoring cutaneous blood perfusion. As an early indicator of inflammation and changes in the microcirculation, LDF has been applied in many fields of clinical medicine and dermatology in healthy skin as well as in inflammatory diseases (17), and also for research purposes in the vulvar skin (5,8,18,19). Monochromatic, coherent light is emitted onto the skin and reflected at different wavelengths by the tissue and by the moving red blood cells in small vessels. The reflected light is detected photoelectrically and a dimensionless output signal is generated, which is proportional to the red blood cell flow. The signal is then processed in a personal computer, and the perfusion level can be displayed and calculated in a color-coded manner on the screen. Areas of interest can be defined and analyzed separately. By using a Laser Doppler Perfusion Imager (LDPI), the disadvantage of placing the probe directly on the skin can be avoided. Furthermore, larger areas of up to 12 cm^2 can be mapped (18). However, in the genital area, scanning larger areas is difficult, as the vulvar skin is not flat and, therefore, not parallel to the probe, which can lead to artifacts (18). The laser Doppler technique has been used to quantify the irritant response of the vulva to sodium lauryl sulfate (SLS) in an experimental setting. By using measuring intervals of 45 seconds with a sampling rate set at one measurement per second, a higher baseline but a lower blood flow increase of the vulvar skin was detected as compared to the forearm skin after exposure to SLS. The sensitivity for detecting changes of the relative blood flow was higher compared to visual scoring (7,8). In lichen sclerosus lesions, the perfusion was found to be elevated and even increased after mechanical alteration, due to scratching, mast cell degranulation, histamine release, and reactive vasodilatation (20). In epithelial tumors, such as the vulvar squamous cell carcinoma, increased cutaneous perfusion was detected using LDPI, which was attributed to neoangiogenesis with a lack of autonomic control (21). This method is relatively time consuming and easily influenced by environmental as well as individual-related factors (22). Constant measurement conditions, such as room temperature and relative humidity, must be maintained, as well as rest periods for the subjects (at least 20 minutes) prior to the measurements.

Transepidermal Water Loss

Disturbance of the epidermal barrier function, which is maintained mainly by corneocytes and stratum corneum lipids, occurs with increased transepidermal water loss (TEWL). This phenomenon occurs early in irritant reactions and precedes visible skin changes. Accordingly, the TEWL is a very sensitive parameter and has become one of the most important bioengineering methods. Measurement of the TEWL has been used in several studies on the vulvar skin, mainly to quantify irritant contact dermatitis (2,23,24). Different methods for TEWL measurements are available. In general, the more common open-chamber devices, such as the Tewameter® (Courage & Khazaka, Cologne, Germany), and the Evaporimeter® (Servo Med, Stockholm, Sweden) have become much more established, as compared to the closed-loop systems (25). The open-chamber methods utilize a cylindric probe that is integrated in a hand piece and equipped with a pair of sensor units (hygro sensors coupled with thermistors). When placed onto the skin, the probe measures the continuous water vapor gradient from the skin surface. Ideally, the probe should be handled in a horizontal plane position, which is difficult to achieve on the vulvar skin. In contrast, the closed system is designed to be applicable in different positions (25). However, the main drawback of this method is the tendency to occlude the skin, thus causing artifacts. Furthermore, continuous measurements are not possible with this method (26).

Baseline values of the TEWL were found to be significantly higher on the vulva compared to the forearm skin (27). Age-related differences were observed between pre- and post-menopausal women, as the TEWL was significantly lower in postmenopausal compared to premenopausal women (28). In general, significant intra- and inter-individual variations of the TEWL are well known, not only in the genital area. As the water evaporation from the skin is also influenced by thermoregulative requirements of the individual and sweat gland activity, it is of utmost importance to exclude disturbing variables by thoroughly following the guidelines of the European Society of Contact Dermatitis on the measurements of TEWL (26). TEWL can only be measured after an appropriate waiting period for the postocclusion water loss to subside (9).

Skin Hydration Measurement

Skin dryness is related to the water content of the stratum corneum. The stratum corneum hydration interacts with the barrier function, permeability, and mechanical properties of the skin and is related to the water-binding capacity of the stratum corneum lipids (29). Objective quantification of skin hydration by bioengineering tools has gained wide popularity, as it provides fundamental information of the skin function and is comparatively easy to perform. Three electrical methods for the skin hydration measurements are used currently, based on capacitance, impedance, and conductance measurements (30). The Corneometer® (Courage & Khazaka, Cologne, Germany) is based on a capacitance measurement. Two metal plates with an electric field in between are integrated in the electrode surface. Capacitance is the capability to store the electrical charge that is built up by the electron excess at one plate and an electron deficit at the other plate. It is influenced by the dielectric constant of the material between the plates, which changes with water content. The device estimates the water content in the epidermis up to an approximate depth between 60 and 100 μm (29). The Corneometer CM 825® is the most recent version. The Skicon® principle is based on the conductance measurement of a fixed high-frequency current of 3.5 MHz with a probe consisting of two concentric electrodes (I.B.S. Hamamatsu-shi, Japan). It measures more superficial depths as compared to the Corneometer. The Nova Dermal Phase Meter® (Nova Technology Corporation, Gloucester, Massachusetts, U.S.A.) is an impedance-based capacitance instrument (30). Fluhr et al. (31,32) have undertaken comparative and systematic studies of five instruments.

In order to gain accurate and reliable results with any of the devices, a considerable number of individual and environmental factors must be recognized. Dependence of the position and pressure exerted on the probe must be considered. Because of occlusion, values can increase in repeated measurements. Thus, waiting periods of at least five seconds are recommended. In addition, environmental conditions must be considered; constant room temperature and relative humidity should be ascertained (30).

Capacitance measurements with the use of the Corneometer have had widespread application, as does the measurement of the TEWL, in studies of vulvar skin physiology and experimental contact dermatitis (2,5,7,8,23,24,27). Baseline capacitance values of unaffected, healthy skin were found to be significantly higher at the vulva as compared to the forearm. However, reactivity of female genital skin after exposure to typical detergent irritants such as SLS was not higher as compared to the forearm (28). Age-related differences were detected in pre- and post-menopausal vulvar skin. The dehydrating capacity of SLS was less pronounced in postmenopausal as compared to premenopausal women (27).

Skin Surface pH

In general, the pH value reflects the free hydrogen ion concentration of aqueous solutions. However, as the skin is not an aqueous solution, the surface pH, which is recorded in a semihydrophobic milieu, most likely represents the combined acidity of exposed corneocytes, lipids, and water-soluble compounds (33). The surface pH, which is related to the term "acidic mantle of the skin," is influenced by many exogenous and endogenous factors, such as free fatty acid presence on the surface, desiccation, sweating, water content, bacterial count (1), and environmental factors such as temperature and air humidity. Its role has been more understood in recent years. Surface pH has been shown to be regulated by the generation of free fatty acids (34) and itself contributes to the regulation of epidermal permeability barrier homeostasis, stratum corneum integrity (35), and antimicrobial defense (34). In healthy skin, pH values range between 4.5 and 6.0, and turns alkaline in the presence of ammonia, which is the degradation product of sweat with bacteria. While values between 4.0–5.0 are supposed to prevent occurrence and growth of microorganisms, elevated values can promote bacterial colonization (36). The pH of the vulva was described to be more acidic, ranging from 3.8 to 4.2 during the menstrual cycle (33). However, in other bioengineering studies, significant differences between baseline pH values of the vulva and the forearm were not confirmed (7); in fact, the values obtained on vulvar skin tended to be even higher (23). The stratum corneum pH is altered by inflammation, dryness, and irritant-induced skin changes (7). After standardized trauma with tape stripping, vulvar skin surface pH decreased immediately but recovered more quickly than that of the forearm skin (24). The glass electrode technique using a pH-Meter® (Courage & Khazaka, Cologne, Germany) has gained widespread acceptance for measurement of skin surface pH (36). The device must be calibrated prior to measurements using standard buffers and must be rinsed with distilled water after each measurement. It must be realized that a surplus of water on the electrode as well as an electrode that is too dry affects the results. In addition, no residues of cosmetics must be left on the skin (33).

MEASURING MECHANICAL PROPERTIES

In vivo quantification of mechanical skin properties remains difficult. Several techniques have been developed, including tensile, torsional, indentation, suction, and vibration tests, which makes it difficult to compare results (37). The Cutometer® (Courage & Khazaka, Cologne, Germany) is a suction device, which applies a vacuum on the skin surface in a test area of only 3 mm^2 by using a hand-held probe. The method is suitable to monitor therapy and/or progression of connective tissue diseases such as scleroderma, and has been used in cosmetology for efficacy quantification of antiaging products (38,39). When comparing the elasticity parameters of the forearm and the vulvar skin, the ratio between viscous deformation (Uv) and elastic deformation (Ue) and the biological elasticity, i.e., the ratio between immediate recovery (Ur) and total deformation (Uf), were both significantly lower in the vulvar than in the forearm skin. Age-related differences were similar on both sites (40). The frictional properties of the vulvar skin are of interest due to its relation to eventual frictional trauma and resulting lichenification. Using a Newcastle Friction Meter (Design Unit Department of Mechanical Engineering, Newcastle University, Newcastle-upon-Tyne, U.K.) with an annular Teflon ring rotating at constant velocity, the friction coefficient of the vulvar skin was found to be higher than on the forearm skin, due to higher hydration levels of vulvar stratum corneum (28).

CONCLUSION

In conclusion, detection and investigation of clinical and subclinical vulvar changes, such as in irritant contact dermatitis, can be accomplished by using noninvasive bioengineering methods to monitor early inflammatory changes. LDPI and measurement of color reflectance can be recommended initially to assess irritant reactions on vulvar skin, and combination of different methods might be useful (7).

REFERENCES

1. Elsner P, Maibach HI. Microbiology of specialized skin: the vulva. Semin Dermatol 1990; 9:300.
2. Elsner P, Wilhelm D, Maibach HI. Sodium lauryl sulfate-induced irritant contact dermatitis in vulvar and forearm skin of premenopausal and postmenopausal women. J Am Acad Dermatol 1990; 23:648.
3. Farage M, Maibach HI. The vulvar epithelium differs from the skin: implications for cutaneous testing to address topical vulvar exposures. Contact Dermatitis 2004; 51:201.
4. Bauer A et al. Vulvar dermatoses—irritant and allergic contact dermatitis of the vulva. Dermatology 2005; 210:143.

5. Elsner P, Maibach HI. Cutaneous responses to topical methyl nicotinate in human forearm and vulvar skin. J Dermatol Sci 1991; 2:341.
6. Frosch PJ, Kligman AM. The soap chamber test. A new method for assessing the irritancy of soaps. J Am Acad Dermatol 1979; 1:35.
7. Elsner P, Wilhelm D, Maibach HI. Multiple parameter assessment of vulvar irritant contact dermatitis. Contact Dermatitis 1990; 23:20.
8. Wilhelm D et al. Evaluation of vulvar irritancy potential of a menstrual pad containing sodium bicarbonate in short-term application. J Reprod Med 1991; 36:556.
9. Warren R et al. Transepidermal water loss dynamics of human vulvar and thigh skin. Skin Pharmacol Physiol 2005; 18:139.
10. Serup J. Bioengineering and the skin: standardization. Clin Dermatol 1995; 13:293.
11. Pierard GE. EEMCO guidance for the assessment of skin colour. J Eur Acad Dermatol Venereol 1998; 10:1.
12. Kollias N. The physical basis of skin color and its evaluation. Clin Dermatol 1995; 13:361.
13. Fullerton A et al. Guidelines for measurement of skin colour and erythema. A report from the Standardization Group of the European Society of Contact Dermatitis. Contact Dermatitis 1996; 35:1.
14. Uhoda E et al. Skin weathering and ashiness in black Africans. Eur J Dermatol 2003; 13:574.
15. Kimbrough-Green CK et al. Topical retinoic acid (tretinoin) for melasma in black patients. A vehicle-controlled clinical trial. Arch Dermatol 1994; 130:727.
16. Elsner P. Chromametry. Hardware, measuring principles and standardisation of measurements. In: Berardesca E, Maibach HI, eds. Handbooks of Skin Bioengineering. Cutaneous Blood Flow and Erythema. Boca Raton: CRC Press, 1994.
17. Eun HC. Evaluation of skin blood flow by laser Doppler flowmetry. Clin Dermatol 1995; 13:337.
18. Saravanamuthu J et al. A new technique to map vulva microcirculation using laser Doppler perfusion imager. Int J Gynecol Cancer 2003; 13:812.
19. Jackson AE et al. Assessing vulvar lesions. Laser-Doppler flowmetry as a possible technique. J Reprod Med 1994; 39:953.
20. Greaves MW, Wall PD. Pathophysiology of itching. Lancet 1996; 348:938.
21. Jain RK. Determinants of tumor blood flow: a review. Cancer Res 1988; 48:2641.
22. Bircher A et al. Guidelines for measurement of cutaneous blood flow by laser Doppler flowmetry. A report from the Standardization Group of the European Society of Contact Dermatitis. Contact Dermatitis 1994; 30:65.
23. Elsner P, Maibach HI. The effect of prolonged drying on transepidermal water loss, capacitance and pH of human vulvar and forearm skin. Acta Derm Venereol 1990; 70:105.
24. Wilhelm D, Elsner P, Maibach HI. Standardized trauma (tape stripping) in human vulvar and forearm skin. Effects on transepidermal water loss, capacitance and pH. Acta Derm Venereol 1991; 71:123.
25. Nuutinen J et al. A closed unventilated chamber for the measurement of transepidermal water loss. Skin Res Technol 2003; 9:85.
26. Pinnagoda J et al. Guidelines for transepidermal water loss (TEWL) measurement. A report from the Standardization Group of the European Society of Contact Dermatitis. Contact Dermatitis 1990; 22:164.

27. Elsner P, Wilhelm D, Maibach HI. Effect of low-concentration sodium lauryl sulfate on human vulvar and forearm skin. Age-related differences. J Reprod Med 1991; 36:77.
28. Elsner P, Wilhelm D, Maibach HI. Frictional properties of human forearm and vulvar skin: influence of age and correlation with transepidermal water loss and capacitance. Dermatologica 1990; 181:88.
29. Berardesca E, Borroni G. Instrumental evaluation of cutaneous hydration. Clin Dermatol 1995; 13:323.
30. Berardesca E. EEMCO guidance for the assessment of stratum corneum hydration: electrical methods. Skin Res Technol 1997; 3:126.
31. Fluhr JW et al. Comparative study of five instruments measuring stratum corneum hydration (Corneometer CM 820 and CM 825, Skicon 200, Nova DPM 9003, DermaLab) Part I. In vitro. Skin Res Technol 1999; 5:161.
32. Fluhr JW et al. Comparative study of five instruments measuring stratum corneum hydration (Corneometer CM 820 and CM 825, Skicon 200, Nova DPM 9003, DermaLab) Part II. In vivo. Skin Res Technol 1999; 5:171.
33. Parra JL, Paye M. EEMCO guidance for the in vivo assessment of skin surface pH, Skin. Pharmacol Appl Skin Physiol 2003; 16:188.
34. Fluhr JW et al. Generation of free fatty acids from phospholipids regulates stratum corneum acidification and integrity. J Invest Dermatol 2001; 117:44.
35. Hachem JP et al. PH directly regulates epidermal permeability barrier homeostasis, and stratum corneum integrity/cohesion. J Invest Dermatol 2003; 121:345.
36. Chikakane K, Takahashi H. Measurement of skin pH and its significance in cutaneous diseases. Clin Dermatol 1995; 13:299.
37. Pierard G. A critical approach to in vivo mechanical testing of the skin. In: Leveque JL, ed. Cutaneous Invetsigation in Health and Disease. New York, Basel: Marcel Dekker, 1989:215.
38. Hanau A et al. Noninvasive diagnosis of skin functions. Hautarzt 2003; 54:1211.
39. Habig J et al. Effect of single UVA and UVB irradiation on the surface composition and viscoelastic properties of skin in vivo. Hautarzt 1996; 47:515.
40. Elsner P, Wilhelm D, Maibach HI. Mechanical properties of human forearm and vulvar skin. Br J Dermatol 1990; 122:607.

17

Transepidermal Water Loss Dynamics of Human Vulvar and Thigh Skin

Raphael Warren

The Procter & Gamble Company, Feminine Care Innovation Center, Cincinnati, Ohio, U.S.A.

Michaelle B. Jones

The Procter & Gamble Company, Cincinnati, Ohio, U.S.A.

Peter Elsner

Department of Dermatology and Allergology, Friedrich-Schiller University, Jena, Germany

INTRODUCTION

Transepidermal water loss (TEWL) is considered to be an indicator of the functional state of the cutaneous barrier (1–3). TEWL is believed to be related to irritant sensitivity and has been used to evaluate the clinical condition of the skin. Damage to the skin barrier from skin disease and physical or chemical trauma increases TEWL from an unperturbed baseline value. In addition,

From Skin Pharmacol Physiol 2005; 18:139, S. Karger AG, Basel.

TEWL is affected by environmental factors that include skin temperature, relative humidity of the air, occlusive factors, and mechanical abrasion. Physiological factors, such as cutaneous blood flow, stress, diurnal rhythm, eccrine and sweat gland density, and the thickness and composition of the stratum corneum, affect TEWL as well (4–10).

Vulvar irritant contact dermatitis is difficult to diagnose and irritation from sites used typically for measuring dermatitis (i.e., the forearm) are not predictive for the objective assessment of irritant dermatitis of the vulva (11–13). Previously, we sought to establish a standard procedure for assessing vulvar skin TEWL so that TEWL could be used as an indicator for the integrity and clinical status of vulvar skin.

Vulvar skin represents a unique dermatological region. For example, vulvar skin has a thinner stratum corneum than other skin (5); it can be considered at least semi-occluded (by virtue of garments and skin-on-skin contact) and naturally hydrated tissue (by virtue of garments, and abundance of eccrine and sweat glands, and its proximity to the vaginal orifice) (14,15). Under conditions of occlusion and hydration, TEWL cannot be measured effectively. In these situations, skin surface water loss (SSWL) over a period of time may be a more accurate indicator of the vulvar skin's integrity.

The measurement of vulvar SSWL is particularly challenging due to its semioccluded state and a location that is difficult to assess without causing stress to the individual. This, coupled with the vulva's richly innervated tissue and an abundance of eccrine and sweat glands, made the task of measuring SSWL quite ambitious (16). Previous reports showed that vulvar SSWL (in particular, the midpoint of the labia majora) is considerably greater than the forearm SSWL (15,16).

For this study, we compared the SSWL dynamics of the vulva and the inner thigh, sites that are partially occluded by garments, and for the inner thigh, a site that is closely apposed to the genital skin. We also assessed the influence of age, body-mass index (BMI), and atopy.

EVALUATION OF TRANSEPIDERMAL WATER LOSS

TEWL was assessed in 58 women 18 to 35 years of age, with regular menstrual cycles (25 to 35 days) and a menstrual flow of five or less than five days. Exclusion criteria were the use of immunosuppressive drugs, chemotherapy, anti-inflammatories, antihistamines, or steroids; an active vulvar/vaginal infection; high blood pressure/cardiovascular disease, and pregnancy. Prior to treatment, the participants completed a medical questionnaire that included an atopic dermatitis self-assessment (Table 1) (17) and had their weight and height recorded. Participants received a set of standard cotton panties to wear during the study period and an oil-free, personal cleansing body wash to use in lieu of their normal cleansing product. Participants were asked to refrain from body cleansing within two hours of their clinical visit, from intercourse during the

Table 1 Relationship Between Participant Atopy Status and Vulvar Transepidermal Water Loss Parameter

Parameter	SSWL (AUC) (g/m^2; 0–30 min ± SEM)	TEWL (30 min) (g/m^2-hr ± SEM)
Atopy Status (from Questionnaire)		
Not atopic (Score < 6; $n = 42$)	15.5 ± 1.0	24.2 ± 1.8
Suspected atopy (Score 6–10; $n = 5$)	15.5 ± 4.7	23.7 ± 7.0
Atopic (Score > 10; $n = 7$)	18.5 ± 3.1	28.6 ± 5.7

Note: Participants were considered having atopy if their score was >10 or if participants had been diagnosed with atopy.
Abbreviations: SSWL, skin surface water loss; TEWL, transepidermal water loss; AUC, area under the curve; SEM, standard error of mean.

24 hours preceding their visit, and from drinking any caffeinated beverage on the day of their visit. We did not control all clothing worn, physical activity, or bathroom habits and practices.

Procedure for Measuring Transepidermal Water Loss

To avoid the influence of menstruation and associated humidity and fluid effects on SSWL, the investigators measured TEWL 9 to 11 days post menses. The measurements were taken in a quiet room and under constant environmental conditions (29°C to 32°C at skin surface, ambient at 21°C to 23°C, and 41% to 58% relative humidity) using an evaporimeter over a 30-minute period (data collected after 0, 2, 5, 10, 20, and 30 minutes). Following the vulvar measurements, TEWL measurements were made at an adjoining thigh area. Only data collected from participants with a negative rate of TEWL change ($n = 54$) were used in the statistical analysis.

TRANSEPIDERMAL WATER LOSS FINDINGS

Previously, it has been shown that the SSWL dynamics over time resemble an asymptotic distribution, with a high value immediately after panty removal that gradually declines over time (16). Of the 58 participants enrolled in the study, 54 (93%) expressed a declining SSWL slope (Fig. 1). Their initial mean SSWL value of 46.2 g m^{-2}/hr ± 2.6 (SE) declined gradually and significantly to 24.7 g m^{-2}/hr ± 1.6 (SE) at 30 minutes ($p < 0.001$). Thirty of the 54 participants enrolled in the study used some form of contraceptive medication. This subgroup displayed the same overall SSWL pattern and was not significantly different from the remaining participants not using contraceptive medication [area under the curve (AUC), $p = 0.25$].

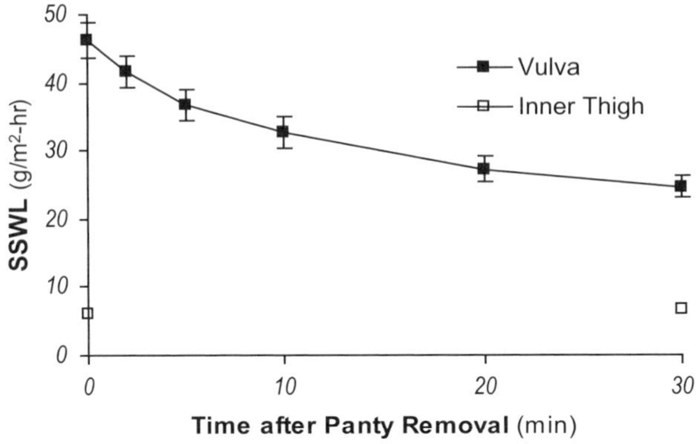

Figure 1 Comparison of vulvar and thigh skin surface water loss. *Abbreviation*: SSWL, skin surface water loss.

Despite being considered a semioccluded region (by virtue of garment and skin-on-skin interactions), the mean values for the inner thigh were generally constant (6 to 7 $g\,m^{-2}/hr$) and significantly less than vulvar SSWL (Fig. 1). These data were more consistent with previously published data for the back, another semioccluded region of the body (5,7). Factors such as garment fit and mechanical abrasion, presence of an insular hair cushion, proximity to the vaginal orifice, abundance of sweat and eccrine glands, and stratum corneum thickness likely contribute to these differences (5,14,15).

The enrolled participant population had a mean age of 26.9 ± 6.4 years standard deviation (SD), a mean BMI of 23.5 $kg\,m^{-2} \pm 4.1$ (SD), and a mean atopic score of 3.5 ± 3.4 (SD). Within the observed range of age and BMI, both age and BMI had minimal effect on SSWL, with age having the least impact. Thus, among age, BMI, and atopic score, there was a trend for atopic score to have an impact on SSWL.

There have been numerous studies showing an increase in TEWL with noneczematous atopy (18). The limited spread of values for atopy, which may have reduced the statistical power of the model calculations, combined with the novel structural and anatomic disposition of vulvar skin, may have limited our ability to detect a stronger atopic effect on vulvar SSWL. Additional analysis of a larger population of atopic individuals is warranted.

CONCLUSION

This study confirmed that the SSWL dynamics for vulvar skin in a large participant sampling and its properties are considerably different from an adjacent semi-occluded inner thigh region. To avoid the influence of the menstrual cycle and associated excess humidity and menstrual fluid, we collected data

9 to 11 days following menstruation. Interestingly, the menstrual cycle has been shown to influence skin reactivity to contact irritants at distal locations (i.e., upper arm) (19). As TEWL is believed to be one parameter associated with skin reactivity, we speculate that the menstrual cycle may similarly affect SSWL dynamics at the vulva.

REFERENCES

1. Wilson DR, Maibach HI. Transepidermal water loss: a review. In: Leveque JL, ed. Cutaneous Investigation in Health and Disease. Non-Invasive Methods and Instrumentation. New York: Marcel Dekker, 1989:113.
2. Leveque JL. Measurement of transepidermal water loss. In: Leveque JL, ed. Cutaneous Investigation in Health and Disease. Non-Invasive Methods and Instrumentation. New York: Marcel Dekker, 1989:135.
3. Rougier A. TEWL and transcutaneous absorption. In: Elsner P, Berardesca E, Maibach H, eds. Bioengineering of the Skin: Water and the Stratum Corneum, Boca Raton: CRC Press, 1994:103.
4. Aly R et al. Effect of prolonged occlusion on the microbial flora, pH, carbon dioxide, and transepidermal water loss on human skin. J Invest Dermatol 1978; 71:378.
5. Ya-Xian Z, Suetake T, Tagami H. Number of layers of the stratum corneum in normal skin-relationship to the anatomical location on the body, age, sex, and physical parameters. Arch Dermatol Res 1999; 291:555.
6. Fluhr JW et al. Effects of prolonged occlusion on stratum corneum barrier function and water holding capacity. Skin Pharmacol Appl Skin Physiol 1999; 12:193.
7. Pinnagoda J et al. Guidelines for transepidermal water loss (TEWL) measurement. Contact Dermatitis 1990; 22:164.
8. Potts RO. Stratum corneum hydration: experimental techniques and interpretation of results. J Soc Cosmet Chem 1986; 37:9.
9. Lavrijsen APM et al. Barrier function parameters in various keratinization disorders: transepidermal water loss and vascular response to hexyl nicotinate. J Dermatol 1993; 129:547.
10. Yosipovitch G et al. Time-dependent variations of the skin barrier function in humans: transepidermal water loss, stratum corneum hydration, skin surface pH, and skin temperature. J Invest Dermatol 1998; 110:20.
11. Britz MB, Maibach HI. Human cutaneous vulvar reactivity to irritants. Contact Dermatitis 1979; 5:375.
12. Elsner P, Wilhelm D, Maibach HI. Sodium lauryl sulfate-induced irritant contact dermatitis in vulvar and forearm skin of premenopausal and postmenopausal women. J Am Acad Dermatol 1990; 23:648.
13. Elsner P, Maibach HI. Cutaneous responses to topical methyl nicotinate in human forearm and vulvar skin. J Dermatol Sci 1991; 2:341.
14. Erickson KL, Montagna W. New observations on the anatomical features of the female genitalia. J Am Med Women's Assoc 1972; 27:573.
15. Elsner P, Wilhelm D, Maibach HI. Frictional properties of human forearm and vulvar skin: influence of age and correlation with transepidermal water loss and capacitance. Dermatologica 1990; 181:88.
16. Elsner P, Wilhelm D, Maibach HI. Physiological skin surface water loss dynamics of vulvar and forearm skin. Acta Derm Venereol 1990; 70:141.

17. Diepgen TL, Fartasch M, Hornstein OP. Evaluation and relevance of atopic basic and minor features in patients with atopic dermatitis and in the general population. Acta Derm Venereol Suppl (Stockh) 1989; 144:50.
18. Fartasch M. Atopic dermatitis and other diseases. In: Elsner P, Beradesca E, Maibach HI, eds. Bioengineering of the Skin: Water and the Stratum Corneum, Boca Raton: CRC Press, 1994:87.
19. Agner T, Damm P, Skouby SO. Menstrual cycle and skin reactivity. J Am Acad Dermatol 1991; 24:566.

18

Vulvar Toxicology

Christina Y. Wang

Department of Occupational and Environmental Medicine, University of California, and Kaiser Permanente, San Francisco, California, U.S.A.

Howard I. Maibach

Department of Dermatology, University of California School of Medicine, San Francisco, California, U.S.A.

INTRODUCTION

The characteristics of the vulva pose various clinical problems with regard to vulvar toxicology. The vulva is a specialized skin with unique morphologic and functional properties, including increased permeability, higher degree of hydration, a proclivity to irritation as characterized by erythema, edema, and/or corrosion (1), and increased blood flow as compared to skin at other sites (2). Many of these qualities may increase the vulva's vulnerability to toxicities leading to dermatitis; however, the pigmented skin and structural qualities of the vulva make clinical diagnosis by physical examination difficult, as vulvar skin erythema is not readily visible. There is wide variation in physical presentation of vulvar dermatologic disease, making it difficult for the physician to ascertain the true diagnosis and etiology.

Because of these unique characteristics, heterogeneity of clinical findings, and difficulty in standardized access to the vulvar skin for controlled laboratory trials, the epidemiological data and the sensitivity and specificity of toxicological methods are poor; thus, researchers and clinicians have relied on clinical observation in order to validate the toxicological methods.

IRRITATION OF THE VULVA

The vulva may be more prone to irritation due to its unique skin characteristics. Water retention is a major function of the stratum corneum. Transepidermal water loss (TEWL), an objective measure of the efficiency and integrity of the stratum corneum, is higher in vulvar skin versus forearm skin, as measured by an evaporimeter (Servo Med Ep 1; Servo Med, Stockholm, Sweden). The mean TEWL in the vulva is 1.42×10^3, whereas in the forearm it is 8.68×10^2, suggesting that the vulvar stratum corneum is more permeable to water. In addition, the vulvar stratum corneum is thinner, measuring 0.02 μm in thickness, whereas the forearm stratum corneum measures 11.2 μm in thickness (3). Higher TEWL in the vulvar skin may mean that it is a less complete barrier and, thus, more prone to the effects of irritants. Skin surface water loss—which may be influenced by occlusion and eccrine sweating, as is vulvar skin/skin occlusion and skin/garment occlusion—is more variable and subject to more increases (or "bursts") in the vulvar skin versus the forearm skin. This is another potential complicating factor for vulvar skin irritation studies (4).

Given the location, pigmentation, and atypical structure of vulvar skin, objective TEWL measurement appears to offer advantages as an indicator of irritant susceptibility versus that of clinical evaluation by visual screening (5). In an attempt to remove the occlusion factor from the vulvar TEWL, researchers used a desiccation chamber to absorb water evaporation from the vulvar and forearm surfaces (6). By drying the vulvar skin, the TEWL and capacitance (a measure of skin hydration) as measured by a capacitometer decreased (Corneometer CM 820 PC®; Courage and Khazaka, Cologne, FRG). The differences in TEWL and capacitance between dried vulvar and forearm skin were diminished but not eliminated. This finding suggests that occlusion alone is not the answer to vulvar skin's higher intrinsic TEWL; there are likely biochemical differences in the stratum corneum of the vulva and forearm.

Although the vulva has a higher baseline TEWL compared to the forearm, tape stripping the skin (to create compromised skin) produces a less intense response in the vulva. This could be due to the fact that the vulva has less of a physiologic barrier function than the forearm, and stripping the vulvar skin does not compromise its stratum corneum as much as the more competent forearm skin. After tape stripping, the vulvar skin capacitance was lower than that of the forearm, reflective of faster healing (7), possibly because of the vulva's inherent increased blood flow (8) and higher epidermal cell turnover rate. Another difference between forearm and vulvar skin is that the vulvar skin has higher extensibility without a comparable increase in the elastic fiber network and retraction, which potentially could allow for the physiological changes needed in childbirth (9). The vulva shows highly effective repair mechanisms during postpartum recovery. The characteristics that allow for such repair may also predispose the vulvar skin to endogenous and exogenous irritation.

Because of the vulva's inherently higher capacitance, or stratum corneum hydration, it has a higher friction coefficient, μ, as measured by the Newcastle Friction Meter (Design Unit, Department of Mechanical Engineering, Newcastle University, Newcastle-upon-Tyne, U.K.). The vulvar skin friction coefficient is 0.66 ± 0.03 and that of the forearm skin is 0.48 ± 0.01 (10). The higher vulvar skin friction coefficient leads to a higher mechanical friction trauma by contact with garment, skin occlusion, sexual activity, and moisture occlusion from incontinence (11) (which increases the moisture, resulting in a higher friction coefficient) (10). This is yet another physiological reason for the vulvar skin's tendency to become irritated.

The vulva's increased TEWL means that its stratum corneum is not as an effective a barrier against water loss as compared to forearm skin; this, in turn, allows for increased absorption of certain compounds. Hydrocortisone 7.7% applied topically penetrated vulvar skin versus 1.3% percutaneous penetrated in forearm skin. Although the labia majora are the embryologic analog of the scrotum, this structure does not approach scrotal permeability at 42% penetration of hydrocortisone (12). Nonetheless, vulvar skin has more than a seven-fold increase in permeability compared to the forearm skin, which could make the vulva more prone to respond adversely to irritants. The vulva showed more irritation response than the forearm when exposed to the chemical irritants, 17% benzalkonium chloride and 20% maleic acid. Using a visual erythema scale on carefully ring-marginated labia majora skin onto which the irritants were applied, maleic acid caused a positive irritation response in 76% of vulvar skin versus 62% of the forearm skin. Benzalkonium chloride caused positive irritation response in 57% of vulvar skin versus 9% of forearm skin. Rapid onset of burning and stinging sensations upon application of the chemical irritants occurred on the vulvar skin but not on the forearm skin (1). However, the vulva is not more susceptible to all irritants. Sodium lauryl sulfate (SLS), an anionic surfactant, did not cause increased reactivity in the vulvar skin compared to the forearm skin, as demonstrated by visual scoring and a lack of a statistically significant increase in TEWL (13). A recent 4-day skin patch test study of menses and venous blood showed that the vulvar skin was less prone to irritation, as assessed by a four-point erythema scale, as compared to the forearm skin (14).

The vulvar skin has higher hydration (higher capacitance), higher TEWL, and a less-efficient water barrier than nonvulvar skin. Because of these characteristics, polar irritants, such as maleic acid and benzalkonium chloride, can better penetrate hydrated vulvar skin. Normal, nonvulvar skin has less hydrated, more lipophilic stratum corneum; thus, polar compounds do not cross as easily. Irritants such as SLS have lipophilic tails, thus, they do not cross the vulvar skin as easily as they do the forearm skin, which is more permeable to small, lipophilic compounds (15). This helps explain the vulvar skin's varied irritant responses to different chemicals.

BIOENGINEERING METHODS OF ASSESSMENT

Visual inspection and scoring of vulvar irritation reactions may lack the sensitivity to recognize all cases of vulvar skin irritation, including low-grade dermatitis. The visual scoring system ranges from 0 to 4: normal skin, 0; slight redness, spotty or diffuse, 1; moderate, uniform redness, 2; intense redness, 3; and fiery erythema and edema, 4 (4,16). Various bioengineering instruments have enabled scientists to ascertain the vulva's unique skin characteristics objectively.

As mentioned previously, the vulva has increased basal cutaneous blood flow, which may aid in the rapid healing of the vulvar skin after trauma, such as tape stripping. Laser Doppler velocimetry has been used to objectively quantify blood flow in vulvar versus forearm skin. A laser Doppler flowmeter detected the frequency shift (Doppler effect) of He–Ne laser light ($\lambda = 632.8$ nm) caused by moving blood cells. Monochromatic light undergoes a frequency shift when reflected by the moving blood cells, while stationary tissue does not change the frequency. The reflected light is collected by two optical fibers to a pair of photo electrodes. The dimensionless output signal is proportional to the cutaneous blood flow. The basal skin blood flow was found to be significantly higher in the vulva than the forearm (8,16).

TEWL, as mentioned previously, is a measure of stratum corneum integrity against water loss. It is measured with an evaporimeter that has a hand-held probe with a 1 cm tail extension to reduce air turbulence around the hydrosensors and metallic shield to minimize contamination. The skin is maintained at a standard temperature throughout the measurement. Essentially, the evaporimeter measures the amount of water that evaporates via the skin surface. The electrical capacitance of the skin is an indicator of stratum corneum water content. It is measured with a capacitometer, which consists of a probe applied to the skin with slight pressure for three seconds. The skin capacitance is expressed as a digital readout (16).

BEHIND THE KNEE TEST

The behind the knee test was developed to assess the frictional effect and mechanical irritant properties of hygiene products that contact specialized skin areas such as the vulva. Test materials are applied daily to the area behind the knee and held in place for six hours by an elastic knee band. Irritation is graded 30 to 60 minutes after test product removal, preferably in the afternoon, and the following morning before the application of the next sample, using the four-point visual scoring system. It was found that two applications of six hours each on intact skin were sufficient to determine the irritant quality of a product. Depending on what type of product and/or reaction is being examined, one can use dry product on intact skin, dry product on compromised (tape stripped) skin, wet product on intact skin, or wet product on compromised skin. There may also be an association between the subject's reported sensory effects, such as pain, burning, or stinging, and the degree of irritation seen on objective scoring (14,17).

VULVAR DERMATITIS

Irritant Contact Dermatitis

A survey of German family physicians, gynecologists, and dermatologists in 1998 revealed that 24% to 38% of patients with noninfectious genital complaints had a diagnosis of vulvar dermatitis, while the incidence was 20% to 30% in Oxford, U.K., in 2000 (2,18). There are three prototypic clinical responses to irritants: acute irritant dermatitis, chronic (cumulative) irritant dermatitis, and sensory irritation. The acute type develops as a result of exposure to a potent irritant and is equivalent to a chemical burn. The cumulative, chronic type results from repeated exposures to weak irritants and can be confused with allergic contact dermatitis (ACD). Sensory irritation is characterized by stinging and burning caused by chemical exposure with no detectable skin changes. All three types can affect the vulva, and some chemicals, such as propylene glycol, can cause irritation as well as sensitization (18,19). The antiviral medication acyclovir, imiquimod, and podophyllotoxin can cause acute to subacute irritant contact dermatitis (2). The more frequent chronic irritant contact dermatitis has both endogenous and exogenous causes. Some endogenous etiologies include obesity, which results in increased moisture accumulation; increased humidity, with resultant increased friction coefficient; and incontinence, with both moisture and ammonia irritants. Some exogenous vulvar irritants include clothing, soaps, spermicides (non-oxynol 9 and benzalkonium chloride), and antiseptic solutions (0.3% chlorhexidine) (2). Overzealous hygienic practices, using irritating soaps and antiseptic wipes, can often cause irritant contact dermatitis in the vulva, as well (18). Wigger-Alberti and Elsner describe 10 subtypes of irritation (20):

1. Acute
2. Acute delayed
3. Irritant reaction
4. Cumulative
5. Traumiterative
6. Exsiccation
7. Traumatic
8. Pustular and acneiform
9. Nonerythematous
10. Subjective

Allergic Contact Dermatitis

ACD is an immunologically mediated inflammatory cutaneous reaction to an allergen in a sensitized individual. Often, differentiating vulvar allergic versus irritant contact dermatitis can be clinically confusing, as the signs and symptoms often overlap (18) and the physical characteristics of vulvar skin make visual inspection and diagnosis difficult. The acute phase of ACD can produce vesiculation and severe pruritus; during this phase, ACD can spread beyond the site of contact, such as to the upper thighs and suprapubic area. The subacute or chronic signs and symptoms are usually less pronounced. Pruritus and burning symptoms are more subdued. The vulva can show changes such as redness, excoriation, scaling, and altered pigmentation with variable lichenification. Secondary infections can occur as well. The histology of ACD is similar to irritant contact dermatitis, although there can be more pronounced spongiosis in acute cases (18).

There is no absolute human predictive test for ACD. Standard animal model assays for skin sensitization include various guinea pig methods and the local lymph node assay (LLNA) in mice. The guinea pig models include an induction phase, in which the test sample is initially exposed to the same skin area, followed by a rest period of at least seven days and then a challenge exposure to a virgin skin site. The LLNA focuses on the induction phase, soon after which the mice are injected with a label and the draining lymph nodes are analyzed for lymph node activation. Epidermal Langerhans cells are thought to take up antigen absorbed percutaneously, travel to the skin site's draining lymph node, and present the antigen to activate T cells, which differentiate into allergen-responsive T lymphocytes (21,22).

As vulvar tissue has been shown to have increased permeability, higher concentrations of allergenic antigens could penetrate the vulva, be available for presentation to the Langerhans cells in the vulvar skin, and cause sensitization, leading to ACD (15). Because of the vulvar skin's increased permeability and decreased barrier function, ACD information obtained from other skin, such as the forearm, cannot be extrapolated with complete confidence to the vulva. There needs to be a more conservative quantitative risk assessment methodology for vulvar contact sensitization (23).

In order to take into account the vulvar skin's increased permeability to potential allergens, a modified human repeat insult patch test (HRIPT) was developed. Standard patch testing, not repeat insult patch testing, involves the application of possible allergens to the normal skin of the back for two days under occlusion with readings taken at days 2 and 4 (24). The original HRIPT involved nine 24-hour applications of patches with 24-hour rest periods in between during the induction phase. The modified HRIPT increased the cumulative exposure duration by 67%, by increasing the number of applications to fifteen 24-hour patch applications (24 hours daily for five days, for three weeks). This increases the sensitivity of the HRIPT to evaluate sensitization in specialized skin, such as the vulva. It is important to maintain the rest periods in the induction phase to increase the effectiveness of the test. Also, the five-day repeated steps parallel use of some products that contact vulvar skin, like feminine hygiene products during approximately five days of menses (25,26).

A study of 144 patients from Sydney, Australia, with chronic vulvar symptoms found that 64% had dermatitis. However, it was difficult to clinically ascertain which of the 64% had allergic versus irritant contact dermatitis. Another study reviewing patch test results of 135 patients with persistent vulvar symptoms found that 47% had at least one positive reaction, with 29% having a clinically relevant positive result. The most frequent sensitizers were ethylenediamine, neomycin, framycetin, and clobetasol propionate (19). Of the 38 patients with clinical vulvar dermatitis in an Oxford vulvar clinic in 1997, 26% had a relevant positive patch test (27). Fragrance mix positive patch test occurred in 11%, with clinical improvement of vulvar dermatitis symptoms with avoidance of perfumed products, presumably including scented feminine hygiene products. Formaldehyde and its releasing preservatives, Quaternium 15 and DMDM Hydantoin accounted for another 11% of positive patch test results (27).

Patch test data from 1008 patients with anogenital complaints registered in the German Information Network of Departments of Dermatology from 1992 to 1997 revealed that almost 48% of patients had positive patch test reactions to 1114 allergens, with a final diagnosis of ACD in nearly 35% (nearly 23% had irritant contact dermatitis) (2). Local anesthetic Dibucaine HCl was found to be a sensitizer in 7.4% and benzocaine in 2.7% of those patients. Framycetin sulfate, a topical antibiotic, sensitized 2.6% and neomycin sulfate 2.1%. The topical antimycotic clotrimazole sensitized 1.8% of patients, and the nonsteroidal anti-inflammatory drug bufexamac sensitized 1.7% (2). With the rising popularity of topical herbal medicaments, some herbal extract, depending on dose, purity, and quality, were found to be allergens in patients with vulvar symptoms. For example, chamomile sensitized 2.9% of patients, tincture of Arnica montana sensitized 2.1%, and propolis sensitized 2.5%; again, degree of sensitization potential may depend on herbal extract dose, purity, and quality of different products (2).

Many consumer products that come in contact with the vulva contain potential allergens. Dark clothing, such as underwear, can carry paraphenylenediamine-containing dye and formaldehyde, and some sanitary napkins may contain formaldehyde, fragrance, acetyl acetone, and methacrylates—all can be potential sensitizers (18). It is important to remember the vulva's specialized skin features, including increased permeability and penchant for irritation, when considering the vast array of allergen-containing products available to women for use on, around, or against the vulva.

The studies referred to previously depend on patch test frequency data and do not provide sufficient detail to determine clinical relevance. Benezra et al. (28) and Ale and Maibach (29) provide algorithms for determining clinical relevance and in reviewing case reports regarding the "degree of likely clinical relevance."

Photoirritation and Photoallergic Dermatitis

Photoirritation, or phototoxicity, is a chemically induced nonimmunologic skin irritation requiring light, with skin response resembling sunburn (30). Photoallergic dermatitis is a subset of photosensitive dermatitis, which results from UV-induced excitation of a chemical applied to the skin. Photoallergic reactions require a period of sensitization. The reactions are usually delayed, manifesting days to weeks or years after the UV exposure (31). To date, there remains a paucity of vulvar experimental and epidemiological data on the two topics, probably due to the relatively sun-protected location of vulvar skin.

CONTACT URTICARIA

Nonimmunologic Contact Urticaria

The contact urticaria syndrome, or immediate contact reactions, comprises a heterogeneous group of inflammatory reactions that appear, usually within minutes, after contact with the eliciting substance. They include wheal and flare, along with transient erythema, and may lead to eczema. Nonimmunologic contact urticaria (NICU) occurs without previous sensitization and is the most common type of immediate contact reaction. This reaction remains localized; it does not spread to become generalized urticaria and it does not cause systemic symptoms. The strength of the reaction usually varies from erythema to an urticarial response, depending on the concentration, the exposed skin area, mode of exposure, and inciting substance (32,33). Animal models allow for identification of substances capable of immediate contact reactions. A substance can be applied to guinea pig ear lobe, with resulting erythema and edema if the substance indeed is capable of causing a contact urticarial response. Measuring changes in the ear lobe thickness with a micrometer caliper is an accurate, reproducible, and rapid method of quantifying edema. Ear lobe biopsies showing marked dermal edema and intra- and peri-vascular infiltrates of heterophilic (neutrophilic in humans) granulocytes are characteristics of NICU in the guinea pig ear (33,34).

The open test can be used to assess for NICU in humans. In this test, 0.1 mL of the test substance is spread on a 3×3 cm area of the skin on the upper back or extensor surface of the upper arm. The test site is observed for 60 minutes. Edema and erythema, or tiny intraepidermal spongiotic vesicles typical of acute eczema indicate a positive result. The test should first be done on nondiseased skin, and if negative, then on affected skin. The use test involves the patient handling the suspected agent as he/she handled it when symptoms occurred (33,35). Unfortunately, there are no vulvar experimental or epidemiological data on this topic.

Immunologic Contact Urticaria

Immunologic contact urticaria, an IgE-mediated phenomenon, consists of local wheal and flare which, in some individuals, eventuates into asthma, allergic rhinitis and/or conjunctivitis, anaphylaxis, and rarely, death. Diagnosis is documented by skin testing, as noted in the previous section (NICU). When extracutaneous signs and symptoms occur, highly diluted solutions are utilized. Amin et al. (36) provide detailed protocols and precautions.

CONCLUSION

The vulvar skin has distinctive morphology and functional characteristics, including increased permeability, higher degree of hydration, and a tendency for irritation from some chemicals. Various bioengineering methods of assessment demonstrate the vulvar skin's difference from other skin, such as forearm skin, in qualities such as capacitance, blood flow, and water loss, which helps explain some of its clinical properties. There have been numerous studies that show the vulva's unique response to various irritants and allergens. Some chemicals produce higher, others lower, degrees of irritation in vulva skin that differs from forearm skin. Future studies should consider the vulva's unique properties and responses, and use the appropriate methods of testing and assessment for this specialized skin.

REFERENCES

1. Britz MB, Maibach HI. Human cutaneous vulvar reactivity to irritants. Contact Dermatitis 1979; 5:375.
2. Bauer A et al. Vulvar dermatoses—irritant and allergic contact dermatitis of the vulva. Dermatology 2005; 210:143.
3. Britz MB, Maibach HI. Human labia majora skin: transepidermal water loss in vivo. Acta Derm Venereol 1979; 59:23.
4. Elsner P, Wilhelm D, Maibach HI. Physiological skin surface water loss dynamics of human vulvar and forearm skin. Acta Derm Venereol 1990; 70:141.
5. Cua A, Wilhelm KP, Maibach HI. Cutaneous sodium lauryl sulphate irritation potential: age and regional variability. Br J Dermatol 1990; 123:607.
6. Elsner P, Maibach HI. The effect of prolonged drying on transepidermal water loss, capacitance and pH of human vulvar and forearm skin. Acta Derm Venereol 1990; 70:105.
7. Wilhelm D, Elsner P, Maibach HI. Standardized trauma (tape stripping) in human vulvar and forearm skin, effects on transepidermal water loss, capacitance and pH. Acta Derm Venereol 1991; 71:123.
8. Elsner P, Maibach HI. Cutaneous responses to topical methyl nicotinate in human forearm and vulvar skin. J Dermatol Sci 1991; 2:341.
9. Elsner P, Wilhelm D, Maibach HI. Mechanical properties of human forearm and vulvar skin. Br J Dermatol 1990; 122:607.
10. Elsner P, Wilhelm D, Maibach HI. Frictional properties of human forearm and vulvar skin: influence of age and correlation with transepidermal water loss and capacitance. Dermatologica1990; 181:88.
11. Margesson LJ. Vulvovaginal dryness and itching. Skin Therapy Lett 2001; 6:3.
12. Britz MB, Maibach HI, Anjo DM. Human percutaneous penetration of hydrocortisone: the vulva. Arch Dermatol Res 1980; 267:313.
13. Elsner P, Wilhelm D, Maibach HI. Sodium lauryl sulfate-induced irritant contact dermatitis in vulvar and forearm skin of premenopausal and postmenopausal women. J Am Acad Dermatol 1990; 23:648.
14. Farage MA. The behind-the-knee test: an efficient model for evaluating mechanical and chemical irritation. Skin Research and Technology 2006; 12:73–82.

15. Farage M, Maibach HI. The vulvar epithelium differs from the skin: implications for cutaneous testing to address topical vulvar exposures. Contact Dermatitis 2004; 51:201.
16. Wilhelm D et al. Evaluation of vulvar irritancy potential of a menstrual pad containing sodium bicarbonate in short-term application. J Reprod Med 1991; 36:556.
17. Farage MA, Meyer S, Walter D. Development of a sensitive test method to evaluate mechanical irritation potential on mucosal skin. Skin Res Technol 2004; 10:85.
18. Margesson LJ. Contact dermatitis of the vulva. Dermatol Ther 2004; 17:20.
19. Kamarashev JA, Vassileva SG. Dermatologic diseases of the vulva. Clin Dermatol 1997; 15:53.
20. Wigger-Alberti W, Elsner P. Contact dermatitis due to irritation. In: Kanerva L et al., eds. Handbook of Occupational Dermatology. Berlin Heidelberg: Springer Verlag, 2000, chap. 11.
21. Klecak G. Test methods for allergic contact dermatitis. In: Zhai H, Maibach HI, eds. Dermatotoxicology. 6th ed. Boca Raton: CRC Press, 2004, chap. 38.
22. Kimber I et al. The local lymph node assay. In: Zhai H, Maibach HI, eds. Dermatotoxicology. 6th ed. Boca Raton: CRC Press, 2004, chap. 41.
23. Farage MA et al. Quantitative risk assessment for the induction of allergic contact dermatitis: uncertainty factors for mucosal exposure. Contact Dermatitis 2003; 49:140–147.
24. Salim A, Powell S, Wojnarowska F. Allergic contact dermatitis of the vulva—an overlooked diagnosis. J Obstet Gynecol 2002; 22:447.
25. Farage MA et al. A modified human repeat insult patch test for extended mucosal tissue exposure. Contact Dermatitis 2003; 49:214.
26. Farage MA, Meyer S, Walter D. Evaluation of modifications of the traditional patch test in assessing the chemical irritation potential of feminine hygiene products. Skin Res Technol 2004; 10:73.
27. Crone AM et al. Aetiological factors in vulvar dermatitis. J Eur Acad Dermatol Venereol 2000; 14:181.
28. Benezra C et al. A systematic search for structure-activity relationships of skin contact sensitizers; methodology. J Invest Derm 1985; 85:351.
29. Ale SI, Maibach HI. Clinical relevance in allergic contact dermatitis, an algorithmic approach. Dermatosen 1995; 43:119.
30. Marzulli FN, Maibach HI. Photoirritation (phototoxicity, phototoxic dermatitis). In: Zhai H, Maibach HI, eds. Dermatotoxicology. 6th ed. Boca Raton: CRC Press, 2004, chap. 17.
31. Modjtahedi SP et al. Cosmetic reactions. In: Zhai H, Maibach HI, eds. Dermatotoxicology. 6th ed. Boca Raton: CRC Press, 2004, chap. 51.
32. Lahti A. Non-immunologic contact urticaria. Acta Dermatol Venereol 1980; 60:1.
33. Amin S, Lahti A, Maibach HI. Contact urticaria and the contact urticaria syndrome (immediate contact reactions). In: Zhai H, Maibach HI, eds. Dermatotoxicology. 6th ed. Boca Raton: CRC Press, 2004, chap. 42.
34. Lahti A, Maibach HI. An animal model for non-immunologic contact urticaria. Toxicol Appl Pharmacol 1984; 76:219.
35. Lahti A, Maibach HI. Immediate contact reactions (contact urticaria syndrome). In: Maibach H, ed. Occupational and Industrial Dermatology. 2nd ed. Chicago: Year Book Medical, 1987:32.
36. Amin S, Lahti A, Maibach HI, eds. Contact Urticaria Syndrome. Boca Raton: CRC Press, 1997.

19

Consumer Research and In-Market Comments

Brigitte Nijs
The Procter & Gamble Company, Schwalbach am Taunus, Germany

INTRODUCTION

Feminine hygiene product development requires real innovation in order to connect "what's needed" and "what's possible," that is, connecting a superior understanding of consumer habits and attitudes with leading-edge technology. That is why research and development, together with marketing and market research, observe consumers using their products at home, look for ways to improve the products, and find ways to simplify the overall in-use experience.

With an opportunity identified, the product development team creates prototypes in the laboratories, working with technologies in product, process, and packaging design. These prototypes are tested with consumers to determine whether the product design works. The cycle of learning is iterative: a design is made in the laboratory, tested with consumers, changed based on what is learned from consumers, and the modified product is retested until it is right, as judged by the consumer. This chapter describes the process of consumer research conducted on feminine hygiene products before the products are marketed and available for women to use.

WHAT DO WOMEN WANT FROM A FEMININE HYGIENE PAD?

First and most importantly, women seek protection: the avoidance of soiling of the underwear and/or outer garments during menstruation (Fig. 1). Why is protection so important for consumers? Today, approximately 50% of all women

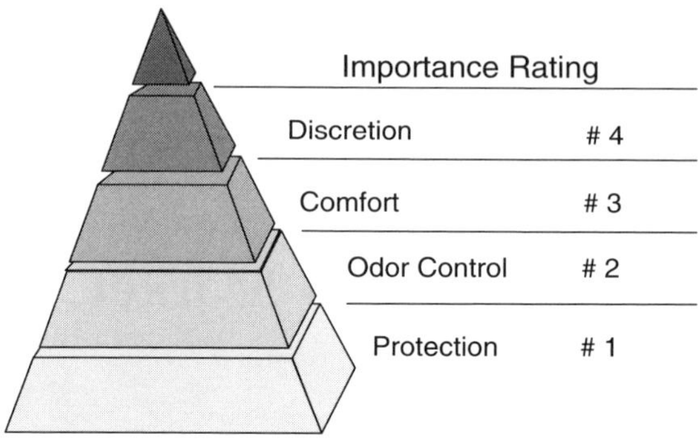

Figure 1 Factors of importance women seek from a feminine hygiene pad. *Source*: Courtesy of Research International Agency. (*See color insert p. 8.*)

experience at least one episode of staining of their undergarments during their menstrual period and approximately 10% of all women experience at least one blood stain on outer garments.

In addition to effective protection, women want to be reassured that wearing the pad will help reduce the malodor that may develop in the vulva area during the menstrual flow. Although the level of odor might not be very high, especially when the woman practices good vulvar hygiene, there is a psychological effect driving women to seek a proper odor control from the pad. It is also important to women that the pad remains comfortable when it is worn over several hours. When both the basic protection performance and the comfort elements are satisfied, women claim that it is important that the pad provides the needed discretion. Women want to continue their regular activities as much as possible during the menstrual period and do not want the pad to limit activity or be noticeable through clothing.

CONSUMER RESEARCH PROCESS FOR FEMININE HYGIENE PRODUCTS

This section describes the process of developing a feminine hygiene product from the early phase of understanding women's habits and practices, the early generation of a novel idea, making prototypes leading to readiness for market, and ensuring that the product is widely available to all women.

Understanding Consumer Habits and Practices

First, a questionnaire is sent to a large number of women asking about their current habits and practices concerning their feminine hygiene routine. Women are asked to clearly list what products they use, how satisfied they are with their current products, and what are their additional hygiene practices along with the use of these feminine hygiene products.

Laboratory Prototyping with Associated Laboratory Testing

Following an in-depth understanding building on these habits and practices and an assessment of the need gaps, the developer begins by creating prototypes of potential products that can better meet the consumers' needs. First, simple laboratory tests are conducted on product parts (e.g., tests of core absorbent properties, product integrity tests) or on the total prototype product (e.g., speed of menstrual liquid absorption) to assess its likely performance in use. As the prototype approaches the final product design, more complex tests are conducted that involve the actual wearing of the product (e.g., leakage protection tests, stay-in-place studies).

Controlled Panel Tests

Once the prototype approaches its final design, first test production runs are initiated to ensure the prototype can be converted into production. During this process of experimental production in the plant, the products are first made for further quality testing with women. At this stage, diary and technical perception testing may be conducted, during which women are supplied with the products and asked to wear them as they normally do. While wearing them, women are asked to keep a diary about their wearing experience: how well the product met their protection expectation and how comfortable the product was during actual use.

Another type of controlled panel test is the clinical test, which is conducted to assess the safety of using the product. The safety assurance program to support major innovations for feminine hygiene products often requires the performance of prospective, randomized, controlled clinical trials under practical conditions of use. The studies often share several common features and standard protocols are developed with the input of respected academic and medical experts. The protocols employ objective, numerical scales for assessing tissue irritation and skin condition of the external and internal genitalia. All clinical studies must be approved by an independent institutional review board and/or by an ethics committee and should be examiner-blinded, utilizing independent academic physicians in obstetrics, gynecology, or dermatology as investigators. Subjects can be recruited from the population at large, and must sign an informed consent form before participating (1).

In-Market Consumer Tests

Different types of in-market consumer tests are undertaken to maximize the success of the new product design and to minimize the risk of consumer dissatisfaction when the product is finally made available to the marketplace.

Product Test

Within this large-scale quantitative test, women are exposed to the product design. They are asked to use the product under regular usage conditions over a menstrual cycle. At the end of the wearing test, women receive a questionnaire about the product, allowing them to rate the different product-performance parameters and also to compare the new product with the one ordinarily use.

Concept and Use Test

This is a pretest market large-scale quantitative technique. In addition to evaluating the pure product performance, product manufacturers test the concept of how to clearly present it to consumers, as well as its "fit" with the overall brand under which it is envisioned to be sold in the market.

Test Market

Prior to a wide market rollout, a new product or product design might be launched first in a test market, allowing the product manufacturer to gain more in-market experience. Typically, for this test, a city with a representative population distribution is selected. Most companies developing feminine hygiene products follow extensive testing programs, as not only do they want to be sure that the new product design fully meets the consumers' needs, they also gather useful information about the safety of using the product.

QUALITY ASSURANCE FOR PRODUCTION OF FEMININE HYGIENE PRODUCTS

While the novel feminine hygiene product is being assessed for safety and effectiveness, the production process is being developed. A good quality production process must ensure that the product and its manufacturing meet several requirements. This applies to clinical studies, normal consumer studies, and market shipment alike.

1. First and foremost, consumers expect a good and functional product that delivers the desired performance. Production should follow good manufacturing practices. This means that high hygiene standards (in building, equipment, and operation) and high manufacturing quality must be provided.
2. On feminine hygiene products, there are numerous regulations worldwide that must be met. Governmental agencies, such as the U.S. Food and Drug Administration (FDA), reserve the right to audit manufacturers for compliance. A good quality system reflects all necessary requirements in written procedures and ensures that regulations are met. These are properly included and documented in the relevant work processes.
3. A growing number of trade customers require a quality certification from the manufacturer. The ISO 9001:2000 certificate is the most common global system. This is the trade's safeguard that manufacturers follow a quality system that has been certified by a third party.

4. In many countries, liability laws have changed, and manufacturers have to provide evidence of their standards in court. Operations must be transparent and the work traceable. Production is allowed only according to approved standards, procedures, and good documentation. Production equipment and processes must be validated for their purpose and only quality materials can be used. The product is released into the marketplace only when it meets all specifications.
5. A consumer-response system is needed to provide the consumer with the means to ask questions or to provide testimonials or comments/complaints. Such a system not only helps to satisfy consumers, but is also a great analysis tool to learn of market successes and failures and to improve internal systems in the manufacture of a product that will provide consumers with the desired experience.

CONSUMER COMMENTS FROM MARKET USE

The process described in this section is based on the experiences of the Procter & Gamble Company with their pads, tampons, and panty liners, but similar processes on handling postlaunch consumer comments are available at other large companies producing feminine hygiene products.

Products are launched in the market typically with the means to contact the producing company included in the package artwork (mostly located on the side or back panel), providing consumers with an easy way to express their experience with the product or marketing. When the consumer contacts the producing company, the consumer comments-handling process is activated within the company.

Consumers contact the producing company for three different reasons:

1. Testimonial. Consumers may provide positive feedback to the producing company. For example, if they are very satisfied with the improved protection that the newly launched feminine hygiene product offers; they often claim that they would also recommend the product to their friends or family.
2. Inquiry. Consumers may ask questions or make requests and/or suggestions. For example, women would like to better understand the differences between the many feminine hygiene products a company sells or they may suggest a design/package improvement.
3. Complaints. Women express dissatisfaction, complaining of a problem or an adverse event. For example, they are unable to locate the product they want to buy or find that the product does not perform to their expectations.

A more in-depth analysis of consumers' comments allows the company to define follow-up actions properly.

CONCLUSION

Innovation and understanding of consumer needs are the keys to developing effective feminine hygiene products upon which consumers can rely. Learning what women want in a feminine hygiene product is the result of thorough and thoughtful consumer research. The process of consumer research, which culminates in the introduction of the product to the marketplace, involves many phases, each guided subsequently by consumer feedback. Throughout the process, manufacturers follow the guidelines of governmental agencies such as the FDA and of third-party trade associations to obtain certification and assure consumers of product safety and manufacturing quality.

This development process, from initial understanding of consumer needs through development of products and safety testing up to final introduction of the new product to market, may take several years, and these development investments are performed to ensure that only quality products reach the market.

REFERENCE

1. Internal Procter & Gamble Procedures on Product Development.

Index

Abscesses
  treatment, 123–125
ACD. *see* allergic contact dermatitis (ACD)
Acne vulgaris
  menstrual cycle, 172
Acrochordons, 123
Acyclovir
  herpes simplex virus, 129–130
Adrenarche, 32
Africa
  menstrual hygiene, 195–196
African Americans
  idiopathic precocious puberty, 33
  incontinence dermatitis, 205
  menstrual protection practices, 191
  vulvar vestibulitis syndrome, 103–104
Afro-Caribbean
  perineal cleansing, 198
Allergic contact dermatitis (ACD), 291–293
5-Aminolaevulinic acid, 121
  vulvar intraepithelial neoplasia, 140
Androgen receptors, 16
Androgens
  lichen sclerosus, 121
Angioedema
  menstrual cycle, 178–179
Antifungal preparations, 230
Antihistamines
  contact dermatitis, 118
APD. *see* autoimmune progesterone dermatitis (APD)
Aphthous ulceration
  menstrual cycle, 173
Arm
  occlusion, 163
Asians
  pubic hair, 32
Atopic dermatitis, 119
  menstrual cycle, 173
Atrophic vaginitis, 68–69
Autoimmune estrogen dermatitis
  menstrual cycle, 177–178
Autoimmune progesterone dermatitis (APD)
  menstrual cycle, 176–177
Azathioprine
  atopic dermatitis, 119
Azithromycin, 127
  Haemophilus ducreyi (chancroid), 126
  Treponema pallidum, 126

Bacterial infection
  treatment, 123–125
Bacterial vaginosis (BV), 80–81
  douching, 200
Barrier creams, 207–208
Bartholin's glands, 103, 124
  anatomy, 2, 6

Baths
  bubble, 217–219
  Sitz, for abscess, 124
Behind the knee test, 290
Benign vulvar nodules or tumors, 123
Benzyl benzoate
  scabies, 135, 136–137
Betamethasone
  contact dermatitis, 118
  vulvar vestibulitis syndrome, 108
Bidet, 198
Biofeedback
  vulvar vestibulitis syndrome, 108
Biophysical variables
  quantitative comparison, 15
Births
  preterm douching, 200
Bleomycin
  molluscum contagiosum, 134
  vulvar neoplasms, 142
Blood perfusion
  cutaneous, 273–274
Blood vessels
  ethnic/racial differences, 242, 243–245
Body perception changes, 260–261
Body splashes, 222
Body washes, 217–219
Breast development, 33
Bubble bath, 217–219
Bulbocavernosus muscle, 7
Burow's solution
  atopic dermatitis, 119
Butoconazole
  vulvovaginal candidiasis, 128
BV. *see* bacterial vaginosis (BV)

Calcipotreine
  psoriasis, 120
Calcium citrate
  idiopathic vulvodynia, 95
Calymmatobacterium granulomatis, 127
Candida albicans, 73–74
Candida (Torulopsis) *glabrata*, 70–71
Candida infection
  vulvar vestibulitis syndrome, 106
Candida vaginitis
  menstrual cycle, 174
Canthridin
  molluscum contagiosum, 134
Carbon dioxide laser
  lichen planus, 123
Castration, 263
  female, 265
CBT. *see* cognitive behavioral therapy (CBT)
CD4+ lymphocytes, 16
CD8+ lymphocytes, 16
Ceftriaxone
  Haemophilus ducreyi (chancroid), 126
  Treponema pallidum, 126
Cellulitis
  treatment, 123–125
Cervical cancer
  douching, 200
Cervical mucus, 16
Chancroid, 126
Chemoradiation
  vulvar neoplasms, 142
Chemotherapy
  vulvar neoplasms, 141
Childhood sexuality
  eradication, 264
  invention, 261
China
  menstrual hygiene, 196
  perineal cleansing, 198
Chlamydia trachomatis strain, 127
Chloasma
  menstrual cycle, 172
Christian values, 263
Cidofovir
  genital warts, 133
  molluscum contagiosum, 134
Ciprofloxacin
  Haemophilus ducreyi (chancroid), 126
Cleanliness products, 217–223
Clitoridectomies, 265
Clitoris (glans clitoridis)
  anatomy, 2, 4
  embryology, 1

Cloaca
  embryology, 1
Clobetasol
  lichen sclerosus, 120
Clotrimazole
  vulvovaginal candidiasis, 128
Cognitive behavioral therapy (CBT)
  vulvar vestibulitis syndrome, 110
Complaints, 301
Concept and use tests
  feminine hygiene products, 300
Condyloma acuminata, 131, 132
Consumer habits
  feminine hygiene products, 298
Consumer research, 297–302
  feminine hygiene products, 298–299
Consumer tests
  feminine hygiene products, 299–300
Contact dermatitis, 117–119
  allergic, 291–293
  irritant, 291
  menstrual cycle, 179
  sanitary pads, 193
Contact urticaria, 294
Controlled panel tests
  feminine hygiene products, 299
Corneocytes
  ethnic/racial differences, 236–242
Corticosteroids
  atopic dermatitis, 119
  lichen simplex chronicus, 123
Corynebacteria, 46
Cosmetic genital surgery, 266–267
Cotton-swab test, 92
Cowper's glands. *see* Bartholin's glands
Crotamiton
  scabies, 135, 136
Cryotherapy
  human papilloma virus, 132
  lichen planus, 123
  molluscum contagiosum, 134
Cups
  menstrual, 227
Curettage
  molluscum contagiosum, 134
Cutaneous blood perfusion, 273–274
Cutaneous epithelium, 12
Cyclic vulvovaginitis
  menstrual cycle, 174
Cystitis
  interstitial
    vulvar vestibulitis syndrome, 107

Dapsone
  lichen planus, 122
Darier's disease
  menstrual cycle, 173–174
Delivery
  vagina/vulva, 35–36
Deodorant sprays
  feminine, 222, 223
Dermatitis. *see also* contact dermatitis
  atopic, 119
    menstrual cycle, 173
  autoimmune estrogen
    menstrual cycle, 177–178
  autoimmune progesterone
    menstrual cycle, 176–177
  diaper, 184, 185
  incontinence, 39, 205–208
  photoallergic, 293–294
  seborrheic, 120
  vulvar, 291–294
Dermatitis herpetiformis
  menstrual cycle, 175–176
Developing world
  menstrual hygiene
    reproductive age women, 194–196
Diabetes mellitus
  vulvovaginal candidiasis, 21
Diaper dermatitis, 184, 185
Diaper rash, 186
Diet
  vulvar vestibulitis syndrome, 107
Dioxin
  tampons, 226
Disposable pads, 226–227
Diva Cup, 224
Donovanosis, 127
Douches, 219–220
Douching, 198–202, 220, 221
  sexuality transmitted diseases, 200, 202

Doxepin
  contact dermatitis, 118
Doxycycline, 127
  lymphogranuloma venereum, 127
  Treponema pallidum, 125
Dusting powder, 222
Dyes
  pubic hair, 229
Dyspareunia
  vulvar vestibulitis syndrome, 108
    introital, 102

Early childhood
  labia majora, 30
  vagina/vulva, 30–32
Eccrine sweat glands, 44
Economy
  industrialized
    demands, 261–262
Ectoparasitic infections, 134–138
Ectopic pregnancy
  douching, 200
Eczematous and papulosquamous vulvar dermatoses, 117–123
Elderly
  vagina/vulva, 36–37
Electrosurgery
  genital warts, 133
  molluscum contagiosum, 134
  vulvar intraepithelial neoplasia, 140
Embryonic ectoderm, 12
Endometrial cycle, 154
Endometriosis
  tampons, 225–226
Enterobius vermicularis
  premenarchal girls, 187
Epidermis, 12
Epithelium
  cutaneous, 12
  nonkeratinized
    vulvar vestibule, 13
  variations, 12–14
  vulvar vestibule, 14
Erosive lichen planus, 79
Erythema quantification, 272–273
Erythromycin
  lymphogranuloma venereum, 127
  Treponema pallidum, 125
Escherichia coli, 21
Estrogen
  menstrual cycle, 169
  receptors, 16
  skin, 168–170
Ethnically/racially different skin characteristics, 236–247
Ethnic differences
  skin surface microflora, 248
Ethnic groups
  pubic hair, 32
Ethnicity
  vulva, 235–252
Europe
  incontinence dermatitis, 205
Evangelical movement, 263

Famciclovir
  herpes simplex virus, 130
Fatty acids
  antimicrobial properties, 46
Female castration, 265
Female genital alterations
  contemporary North American, 266–267
  sociological implication, 255–267
  types, 263–264
Female sexuality control
  19th and 20th century procedures, 264–266
Feminine deodorant sprays, 222, 223
Feminine hygiene pad
  important factors, 297–298
Feminine hygiene products
  quality assurance, 300–301
Feminine hygiene sprays, 198
Feminine suppositories, 222
Femoral artery, 7
Femoral cutaneous nerve, 7
Femoral node dissection
  vulvar neoplasms, 140
Fibroepithelial polyps, 123
Fibroma, 123
Fibromyoma, 123
Fingerprinting techniques
  microbes, 52
5-Aminolaevulinic acid, 121
  vulvar intraepithelial neoplasia, 140

Fluconazole
vulvodynia, 117
Fluocinolone
contact dermatitis, 118
5-Fluorouracil (5-FU)
genital warts, 133
molluscum contagiosum, 134
vulvar intraepithelial neoplasia, 139
vulvar neoplasms, 142
Follicle-stimulating hormone (FSH), 152, 154
menstrual cycle, 169
Folliculitis
vulvar, 205
Fragrances, 222
FSH. *see* follicle-stimulating hormone (FSH)
Fungal infection, 128–129

Gabapentin
idiopathic vulvodynia, 95
vulvodynia, 116
Genital alterations
female
contemporary North American, 266–267
sociological implication, 255–267
types, 263–264
Genital autoinoculation
premenarchal girls, 187–188
Genital hygiene, 183–208
infants, 183–184
premenarchal girls, 184–188
reproductive age women, 188–203
Genital surgery, 264
cosmetic, 266–267
Genital tubercle
embryology, 1
Genital warts
laser surgery, 133
Genital warts (*Condyloma acuminata*), 131, 132
Genitofemoral nerve, 7
Glans clitoridis
anatomy, 2, 4
embryology, 1
Gonadarche, 32
Gonadotrophin-releasing hormone (GnRH), 152, 154, 168
Gram-negative bacteria, 46
Gram-positive bacteria, 46
Granouloma inguinale, 127
Griseofulvin
lichen planus, 122

Habits, consumer
feminine hygiene products, 298
Haemophilus ducreyi (chancroid), 126
Hair. *see* pubic hair
Hart's line marks, 5, 44
Hereditary angioedema
menstrual cycle, 178–179
Herpes gestationis (HG)
menstrual cycle, 175
Herpes simplex labialis
menstrual cycle, 173
Herpes simplex virus, 129–131
HG. *see* herpes gestationis (HG)
Hormonal responsiveness, 16
Human papilloma virus (HPV)
genital warts, 131–132
vulvar vestibulitis syndrome, 106
Hydrocortisone, 37
permeability, 18, 19
Hydrolysis, 218
Hygiene
genital, 183–208
menstrual, 188–194
premenarchal girls, 188
vulvar, 64
products, 217–230
Hygiene pad
feminine
important factors, 297–298
Hygiene products
feminine
quality assurance, 300–301
Hygiene sprays
feminine, 198
Hymen
anatomy, 2, 5
Hyperpigmentation
menstrual cycle, 172

Idiopathic precocious puberty, 33–34
Idiopathic vulvodynia, 85–97
  comorbid conditions, 89–90
  demographics, 89
  diagnosis, 90–93
  etiology, 87
  gynecologic history, 90
  prevalence, 88–89
  psychosocial and sexual aspects, 90
  symptoms, 87
  terminology and history, 85–86
  treatment, 94–96
Ilioinguinal nerve, 7
Imiquimod
  human papilloma virus, 131–132
  molluscum contagiosum, 134
  vulvar intraepithelial neoplasia, 139
Immune cells, 16–17
Immunomodulators
  molluscum contagiosum, 134
Incision
  abscess, 124
Incontinence
  control products, 227–228
Incontinence dermatitis, 39, 205–208
India
  menstrual hygiene, 195
Industrialized economy
  demands, 261–262
Industrialized world
  menstrual hygiene
    reproductive age women, 188–194
Infants
  genital hygiene, 183–184
  labia majora, 30
  vaginal discharge, 183–184
  vagina/vulva, 30–32
  vulvar anatomy, 183–184
Infectious diseases
  treatment, 123–128
Infectious vulvitis
  vulvar vestibulitis syndrome, 104
Inguinofemoral lymph node metastases
  vulvar neoplasms, 141
In-market consumer tests
  feminine hygiene products, 299–300
Inquiry, 301
Interferon
  molluscum contagiosum, 134
Interferon alpha
  genital warts, 133
  vulvar intraepithelial neoplasia, 139
  vulvar vestibulitis syndrome, 105–106, 109
  vulvodynia, 117
Interferon beta
  genital warts, 133
  vulvar vestibulitis syndrome, 109
Interlabial pads, 227
Interstitial cystitis
  vulvar vestibulitis syndrome, 107
Intertrigo, 205
Introital dyspareunia
  vulvar vestibulitis syndrome, 102
Irritant contact dermatitis, 291
Ischiocavernosus muscle, 6
Islam
  pubic hair removal, 203
Islamic societies
  menstrual hygiene
    reproductive age women, 196–197
Itching
  vulvar vestibulitis syndrome, 104
Ivermectin
  scabies, 135, 136, 137–138

Jarisch-Herxheimer, 126

Keratosis follicularis (Darier's disease)
  menstrual cycle, 173–174
Koebner's phenomenon, 119

Labial adhesions
  prepubertal girls, 31–32
Labia majora
  anatomy, 2, 3–4
  blood flow, 14
  contact dermatitis, 67
  embryology, 1
  epithelial thickness with age, 35
  infancy and early childhood, 30
  innervation, 14
  menses, 161
  menses and venous blood, 161

occlusion, 162
permeability, 18–19
Labia minora (nymphae)
anatomy, 2, 4, 44
contact dermatitis, 67
embryology, 1
Labioscrotal swellings
embryology, 1
Laboratory testing
feminine hygiene products, 299
Lactic acid
molluscum contagiosum, 134
Langerhans cells, 12, 13, 14, 16, 17
Laser doppler flowmetry (LDF), 273–274
Laser surgery
genital warts, 133
pubic hair, 229
vulvar intraepithelial neoplasia, 139–140
Latin America
menstrual hygiene, 195
LDF. *see* laser doppler flowmetry (LDF)
LH. *see* luteinizing hormone (LH)
Lichen atrophicus sclerosus (LSA), 72–73
Lichen planus, 80
erosive, 79
treatment, 122–123
Lichen sclerosus, 74, 75, 120–122
Lichen simplex chronicus (LSC), 71–72, 123
Lidocaine
vulvar vestibulitis syndrome, 108
vulvodynia, 116
Lindane
scabies, 134, 135
Lipid content
ethnic/racial differences, 247–249
LSA. *see* lichen atrophicus sclerosus (LSA)
LSC. *see* lichen simplex chronicus (LSC)
Lubricants, 228
Lupus erythematosus
menstrual cycle, 174–175
Luteinizing hormone (LH), 152, 154
menstrual cycle, 169
Lymph node metastases
inguinofemoral
vulvar neoplasms, 141
Lymphocytes, 16
Lymphogranuloma venereum (*Chlamydia trachomatis* strain), 127

Malathion
scabies, 137
Market use
consumer comments, 301
Marsupialization, 124
Mast cell granules
ethnic/racial differences, 249
Masturbation, 256–259
Matrix metalloproteinases (MMP)
menses, 159
Medical authority
changes, 260
Melanocytes, 12
Menarche, 32
mean age, 34
Menopause
vagina/vulva, 36–37
Menses
composition and properties, 155–160
elasticity, 160
images, 158
labia majora, 161
occlusion, 161–163
skin, 160–162
Menstrual cups, 227
Menstrual cycle, 151–155
bacterial populations, 50
hormonal changes, 167–168
skin, 20, 167–170
skin disorders, 172–179
vagina/vulva, 34–35, 36
Menstrual hygiene
reproductive age women, 188–194
developing world, 194–196
industrialized world, 188–194
Orthodox Judaism and Islamic societies, 196–197
Menstrual protection
practices, 190
products, 223–227
alternative, 224, 227

Merkel cells, 12, 13
Methotrexate
  vulvar neoplasms, 142
Mexican Americans
  incontinence dermatitis, 205
  menstrual protection practices, 191
Miconazole
  vulvovaginal candidiasis, 128
Microbes
  adherence, 47
  counts, 49
  host immune mechanisms, 47
  interactions, 46
  moisture, 44–45
  nutrients and inhibitors, 45–46
  pH, 45
Microflora
  ethnic/racial differences
    skin surface, 248
    surface, 247–249
  exogenous, 47–48
  resident *vs.* transient, 48–53
Microorganisms
  vagina/vulva, 51
Mitomycin C
  vulvar neoplasms, 142
Mittelschmerz, 154
MMP. *see* matrix metalloproteinases (MMP)
Mohs microsurgery
  vulvar neoplasms, 141
Moisture, 64
Moisturizers, 228
  atopic dermatitis, 119
Molluscum contagiosum, 133–134
Mons pubis
  anatomy, 2, 3, 43–44
Muslims
  menstrual hygiene, 197

Native Americans
  pubic hair, 32
Necrotizing fasciitis, 125
Newborn
  vulva
    anatomy, 30
Nonkeratinized epithelium
  vulvar vestibule, 13
Nylon underwear
  vulvovaginal candidiasis, 193–194
Nymphae
  anatomy, 2, 4, 44
  contact dermatitis, 67
  embryology, 1
Nystatin
  vulvovaginal candidiasis, 128

Odor-control products, 217–223
Ointments
  contact dermatitis, 118
Older women
  genital hygiene, 204–208
  perineal hygiene, 205
Oophorectomy, 265
Orthodox Judaism
  menstrual hygiene
    reproductive age women, 196–197
Ovarian cancer
  talc powders perineum, 203
Ovarian cycle, 152–154
Oxalates
  vulvar vestibulitis syndrome, 107
  vulvodynia, 117

Padette interlabial pad, 224
Pads
  disposable, 226–227
  feminine hygiene
    important factors, 297–298
  interlabial, 227
  liners
    vulvovaginal candidiasis, 193–194
  sanitary, 193
Pain
  vulvar
    diseases causing, 77–80
    self-reported descriptors, 91
Pantyhose
  vulvovaginal candidiasis, 193–194
Panty liners, 190, 194, 226–227
Paraurethral glands. *see* Skene's glands
Paroxetine
  idiopathic vulvodynia, 95
PCT. *see* porphyria cutanea tarda (PCT)
PDT. *see* photodynamic therapy (PDT)

Pelvic floor muscles rehabilitation
vulvodynia, 117
Pelvic inflammatory disease (PID), 202
douching, 200
Penicillin G
Treponema pallidum, 125
Penis
embryology, 1
Perineal muscle, 7
Perineum
powders, 202–203
routine cleansing, 197–199
Permethrin
scabies, 134, 135, 137
Phenol
molluscum contagiosum, 134
pH gradient
ethnic/racial differences, 246, 247
pH surface, 276–277
Photoallergic dermatitis, 293–294
Photodynamic therapy (PDT), 121
Photoirritation, 293–294
Physician/priest
new body, 260
PID. *see* pelvic inflammatory disease (PID)
Pinworm (Enterobius vermicularis)
premenarchal girls, 187
Pituitary hormones
menstrual cycle, 169
Podofilox
human papilloma virus, 131
Podophyllin
human papilloma virus, 132
Porphyria cutanea tarda (PCT)
menstrual cycle, 175
Postmasturbation disease, 259–263
Postmenopausal atrophic vulvovaginitis, 37
Powder
dusting, 222
talc
perineum, 203
Precocious puberty
idiopathic, 33–34
Pregnancy
ectopic
douching, 200
vagina/vulva, 35–36
vulvovaginal candidiasis, 21
Premenarchal girls
aberrant hygiene practices, 188
genital autoinoculation, 187–188
genital hygiene, 184–188
Premenstrual syndrome, 171
Premoistened wipes, 222
Preterm births
douching, 200
Priest/physician
new body, 260
Product tests
feminine hygiene products, 299–300
Progesterone
lichen sclerosus, 121
menstrual cycle, 169, 170–171
receptors, 16
Prothrombin activator complex
menses, 158–159
Pruritus vulvae
menstrual cycle, 174
Psoralen
psoriasis, 119
Psoriasis, 119–120
menstrual cycle, 172–173
Pubarche, 32
Puberty
idiopathic precocious, 33–34
vagina/vulva, 32–34
Pubic hair
development, 32
laser surgery, 229
removal, 203
products, 228–229
Pudendal arteries, 7
Pudendal nerves, 7
Pudendum. *see* vulva

Racial differences
skin surface microflora, 248
Racially different skin
characteristics, 236–247
Radiotherapy
vulvar neoplasms, 141
Rash
diaper, 186
Religious fervor, 262–263

Research
  consumer, 297–302
    feminine hygiene products, 298–299
Restraining techniques, 264
Retinoid
  lichen planus, 122
  psoriasis, 120
Rosacea
  menstrual cycle, 172

Salicylic acid
  molluscum contagiosum, 134
Sanitary pads, 193
Scabies *(Sarcoptes scabiei)*, 134–138
  treatment, 135
Scrotum
  embryology, 1
Sea sponges, 224, 227
Sebaceous glands, 44
Seborrheic dermatitis, 120
Sex characteristics
  onset, 33
Sex hormones
  skin, 168–171
Sexuality
  childhood
    eradication, 264
    invention, 261
  female control
    19th and 20th century procedures, 264–266
Sexuality transmitted diseases (STD)
  douching, 200, 202
Sexual response
  innervation, 14
Sexual steroid hormones
  menstrual cycle, 169
Shaving
  pubic hair, 228–229
Sitz baths
  abscess, 124
Sjogren's syndrome, 71
Skene's glands
  anatomy, 2, 6
Skin
  color
    measurement guidelines, 273
    reflectance, 272–273
  disorders
    menstrual cycle, 172–179
  elastic recovery and extensibility
    ethnic/racial differences, 242, 246
  erythema
    measurement guidelines, 273
  hydration
    ethnic/racial differences, 236
    measurement, 275–276
  irritation, 19–20
  menstrual cycle, 20, 167–170
  physiologic parameters, 38
  surface microflora
    ethnic/racial differences, 248
  surface pH, 276–277
  vulvar
    epithelial structure, 13
    microbiology, 20–22
Skinning vulvectomy
  vulvar intraepithelial neoplasia, 140
Skin surface water loss (SSWL), 282
SLS. *see* sodium lauryl sulfate (SLS)
Soaps, 217–219
  making, 218–219
Sodium lauryl sulfate (SLS), 20, 161
Spinnbarkeit test, 160
Splashes, 222
Sponges
  sea, 224, 227
SSWL. *see* skin surface water loss (SSWL)
Staphylococcus aureus, 21
STD. *see* sexuality transmitted diseases (STD)
Steroid hormones
  sexual
    menstrual cycle, 169
Stress urinary incontinence
  hygiene challenges, 204
Sulfur
  scabies, 135, 136
Suppositories
  feminine, 222
Surface microflora
  ethnic/racial differences, 247–249
Surgical genital procedures, 264
Sweat glands
  eccrine, 44
Syphilis, 125–126

Tacrolimus
atopic dermatitis, 119
lichen planus, 122
lichen sclerosus, 121
Talc powders
perineum, 203
Tampons, 189, 190, 224
absorbency ratings, 192, 225
FDA regulation, 192
Tazarotene
psoriasis, 120
Teraconazole
vulvovaginal candidiasis, 128
Testimonials, 301
Test market
feminine hygiene products, 300
Testosterone
permeability, 19
Tetracycline
Treponema pallidum, 125
TEWL. *see* transepidermal water loss (TEWL)
Thrombin
menses, 159
Tinea, 205
Tioconazole
vulvovaginal candidiasis, 128
Tissue hydration and barrier function, 17–18
T lymphocytes, 17
Toilet habits
premenarchal girls, 186
Torulopsis, 70–71
Towelettes, 222
Toxic shock syndrome (TSS), 191–195, 191, 225
Transepidermal water loss (TEWL), 17–18, 20, 45, 274–275, 281–285
atopy, 283
ethnic/racial differences, 236, 237–241
evaluation, 282–283
finding, 283–284
measuring, 283
vulvar *vs.* forearm skin, 288
vulvar *vs.* thigh skin, 284
Treponema pallidum (syphilis), 125–126
Tretinoin cream
molluscum contagiosum, 134
Triamcinolone acetonide
contact dermatitis, 118
vulvodynia, 117
Trichloroacetic acid
human papilloma virus, 132
molluscum contagiosum, 134
Trichomoniasis vaginalis, 81
Tricyclic antidepressants
idiopathic vulvodynia, 95
vulvar vestibulitis syndrome, 108
vulvodynia, 116
Trimethoprim-sulfamethoxazole, 127
TSS. *see* toxic shock syndrome (TSS)
Tubercle
genital
embryology, 1
Tumors
benign, 123
Turks
pubic hair removal, 203

Ulcers, 79–80
Ultraviolet radiation
psoriasis, 119
Underwear
nylon
vulvovaginal candidiasis, 193–194
Urethra
anatomy, 5
Urethral orifice
anatomy, 2
Urge urinary incontinence
hygiene challenges, 204
Urinary incontinence
hygiene challenges, 204–205
stress
hygiene challenges, 204
urge
hygiene challenges, 204
Urinary tract infections
sanitary pads, 193
Urogenital tract
female
embryologic derivation, 12

Urticaria
  contact, 294
  menstrual cycle, 178–179
Use tests
  feminine hygiene products, 300
Uterine bleeding
  hygiene challenges, 204

Vagina
  changes throughout life, 27–39
  from infancy to old age, 28–29
  irritative symptoms normalcy, 60
  microbial shifts
    tampons, 225
Vaginal creams, 229
Vaginal discharge, 66
  characteristics, 58–59
  diseases causing, 80–81
  infancy and early childhood, 30
  infants, 183–184
Vaginal epithelium
  infancy and early childhood, 30
  permeability, 19
Vaginal introitus
  infancy and early childhood, 30
Vaginal odor
  characteristics, 59
Vaginal orifice
  anatomy, 5–6
Vaginal symptoms, 57–61
Vaginal ulcers
  tampons, 225
Vagina/vulva
  infancy and early childhood, 30–32
  menstrual cycle, 34–35, 36
  microorganisms, 51
  puberty, 32–34
  reproductive years, 34–36
Vaginitis
  atrophic, 68–69
  Candida
    menstrual cycle, 174
Valacyclovir
  herpes simplex virus, 130
Values
  Christian, 263
Venlafaxine
  idiopathic vulvodynia, 95
Venous blood
  labia majora, 161
  skin, 160–162
Vestibular bulbs
  anatomy, 2, 6
Vestibular erythema
  vulvar vestibulitis syndrome, 102
Vestibular pain
  measurement, 102
Vestibule
  anatomy, 2, 5
  vulvar, 44
    permeability, 19
Vestibulectomy
  vulvodynia, 117
Vestibulitis
  vulvar, 77–80
Vestibuloplasty
  vulvar vestibulitis syndrome, 109–110
Victorian ideals, 262–263
VIN. *see* vulvar intraepithelial neoplasia (VIN)
Viral infection, 129–134
Virginity
  tampons, 226
Vulva. *see also* vagina/vulva
  adult
    anatomy, 2
  anatomy, 1–7, 43–44, 65
    infants, 183–184
  bioengineering methods, 271–277
  blood flow and innervation, 14–15
  blood supply, 7
  burning
    diseases causing, 66–71
  changes throughout life, 27–39
  common diseases, 63–81
  contact dermatitis, 66–68
  diseases
    assessment, 63–64
  diseases causing itching, 71–76
  embryology, 1–2
  ethnic differences, 235–252
  hygiene, 64
    products, 217–230
  from infancy to old age, 28–29
  innervation, 7

irritation, 288–289
assessment, 290
lesions
biopsy, 66
lymphatic drainage, 7
microbial ecology, 43–54
microbial growth and diversity, 44–48
microflora, 48–53
muscles
anatomy, 6–7
newborn
anatomy, 30
physical examination, 64–66
prepubescent, 31
tissue structure and physiology, 9–22
Vulvar dermatitis, 291–294
Vulvar folliculitis, 205
Vulvar intraepithelial neoplasia (VIN), 69–70, 71, 121, 138–140
laser surgery, 139–140
Vulvar neoplasms, 138–142
invasive, 140–142
treatment, 138
Vulvar pain
diseases causing, 77–80
self-reported descriptors, 91
Vulvar skin
epithelial structure, 13
microbiology, 20–22, 20
Vulvar therapies
evidence *vs.* testimony, 115–143
Vulvar toxicology, 287–302
Vulvar vestibule, 44
permeability, 19
Vulvar vestibulitis, 77–80, 78, 79
Vulvar vestibulitis syndrome (VVS), 101–111
antifungal and antiviral agents, 108–109
biofeedback, 108
definition and characteristics, 101–103
differential diagnosis, 104
etiology, 105–107
genetic predisposition, 105–106
infection causing, 106
management, 107–110
neuropathy secondary to inflammation, 105–106
physical causes, 107
prevalence and patient demographics, 103–104
primary vs. secondary, 102–103
psychosexual dysfunction, 107
supportive and multimodal approaches, 109
surgery, 109–110
symptom relief, 108
Vulvectomy
skinning
vulvar intraepithelial neoplasia, 140
vulvar neoplasms, 140
Vulvitis
infectious
vulvar vestibulitis syndrome, 104
Vulvodynia, 115–117. *see also* idiopathic vulvodynia
diagnostic algorithm, 93
treatment, 96
Vulvovaginal candidiasis (VVC), 21
pregnancy, 21
treatment, 128
Vulvovaginal epithelia
vs. exposed skin, 10–11
Vulvovaginitis
cyclic
menstrual cycle, 174
postmenopausal atrophic, 37
yeast, 76
VVC. *see* vulvovaginal candidiasis (VVC)
VVS. *see* vulvar vestibulitis syndrome (VVS)

Warts
genital, 131, 132
Washes, 217–219
Waxing
pubic hair, 229
Wellness centers, 264
Wet wipes, 198
Wipes
premoistened, 222
Word catheter
abscess, 124

Yeast vulvovaginitis, 76